HISTORY OF SYPHILIS

HISTORY OF SYPHILIS

Claude Quétel

Translated by Judith Braddock and Brian Pike

The Johns Hopkins University Press
Baltimore

English translation © Polity Press 1990
First published in France as
Le Mal de Naples: histoire de la syphilis
© Editions Seghers, Paris, 1986
All rights reserved
Printed in Great Britain

This translation first published in hardcover, 1990
Johns Hopkins Paperbacks edition, 1992

The Johns Hopkins University Press
701 West 40th Street
Baltimore, Maryland 21211-2190

Library of Congress Cataloging-in-Publication Data
Quétel, Claude, 1939–
[Mal de Naples. English]
History of syphilis / Claude Quétel; translated by Judith
Braddock and Brian Pike.
p. cm.
Translation of : Le mal de Naples.
Includes bibliographical references (p.
ISBN 0–8018–4089–9   ISBN 0–8018–4392–8 pbk.
1. Syphilis—History. I. Title.
RC201.4.QBS13   1990   90–4267
614.5'472'09—dc20   CIP

Contents

Acknowledgements

The publisher and author are grateful to the following for permission to use and for their help in supplying photographs: Bibliothèque Municipale de Caen (Plates 5, 12, 18, 19, 20); Bibliothèque Nationale, Paris (Plates 4, 6, 7, 8, 9, 10, 15); National Archives and Records, Washington (Plates 16, 17); Private Collections (Plates 1, 2, 3, 11, 13, 14, 20). All other photographs are provided by the author.

Introduction: Syphilis as a Cultural Phenomenon

According to the famous definition given by Bichat, the late-eighteenth-century French anatomist and physiologist, life is to be understood in terms of the set of functions which ward off death. If this is so then health, by analogy, cannot be defined without sickness – the absence of the one defines the other. Moreover, it is no accident that in recent decades the interest of researchers whose concern is the study of man has shifted from the first of these oppositions (life–death) to the second (health–sickness). Historians, philosophers, sociologists and doctors have switched from historical demography and scholarly studies of death to a new area, the history of health and sickness. No longer do we have the traditional history of medicine, century by century from Hippocrates to Pasteur, or subject by subject (until recently, any medical treatise written by a reputable authority was expected to begin with a chapter devoted to historical matters); what we have now are quantitative investigations and a desire to contribute to the history of civilization. However, the absence of a proper international research effort has meant that the promise of this rich field of history has scarcely been realized. One of the best illustrations of this fact is the current state of the historical epidemiology of the world.

In many countries (though not in France) medical studies have come to incorporate the new style of history of medicine, with its new aims and methods. This has encouraged, and in turn been encouraged by, the evident interest in these matters shown by the general public. Of course, these are not mere chance developments: today, problems to do with health and medicine are more acute than ever before, because we simply refuse to accept ageing, illness, suffering and death. This anguish which afflicts our de-Christianized societies, this headlong rush in which we daily demand more in the way of medicine and social support, have naturally generated an increasing curiosity about medical matters. 'He who sees things develop from their origin sees them better', said Aristotle. Health problems have a history, and that history can contribute to the development of new ways of living, suffering and dying. Who, for example, would deny that the history of psychiatry, particularly since it is one of dead ends and mistakes, serves as a powerful lesson in modesty and prudence for its practitioners (not to mention the patients!)?

Many fields of exploration have opened up in the last twenty years – not just historical epidemiology, as already mentioned, but also medical anthropology, ethnomedicine, psychohistory, and multidisciplinary studies of the concept and the politics of health, and the professions and bodies of knowledge relating to it. Even the most traditional areas of the history of disease, therapeutics and hospitals, have been opened up to economic, sociological, juridical, philosophical and literary investigation. In any case, these studies – which still seldom involve international comparisons – are, because of their multidisciplinary character, best placed firmly in a sociohistorical perspective. What historian of tuberculosis would nowadays dare to settle for giving a history of the disease *stricto sensu* without seeking to gauge its impact on a society as a whole, or on literature, and without attempting to portray the way of life, moral code and fantasies of that micro-society, the sanatorium?

In fact nothing is more revealing of a society than the history of its diseases, particularly the 'social' diseases (as they were still called in the fifties): alcoholism, tuberculosis, insanity, syphilis, and so on. Besides, these diseases form a family: one leads to another, and there's certainly no law against having them all at once. But the one which is most a part of our culture, the one which has terrorized people the most, the one which has had the greatest influence on morality and literature, is unquestionably syphilis. It killed fewer people than tuberculosis, or even alcoholism, and it was less feared than any form of psychosis, and yet it was the disease which caused the most, and the blackest, ink to flow.

Syphilis, then, is of great interest to the historian of medicine, and even the doctor (it is a serious disease which has by no means disappeared) but its five centuries of eventful existence make it of even greater interest to historians of the new school, those whose concern is the history of attitudes, of sexuality, of those trifles which characterize man: his preferences in food, smells, clothing . . . During the last half-millennium syphilis was queen of the venereal diseases, until being dethroned by a newcomer, AIDS, of which I will say more in the conclusion – not as an arbitrary concession to contemporary concerns (a 'disease' which afflicts many present-day historians), but because there are striking similarities in their epidemiologies and in the responses which have been made to them.

First, though, we should reflect on the notion of 'venereal disease'. The words we use in this context are particularly important, all the more so because they are frequently being changed. In fact they are capable of revealing a good deal about the societies which use them. Take the most serious, the dreaded syphilis, and the most widespread, our old friend gonorrhea. These two, which are popularly christened 'the pox' and 'clap', as if to tame them, have been practically the only diseases of the human race to be named according to the means by which they are transmitted: venereal (*'c'est Vénus tout entière à sa proie attachée'* – Phèdre). The word carries connotations of both sex and sin. One is punished by the very means in which one has transgressed. Nowadays, when we are increasingly unwilling to blame anyone for anything, we talk of 'STD' (Sexually Transmitted Disease). Thus the sexual element is hypocritically concealed in an abbreviation (that late-twentieth-century semantic equivalent of leprosy), and relegated to the role of an innocent vector: the disease is transmitted by sex, just as malaria is transmitted by mosquitoes. One does not become infected through careless-ness, or ignorance of elementary preventative measures, and certainly not as a just punishment for having sinned, but by a trick of fate.

It is easy to change words, but less easy to change attitudes, and despite the revolution in sexual morality, syphilis remains a shameful disease. If you doubt this, you need only go to a medical laboratory and watch the expression on the face of the receptionist when someone comes in and asks for a Bordet-Wassermann test (not to mention when someone asks for an HIV bloodtest!). Until recently it would have been bad form for a dermatologist in a provincial town to greet a patient in a public place; it would have set tongues wagging. We find this amusing nowadays, for today's dermatologist is more often concerned with sunburn and hair-loss than with the pox or clap. Indeed, to be greeted by him can even increase one's social standing, for it suggests that one takes good care of oneself and one's appearance. Gone are the days when the plaque outside a doctor's surgery would boldly proclaim 'dermato-venereology'. But dermatologists themselves know how difficult, if not impossible, it is to persuade a sufferer from venereal disease – sorry, STD – to warn his or her partners. And, of course, everyone nowadays knows that syphilis, like gonorrhea, can be completely cured with a few injections of antibiotics. Imagine what things were like when there was no known cure!

Until a few years ago, before the arrival of the terrifying disease AIDS, syphilis was the most serious of the venereal diseases (I hope the reader will pardon me for persisting in referring to them in this way). But the fear it aroused, like the vehemence of the medical and political writings to which it gave rise, makes it something more than that: a social and cultural phenomenon extending far beyond the domain of health alone. In the present work we will be concerned as much with recounting the history of that great fear as with the history of the disease and its treatments. The terror began in Europe with the appearance, at the very end of the fifteenth century, of a new disease which was more horrifying than leprosy and the plague – because of its novelty, its profusion of symptoms, its extreme contagiousness, the suffering it caused, and the fact that (in the early years, at least) it was often fatal. From this time onwards, the abundance of medical writings, hospital archives, and the autobiographical accounts of sufferers like Grunpeck or Hutten give us a good understanding of the symptoms and the epidemiology of this disease which went under various names, but whose sexual character was immediately perceived by its contemporaries. The speed with which the epidemic spread in Europe soon led to exclusion measures and accusatory writings in which the unfortunate pox-sufferers were made objects of public obloquy. Clearly this was the way in which God had chosen to punish them for their depravity.

In the sixteenth century the 'great pox' took a firm hold in Europe, becoming more widespread as it decreased in virulence. There also began a rather hesitant controversy, which was to continue into the twentieth century, as to whether or not syphilis had been imported from the Americas in Christopher Columbus's caravels. Medical treatises were already giving detailed descriptions of syphilis (no-one yet called it by this name, though the word comes from a poem by Fracastor dated 1530), its symptoms and its epidemiology. Prophylactic measures involving the identification of 'high-risk' groups (notably prostitutes) were sketched out. The struggle to find a treatment began with the introduction of those formidable panaceas mercury and gaiac, which were initially in competition with each other but were later used in combination. As for the literature of the time, it seized on a theme which provided ample opportunities for social satire or for moralizing in the narrow sense of the word.

Reactions to 'the venereal disease', a term which covered both syphilis and gonorrhea (the second of which was considered to be one of the manifestations of the first), were different in each of the two centuries which followed. In the seventeenth century a moralizing approach was adopted; the temptations of the flesh are to be shunned, and so much the worse for pox-sufferers, to treat whom is simply to encourage their lecherous ways, according to some authors. Attention should be directed instead to the wife or child infected by the debauchee. During the course of the eighteenth century, however, moral considerations were gradually supplanted by medical ones. Morality, religious or otherwise, is one thing and disease is another; the pox is a disease, and therefore it must be treated. Mercury reigned supreme at the time, but doctors had to reckon with the prodigious activities of empirics and charlatans. The eighteenth century was also one of intense theoretical endeavour, a time of great controversy between the proponents and detractors of the parasitic theory, a theory which replaced a chemical theory that developed from the all-powerful theory of humours. Important clinicians appeared, men like John Hunter of London, or Balfour of Edinburgh, the first to pose a serious challenge to the 'unicist' theory, the theory that a single venereal 'virus' or poison is responsible for a variety of different symptoms. The eighteenth century was a century rich in contradictions, a time at which licentiousness and the pox went hand-in-hand, but also a time at which venereal disease in new-born children became a problem on a national scale.

Although the nineteenth century was the century of medicine *par excellence*, syphilis (from this point onwards referred to as such) made substantial inroads at first. Despite the work of Ricord, who distinguished between syphilis and numerous other venereal diseases, notably gonorrhea, and who put an end to the physiological doctrines of Broussais, treatment seemed to have reached an *impasse*. Mercury began to fall from favour because of doubts as to its efficacy and the fact that it was shamelessly exploited by charlatans; Auzias-Turenne's curious attempt to develop a 'syphilization' analogous to immunization fell into disgrace, and syphilis continued to spread amongst all classes of society. Already, as with AIDS, there was a single line of defence, albeit a fragile one: the male contraceptive, which was invented in England.

The three major stages of syphilis had been well-described very early on, but not until the late nineteenth century, the era of Fournier, do we see an advance beyond this. Progress was made in basic research – it was Fournier who, amongst other things, identified the syphilitic origin of tabes, and subsequently of general paralysis – and also in the setting up of prophylactic measures of the sort which doctors had been demanding since the sixteenth century. A new subject, syphilology, was born, with university chairs, national and (soon) international societies, and conferences. From this point onwards, a whole department of medicine began to open up, supported by a body of campaigning literature aimed at evoking a general fear of the 'venereal peril'. The institution of marriage and the preservation of one's line became the stakes in an immense moral crusade which was to develop throughout Europe. It was set in motion in a most masterful style with a play which it would be amusing to revive one day, '*Les Avariés*' ['The Rotting Ones']. At the same time, following on from Pasteur's work, experts embarked on the laborious task of discovering more about 'microscopic animals'. After a good deal of trial and error, there was a major event in the history of syphilis when, in 1905, Schaudinn and Hoffmann drew attention to the pathogenic agent of syphilis, a pale-coloured treponema. Five years later, Ehrlich created Salvarsan, also known as '606', thus inaugurating the era in which syphilis was treated with arsphenamines, and putting an end to the increasingly disputed reign of mercury. It was undoubtedly the great turning point in the history of syphilis.

From this point on, a number of questions merited separate treatment because of their importance and, even more so, because of their specificity. There is, for example, the fascinating subject of the connections between syphilis and madness, and also between syphilis and degenerescence (imbecility). Never before has a disease threatening the human race produced such a degree of theoretical elaboration. Following on from Fournier's important discovery that general paralysis is one of the tertiary stages of syphilis, theories of degenerescence ('an unhealthy deviation from an ideal primitive type') which had been in vogue since Morel gave way to the powerful myth of hereditary syphilis. This grew so attractive that, in the aftermath of the First World War, the idea of degenerescence began to be criticized. Thus was born the notion of the 'hérédo', a person of impaired intelligence, except in those rare instances in which syphilis chanced to produce a genius. It is a pity that no-one has traced the influence of this theme in literature – Maupassant's 'GPI', for example, or that marvellous pivotal point in a novel by Huysmans: 'There is nothing but syphilis, reflected Des Esseintes . . .'.

Another favourite theme is the relationship between syphilis and prostitution (not forgetting the effect of the latter on the state of health of the armies). Ought there to be medical surveillance of prostitutes, those 'treponema machine-guns', as one old army doctor jestingly called them shortly after the First World War?

This was the crux of the fierce debate which set the proponents of a more or less strict regime of control (some went as far as proposing to make infection a criminal offence) at odds with those 'laisser-faire, laisser-passer' modern physiocrats who were sufficiently realistic to believe that medical surveillance would only increase clandestine prostitution. After the flood of regulatory measures which engulfed Europe in the first half of the nineteenth century, each country reacted according to its own temperament; the sacrosanct ideal of individual liberty led the English to abolish their rather mild measures, whereas the French moved towards a complex, rule-governed system. After the Second World War, the liberalization of moral codes and the emergence of new high-risk groups (homosexuals in particular, but also commercial travellers, club holidaymakers, university students etc.) led to the abandonment of all discriminatory prophylactic measures – a move which the spread of AIDS is now calling into question.

Fear of syphilis reached a peak during the first half of the twentieth century, particularly during the inter-war period. Syphilis was everywhere, and to defend against it the number of dispensaries was increased and the propaganda campaign was stepped up: pamphlets, posters, radio, the theatre and the cinema were actively used to frighten people. As for literature, it reveals the extent to which an entire generation became obsessed by this great fear; Julien Green relates that his sister Eléonore insisted on wearing gloves whilst reading *Bubu de Montparnasse* because it was about syphilis. Never before had medicine and moralizing been so closely entwined: taking precautions against syphilis was primarily a matter of moral hygiene. 'Fear of the pox is the beginning of wisdom', a doctor wrote in 1918. Admittedly arsenical compounds (notably the celebrated neoarsphenamine) proved effective to a certain degree, at least as far as the treatment of the primary and secondary stages was concerned, but the newly-introduced serological tests proved, alas, that syphilis is a disease which can lie dormant, and that an apparent recovery from it is always questionable.

The sudden evaporation of this terror just after the Second World War, thanks to the miraculous new antibiotics, is a social phenomenon at least as astonishing as what went before it. There was, in fact, an instantaneous shift from a frenzy of fear to a complete lack of concern. From this point onwards, all that was required to destroy this fragile treponema (so fragile that it is impossible to produce a laboratory culture of it and, therefore, a vaccine) was a few hefty doses of penicillin; consequently syphilis became no more than an unpleasant memory, and folk could resume their depravities without fear. It was this lack of concern which led to the upsurge of syphilis in the sixties. Venereal diseases, like road accidents, always happen to other people. But to think like this is clearly to overlook the protean and insidious nature of syphilis which has been so well illustrated over the centuries. Today, atypical forms and unobtrusive symptoms can mislead even doctors themselves, and sometimes it is only years later that a routine blood test chances to reveal a syphilitic. Fear of admitting to one's partner that one has the disease, the failure of doctors to notify it, and the lack of information about it (surprising in an age when we are constantly bombarded by the media) all conspire to ensure the continuance of a disease which is still unacceptably widespread today. So syphilis cannot be relegated to some museum of outlandish diseases; and it is on this point, no longer a historical matter but a medical one, that this book concludes.

Syphilis has had five centuries of colourful history, sometimes horrifying and often amusing, a mixture of myth and medicine. Thousands of medical works have been devoted to it in the course of its history, and it occupies a unique position in literature. It is hardly surprising, then, that syphilis is a topic of consuming interest. How could this disease, steeped in fantasies and horrors, so very revealing of the moral behaviour of all the societies it has cut through with impunity, fail to enthral the historian? Of all diseases, syphilis is the most social, in every sense of the word. More than any other it has provoked, and continues to provoke, changes in society, cultural responses which have a completely different character from medical ones. It is also the disease most adept at surviving in human communities; we do not like it, of course, but it seems to like us. Unlike AIDS (to which I will return in the conclusion), with which we play double-or-quits to decide if we survive or if it does, syphilis does not kill. It has lulled us into a state in which we no longer fear it, a state in which we even overlook it. It endures.

1

A Terrifying Affliction (1495–1519)

Charles VIII's Italian campaign

On 1 September 1494, the king of France, Charles VIII, entered Italy at the head of an army consisting largely of mercenaries: Flemish, Gascons, Swiss and even Italians and Spaniards. This was a military exercise of which Machiavelli was later to observe that 'it needed no more effort than to mark the dwellings required as billets with chalk.' On the last day of the year the French army entered Rome, newly abandoned by the Spanish and Neapolitan troops. There it remained for almost a month, making merry and leading a life of unrestrained debauchery.

So it was an army of loose morals and loose discipline which made its way towards Naples on 28 January, closely followed by a troop of beggars and prostitutes, and, at a more respectful distance, those enemy troops reluctant to do battle. On 22 February 1495, the French army entered Naples unopposed. The garrison of Naples consisted of only a thousand men: Italians and Germans, but mainly Spaniards. The local population, accustomed to such events, at first fraternized with the new occupiers, who immediately yielded to the delights of Naples, having sampled those of Rome only a few weeks before.

It was not until 12 May that the King of France made his ceremonial entrance into the city, dressed as a Byzantine emperor and riding in a chariot drawn by four white horses. A week later, however, Charles VIII was forced to leave the city post-haste, not only because a relieving Spanish army had just landed in Sicily, but also because the situation in Naples had become untenable. His mercenaries had behaved so badly during the two and a half months of occupation that the beginnings of a change of sympathy on the part of certain Italian princes and the enthusiasm of the populace had been transformed into open hostility. 'They had hoped,' writes Commynes, 'to find the French all saintliness, faith and goodness; but there was nothing but disorder, pillaging and debauchery.'

Instead of a lasting conquest, the French carried away with them the germ of the Renaissance. But Charles VIII's soldiers had picked up another far less pleasant germ in the course of their debauches, the germ of a new and terrible disease, so new that it was as yet nameless. The French called it 'the Neapolitan sickness', while the Italians called it 'the French sickness'.

The first descriptions of the disease date from the battle of Fornovo (5 July 1495), where every ounce of *furia francese* was required to break the lines of the allied troops. Cumano, military doctor to the Venetian troops who pursued Charles VIII in his retreat in the aftermath of Fornovo and besieged the Duke of Orléans in Novara, relates that he saw

several men-at-arms or footsoldiers who, owing to the ferment of the humours, had 'pustules' on their faces and all over their bodies. These looked rather like grains of millet, and usually appeared on the outer surface of the foreskin, or on the glans, accompanied by a mild pruritis. Sometimes the first sign would be a single 'pustule' looking like a painless cyst, but the scratching provoked by the pruritis subsequently produced a gnawing ulceration. Some days later, the sufferers were driven to distraction by the pains they experienced in their arms, legs and feet, and by an eruption of large 'pustules' (which) lasted . . . for a year or more, if left untreated.[1]

Benedetto, another Venetian doctor who also served at Fornovo, paints his own grim picture of the new disease:

Through sexual contact, an ailment which is new, or at least unknown to previous doctors, the French sickness, has worked its way in from the West to this spot as I write. The entire body is so repulsive to look at and the suffering is so great, especially at night, that this sickness is even more horrifying than incurable leprosy or elephantiasis, and it can be fatal.[2]

He also saw sufferers who had lost their eyes, hands, noses, or feet. Elsewhere, during the autopsy of a woman infected with the French sickness, he observed bones that were tumerous and suppurated to the marrow beneath, though the periosteum remained intact. This new plague (in the indeterminate sense of that era),[3] whose sexual character had immediately become evident, is mentioned as early as 1495 and 1496 in most of the towns of Italy in terms which testify to the horror which it evoked everywhere it struck.

A doctor in Verona, himself infected with the *Mal Franzoso*, bears witness to the sufferings he endured: 'These pains are more violent towards evening; sufferers feel as if their bones are broken and distended, and they experience a good deal of difficulty in moving them.'[4]

Italian doctors everywhere emphasized the suffering inflicted by the French disease. One of the most important, Leoniceno, the famous professor of medicine at Ferrara, writes that the 'pustules' which first appear on the 'privy parts', and then spread over the whole body, particularly the face, 'are not only repulsive in appearance . . . but also produce great suffering most of the time.'[5] He also discusses at length the idea that the French disease is a form of leprosy, but concludes against it.

The epidemic in Europe

The first Italian war had brought subjects of all nationalities into contact with one another. Charles VIII's mercenaries, who were demobilized during the summer of 1495, were to spread the new disease when they returned to their respective countries.

France was the first to be affected, as many chronicles testify. For example, Jean Molinet, native of Boulonnais and official historian of the house of Burgundy, records 'the trip to Naples made by King Charles of France, the eighth of his name'. Here is how he ends the chronicle:

Finally he conquered the great pox, a violent, hideous and abominable sickness by which he was harrowed; and several of his number, who returned to France, were most painfully afflicted by it; and, since no one had heard of this awful pestilence before their return, it was called the Neapolitan sickness; some called it 'les grosses pocques', others 'la grande gorre', others 'la pancque denarre', and yet others 'les fiebvres Sainct-Job.'[6]

Jean Molinet was not fond of the French for he had lost his property when Artois was annexed to France. It is most probably for this reason that he generously attributes the new disease to Charles VIII, something which no other chronicle mentions. It is, however, interesting to note the appearance of the term 'pox', soon to become popular, and also that a link is made between the Italian campaign and the appearance of the new disease in France. Likewise, the commentaries of the University of Manosque mention that in 1496 the disease of 'las bubas' (the name the Spaniards used to refer to the Neapolitan sickness) had been spread from Romans in Dauphiné as far as Provence by men-at-arms in the service of the King and the illustrious Duke of Orléans.[7]

The Neapolitan sickness did not confine itself to southern

France, however, but left its mark on the towns through which the mercenaries passed. In Lyons an agreement was made on 27 March 1496 between the city magistrates and the King's officers to expel from the city 'persons afflicted with the great pox, lepers and other diseased and contagious wretches who came to this town a few days ago and whom His Majesty the King wishes to have removed from the city to avoid contagion and, with God's help, keep the said city in good health'.[8] In Besançon in April the municipal authorities granted compensation to several people afflicted with 'what is known as the Neapolitan sickness'.[9]

Geneva too stood at this European crossroads. As early as January 1496 the Genevan city magistrates publicly forbade outsiders infected with the pox (*de infectis gorre*) to enter the city, and those victims already within were forbidden to circulate.[10] In a few months the whole of Switzerland was affected by the epidemic, as is shown by a Confederation edict dated 17 May 1496 which sets out the measures to be taken against the contagion carried by men from the wars afflicted with 'foul spots'.[11]

Paris was affected by the autumn of 1496 at the latest, as we are informed by a ledger at the Hôtel-Dieu where it is recorded that the Prioress, sister Jeanne Lasseline, drew from her account a sum of 80 Parisian livres for those suffering from 'the great pox of Naples', [ditto] 420 livres 'to replace most of the aforesaid sheets and blankets which have been ruined and can no longer be used'.[12]

In the last months of the year, pox-sufferers flocked in ever-increasing numbers to the Hôtel-Dieu, where attempts were made to turn them away on the grounds that 'this is the most dangerous of maladies', and that victims 'cannot be admitted as if it were a sort of leprosy by which honest people can be afflicted'.[13] The destitute pox-sufferers were consequently obliged to withdraw to a spot near the cathedral cloisters where they erected small shacks. But the fear of contagion was such that a plan to create an establishment outside Paris was drawn up, and the normally miserly canons of Notre-Dame raised money amongst themselves so as to be rid of such dangerous neighbours as quickly as possible.

The pox also broke out further north, from 1497 onwards. Phillipe de Vigneulles, a chronicler from Metz writes that in the year 1497 'the news reached the nobles of the city of Metz that certain men-at-arms and riff-raff were coming down into Lorraine and wanted to stay in the area of Metz. These were not folk in the service of any prince, but a motley band of ruffians, who had come together during the wars, and of whom a number were afflicted with the malady known as the Neapolitan sickness or the pox ('la gorre'), which is worse than leprosy ('mésailerie')'.[14]

Although by 1497 almost the entire kingdom was affected by the epidemic, certain towns were particularly badly hit, to such an extent that they lent their names to the pox: 'peste de Bordeaux', 'mal de Niort', 'mal du carrefour de Poitiers', 'gorre de Rouen'.

But it was in the Empire that the Neapolitan sickness, rechristened the French sickness, was most widely remarked. From 1495 onwards the first cases broke out in Nuremburg and Strasbourg. In the latter a disease is mentioned which no one had seen until then, an 'unheard-of' disease which the lansquenets (German mercenaries) brought back from the war. Soon there were public processions and from the heights of their pulpits the cathedral preachers denounced, often in vivid terms, the morals of the age which had allowed this new plague to spread.

On the other side of the Rhine, the path taken by the pox in Germany and the terror it inspired are recorded in municipal edicts, local chronicles, half-medical and half-satirical poems in which the lansquenets and the French disease are held to be inextricably linked, and even, despite the fact that publishing was in its infancy, entire treatises.[15] From 1496–7 onwards, German towns lamented, one after the other, the outbreak of the Bösen Blattern (literally: malignant smallpox) which came from France and Italy.[16]

No testimony is more valuable than that of visual images. It is to Sebastian Brant, famous since the publication of *The Ship of Fools* (*Das Narrenschiff*) in 1494, that we owe one of the first pictures of the pox (and Dürer – see chapter 2). It illustrates his poem *De pestilentiali scorra sive mala de Franzos, Eulogium*, which was published at the end of September 1496. In an age when so few people could read, this outstanding man of letters understood the power of the visual image, and in fact the *Narrenschiff* owes much of its success to the extended series of woodcuts which he had commissioned from Dürer. In the *De pestilentiali* . . ., a unique woodcut shows us the Virgin Mary, on a throne of clouds, with the Infant Jesus on her knee. With her right hand she is about to place the imperial crown on the head of Maximilian of Hapsburg, who is surrounded by his men-at-arms. On the other side a group of entreating pox-sufferers covered in pustules receive beams of light from the Infant's left hand. It is impossible to say for certain whether this is a punishment or a cure. (And why should it not be both, each in its turn?).

There are two other German votive pictures dating from before 1600, one invoking Saint Méen against the French disease, the other Saint Denis. Figures densely covered with pustules are on their knees calling upon the saint. A short prayer appears at the

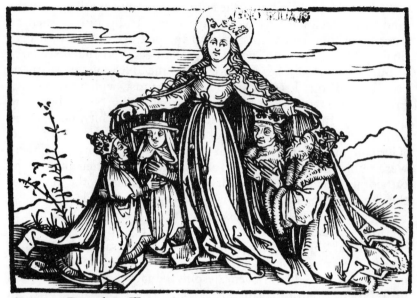

Carmen Dicolon Tetraſtrophon ex ſapphico endeca ſillabo et adonio dimetro F Conradi R C ad clemenʒiſſimá dominá noſtram Mariam ut nos a gallico morbo intactos preſeruet incolumes

PLATE 1 Syphilis (here called 'the French sickness') was a terrifying calamity which spared neither princes nor prelates; the Virgin Mary's protection against it was frequently invoked. (Conrad Reiter, *Mortilogus*, 1508; private collection)

foot of each picture. The first asks by the grace of the holy confessor Minus (Saint Méen) for a merciful protection against the terrible French disease 'by the chastity of our Lord – Amen'; the second appeals to Saint Denis in the following terms: 'O holiest of the Fathers and most mighty protector, Saint Denis, worthy bishop and martyr; heavenly guide, apostle of France and powerful sovereign of the German people, deliver me from the terrible disease called the French disease of which you have cured a throng of Christians in France . . . Deliver me from this most dreadful disease, O most clement Saint Denis.'[17]

Whilst sufferers awaited the intercession of the Virgin Mary and the Saints, the first medical depictions were appearing. Thus, in a medical treatise on the French disease which appeared in Vienna in 1498[18] a woodcut shows us a couple suffering from the pox and covered in pustules. One doctor is examining the urine of the wife whilst, on the other side of the bed, another doctor is applying an ointment to the legs of the husband with a spatula.

Less than ten years after the outbreak of the Neapolitan disease at the battle of Fornovo, then, the whole of Europe was affected by the epidemic. As early as 1496 Brant wrote in his poem that this disease which had invaded Italy and then slipped over the Alps had already reached Germany, Istria, Thrace and Samartia. It is hard to say if the pox had already gained the Don by this date, but it can be seen in England from 1497 onwards, probably carried from Bordeaux to Bristol (where it was for a time known as 'Bordeaux sickness'). Also in 1497, the pox appeared in Scotland under the name *grandgor*, which shows its French origin well enough. A proclamation of King James IV recorded in the registers of the Edinburgh City Council, and dated 22 September 1497, stipulates that patients afflicted with 'grandgor' be confined until they have completely recovered. It is framed as follows:

It is the will of our Sovereign Lord and the Order of Lords of his Council and made known to the Provost and Bailiffs of this place, that the following Proclamation be executed in order to preserve the King's subjects from the great danger of infection by this contagious disease called Grandgor, which has appeared here, and from the great harm which might result therefrom to his Subjects and the Inhabitants of this place; in particular we order and require that, by the efforts of the aforementioned Authorities, all classes of people residing within the boundaries of this place who are infected with, or who have been infected with, and have not been cured of, the aforementioned contagious disease called the Grandgor, should leave this Town and present themselves at ten o'clock in the morning on the beach at Leith, where they will find made ready in the port boats which will be assigned to them by Officers of that place, and will be provided with victuals, and which will transport them to Inch (an island in the Firth of Forth) where they must remain until God restores their Health. And all other persons who take it upon themselves to cure the said contagious disease and who employ the remedy for it must go with them so that none of these people who carry the remedy about them can use the said remedy within the boundaries of this place, nor experiment with it in any wise whatsoever. And anybody who is found to be infected, and who does not go to Inch, as has been set out here, by sunset on *Monday*, and also the aforementioned people who carry the said Health-giving remedy about them if they wish to use it, each and every one of them will be branded on the cheek with a red-hot Iron, so that they may be recognized in future, and if any of them remain they will be exiled without remission.[19]

These severe measures were not put into practice, but they do give a clear indication of the fear which the new disease inspired.

Northern and central Europe were affected a little later, between 1499 and 1502. No-one knows for sure whether the pox arrived in Denmark in 1495 or 1496, but the chronicles of the King of

Denmark mention that 'In the summer (1495) a very great contagion, commonly known as French scabies (*gallica scabies*), previously unknown to the Germans and the Danes, and indeed never before heard of, killed many thousands of men; because of our sins it wormed its way surreptitiously into all countries, with the result that nowadays there is no other sickness which is more common'.[20]

Each newly affected country lost no time naming the new disease after the neighbour which it suspected, usually with good reason, of having been the source of contamination. The following gives an idea of the variety of names: the Muscovites referred to it as the Polish sickness, the Poles as the German sickness, and the Germans as the French sickness – a term of which the English also approved (*French pox*) as did the Italians (which presented certain difficulties). The Flemish and Dutch called it 'the Spanish sickness', as did the inhabitants of North–west Africa. The Portuguese called it 'the Castillian sickness', whilst the Japanese and the peoples of the East Indies came to call it 'the Portuguese sickness'. Only the Spanish, oddly enough, did not call it anything.

Joseph Grunpeck, a 'privileged' witness

A young, intelligent and ambitious scholar from Augsburg, just out of university, published a short pamphlet at the end of 1496 grandiloquently entitled: *A treatise on the pustular epidemic 'Scorre', or the French sickness, containing details of its origin and of the remedies for it, composed by the venerable master Josephus Grunpeck of Burckhausen, following certain poems by Sebastian Brant, professor of civil and canon law.*[21] In it Grunpeck reproduces Brant's poem and its illustration, which has undergone slight modifications, although it would be rash to guess at the intentions behind this. The groups have drawn closer together, the emperor on the left and the pox-sufferers on the right are kneeling, whilst in the foreground lies a pox-victim who is undoubtedly either dead or in a very bad way. Are we to interpret this as a subtle attempt to link the group of victims with the great men of this world? Perhaps not. But it certainly indicates the desire to put the spotlight on the new disease, to dramatize it.

Grunpeck's text makes rather disappointing reading for the historian of medicine as the first nine of its ten chapters are devoted to astrological matters. They show the extent to which the conjunction of the planets, particularly that of Saturn and Jupiter, was to play an important role in explaining the origins of the new disease. Only the tenth chapter contains a few factual observations, and rather dull ones at that: the pox is contagious; one must avoid the public baths during an epidemic; corrupted air must be purified by burning myrrh, incense or juniper berries; the patient must be dieted, given laxatives and rubbed with mercurial ointment.

But the merit of Grunpeck's publication lies elsewhere: it is the oldest printed work to deal with syphilis. The *tractatus* was, moreover, an immediate success, and numerous editions in Latin and German appeared in the years that followed.

In 1498 Grunpeck was in Rome where he was able to study at close hand cases of the pox in soldiers of the Empire who had themselves come to join in the Italian imbroglio. Not long after, he became canon and private secretary to the emperor Maximilian, whom he accompanied on his numerous trips. But Nemesis, who delighted in visiting the disease on those who were too fortunate, already had her eye on the clerk of Augsburg who had so quickly become a person of note. At a banquet which, he later remarked with bitter irony, was attended by Venus as well as by Bacchus and Ceres, he caught the pox himself.

The account of his illness is one of the finest and most terrifying ever written on syphilis.[22] In his now famous introduction Grunpeck powerfully conveys the horror and gravity of the situation in these closing years of the fifteenth century. 'In recent times I have seen scourges, horrible sicknesses and many infirmities afflict mankind from all corners of the earth. Amongst them has crept in, from the western shores of Gaul, a disease which is so cruel, so distressing, so appalling that until now nothing so horrifying, nothing more terrible or disgusting, has ever been known on this earth.'

At first Grunpeck concealed his illness from his friends and his entourage, but his pallor gave him away and, when questioned, he was obliged to own up to his misfortune. Immediately, he adds, 'my very dear friends turned their backs on me as if some pursuing enemy had his sword at their throats, without giving a single thought to the obligations of human fellowship and friendship.' There follows a long, detailed and rather exaggerated description of the effects of the disease: 'the disease loosed its first arrow into my Priapic glans which, on account of the wound, became so swollen that both hands could scarcely encircle it'. The swelling of the glans was followed by an abscess from which a putrid-smelling pus flowed for four months. The suppuration spread over the entire penis and scrotum, which were extensively and deeply ulcerated. He also experienced intense pains in his head and his bones. Soon pustules (*verrucae*) appeared all over his body.

Since the potions, lozenges, powders and pills of the most illustrious doctors were no more effective in curing him than the measures he prescribed in his treatise of 1496 he resorted in desperation to surgeons, lay doctors and, finally, to charlatans. These last, he adds, 'were already everywhere in the provinces, in the towns, in people's homes, to the ruination of mankind, vying with each other in the presence of their patients to make a dishonest penny. I deferred to their ignorance, to their dubious and painful experiments.'

One of these charlatans, a former darner who found medicine more lucrative than his previous trade, managed to blanch[23] his pox after having rubbed him with mercurial ointment twice a day in front of a hot oven. Grunpeck believed himself to have been cured, and rode off to join the Emperor. The pains, alas, soon returned, and were so intense in his legs that he was unable to ride a horse. Gradually, tubercules 'almost as hard as stones' appeared on the fleshy parts of his legs.

Once more Grunpeck had to put up with the indifference of doctors who, as he wrote, 'laden with honours, and renowned for their titles and their knowledge, unwilling for the bad odour to offend a sense of smell accustomed only to perfumes, or to contaminate fingers always warm from constant contact with large sums of gold by touching sordid ulcers, overwhelmed me with their attentions for the span of ten months.' There follows a fierce diatribe against those doctors and apothecaries 'who seek their remedies on Mount Caucasus and in the Caspian Alps, gather them on the banks of the Nile and the Ganges, and borrow them from the Samartians and the Scythians', but end up by admitting their ignorance. 'Wrapped up in the dark obscurity' of these errors and 'plunged into a torrent of suffering' Grunpeck sensed that he would never again 'climb onto the banks of health.'

Once again Grunpeck resorted to untrained doctors and charlatans, writing that 'by the Divine will it has been decreed that only louts and uneducated folk can cure this disease.' And, in fact, after two more years of suffering,

these uncouth men, whoever they were, cesspool emptiers, rubbish collectors, undertakers, cobblers, reapers or menders, had to lance the tubercules, those harbingers of countless horrible and incurable wounds, and thus drive away or suppress the consumption with pills, ointments, creams or some other such medicine; and it is undoubtedly due to the zeal, industry and application of these men . . . that I, afflicted for the second time, and very severely at that, with this illness, recovered my forces sufficiently to resume my usual activities and satisfactorily perform my function of secretary and gentleman in the service of the King.

Further on, Grunpeck leaves off the account of his own misfortunes for a moment to paint a horrifying picture of those of Maximilian's soldiers, tortured by the French disease, whom he had had the opportunity to observe during the war:

Some are covered from the head to the knee with a rough scabies dotted with black and hideous lumps, which spares no part of the face (except the eyes), the neck, the chest or the pubis. They had become so filthy and repugnant that, left in the open air on the battlefield, they hoped to die . . . . Some, instead of bemoaning their painful plight, invited others to laugh and mock at their misfortune. Others, by contrast, moaned and wept and uttered heartrending cries because of the ulceration of their male organ.

Elsewhere, Grunpeck emphasizes the seriousness of the French sickness, which produced renewed attacks of pain in the veins, arteries, limbs and joints despite the fact that 'all the external scabs had disappeared due to the longstanding nature of the sickness and the healing properties of the medicines.'

Grunpeck himself, however, was to survive his illness a long time, for we meet him again at the age of eighty-one, writing a *Prognostication* on Charles the Fifth.

The Spanish doctors (1497–1502)

However, apart from Grunpeck's account, the merit of which lies in his personal testimony, it was the Spaniards rather than the Germans who, in the very last years of the fifteenth century, produced the first great medical treatises on the new disease.[24] As we shall see, there is a very good reason for this.

Gaspar Torella, who was born into a family of doctors in Valencia in 1452, had studied medicine at Montpellier. Not just a brilliant doctor but a great man of letters and a talented mathematician, Torella also had the honour and the benefit of the protection of Rodrigo Borgia, the archbishop of Valencia. First Torella received a bishopric from his already powerful protector (and was immediately obliged to enter holy orders). Then when Rodrigo Borgia became pope in 1492, taking the name of Alexander VI, Torella followed him to Rome. It was there in 1497 that he published his first work on the 'unknown sickness'.[25] He dedicated it to Caesar Borgia, then dean of Valencia.

The previous year ('*anno elapsus* 1496'), he relates, many people fell victim to a cruel sickness, as many in Italy as beyond the mountains . . . Though we need not go into the niceties of a dissertation peppered with quotations from Galen and Avicenna, we should note the observations which Torella appends relating to five patients he claims to have cured during the months of September and October 1497. The first, he relates, was a young man of twenty-four, Nicolas Valentius, who had had sexual relations in August with a woman who was infected with *pudendagra* (one of the many names he gives the disease). Valentius was infected, and an ugly-looking ulcer appeared on his penis, accompanied by a certain hardening of the tissues (*quadam duritie*) which spread 'like the spokes of a wheel, towards the groin'. In six days the ulcer had partly healed over but the patient experienced dreadful pains, especially at night, in the head, neck, shoulders, arms and legs. After ten days the same areas became covered in scabby pustules. The pains and eruptions persisted until 8 October. In four months Valentius, who had undergone a rather complicated course of treatment, recovered completely. He had nodes on all of his limbs; these had appeared recently, but disappeared with the use of purges, blood-lettings, sudations (sweatings), resinous frictions, pills of celandine and aloe. Thus as early as 1496 a first complete case history of syphilis had been recorded.

In a second treatise by Torella, published in 1500[26] and written, according to the fashion of the time, in the form of a dialogue between patient and doctor, it is said that that part of the skin which is in contact with the pus of the *pudendagra* is contaminated. It is usually the genital organs, but another part of the body can just as easily be affected. Thus an infected wet nurse can infect a baby's mouth or face. Conversely, unweaned infants who are themselves infected could give it to several nurses. And, he adds, 'this malignant substance, by its virulence and its corrupting power, defiles everything it touches and converts it into its own substance.'

Another of Pope Alexander VI's doctors, Pedro Pintor, also came from Valencia. To him we owe two treatises on the new disease, one of which appeared in 1499, the other in 1500.[27] 'From 1494 until the present year,' he writes, 'a certain unknown sickness, characterized by different sorts of pain in different parts of the body, and by various sorts of pustules on the skin, has tortured the human race terribly; in Rome its popular name is *morbus gallicus*.'

We need not go into the lengthy astrological considerations which cause Pintor to identify 1483 as the year when the disease began and 1500 as the year it would end, nor need we pursue at present the delicate question of the origin of the disease; Pintor's writings do, however, also contain interesting clinical notes:

This sickness has a hideous aspect, producing various symptoms and, in most people, very acute pains; in others there are no pains, but instead various forms of pustule, large and small. In some cases they merge, in others they remain separate, sometimes limited to the head and face, sometimes appearing on the abdomen and all the limbs. In many they appear on the thighs and legs and spread over the whole surface of the body; in rare cases a fever develops; but if this happens, it is attributable to a completely different cause. The disease does not develop in childhood, and rarely in old age; it begins in the genital organs, especially the male glans and the female vulva (*'in proeputio capitis virgae et in vulva mulierum'*).

There was therefore a clear awareness of the great variation in symptoms from one patient to another. The same diversity is emphasized as regards the cutaneous eruptions of the secondary stage; the damage to the nose and larynx associated with the tertiary stage is mentioned, and pulmonary syphilis is briefly touched on. Pintor stresses, moreover, the extreme contagiousness of the disease and the fact that coitus with a woman infected with it is the principal cause. He adds that those who have withdrawn from society, such as nuns, are safe from contagion.

It was another Spaniard from Valencia, Juan Almenar, a rich nobleman, astronomer and doctor, who, in 1502, devoted a clear and succinct work to the French sickness;[28] this enjoyed a deserved success, more in Italy, where the first editions appeared, than in his own country. Almenar explains that the French sickness, which he proposes to call *'passio turpis saturnina'* (because it distorts the facial features), is generally transmitted by coitus, but also by kissing, breastfeeding and, much more rarely, corrupt air. Almenar adds piously that it is fitting to diagnose this last means of contamination when the sufferers are members of a religious order.

As well as the usual astrological considerations, Almenar examines the primary ulceration of the penis, the sensations of heaviness in the head, and the pains in the cervix which soon affect the joints and which become worse at night. As for the *pustulae* which then overrun the entire body, he emphasizes that they may take many forms, but the thread of his explanation is lost in the theory of the humours: he attributes small, yellowish or ulcerated *pustulae* accompanied by acute pain to an excess of bile, large whitish ones accompanied by gradually spreading pain to phlegm, and blackish *pustulae* to black bile, etc.

However, the most remarkable figure amongst the Spanish doctors is undoubtedly Francisco Lopez de Villalobos, who in 1498, at the age of twenty-four, published a 2,500-line medical poem in Spanish 'on the pestilential *bubas*'[29] which is the oldest work in Spanish on syphilis. At the time he was only a medical student at the University of Salamanca, but ten years later he was doctor to Ferdinand the Catholic. In 1516 he too left Spain for Italy, where he became doctor to Charles V. He died in 1548, at seventy-five, perhaps poor and undoubtedly disappointed by the ingratitude of the men in high places whom he had served all his life, but who forgot him in his old age.

But what was the *bubas*? It was a hitherto unheard-of pestilence ('*no vista jamas*'). Villalobos seems to have been the first to refer to the new disease by the word *bubas* which, although it had already been used in other senses, was to become popular in this one thenceforward. Villalobos also calls it 'the Egyptian scab', 'because it is as awful as the scab which God sent to punish us and make us repent'. When the *buba* appears on the male member, and especially if it is painless, hard and blackish, and accompanied by headaches and a feeling of heaviness in the shoulders, and if the sufferer cannot sleep, but experiences instead senseless and fleeting dreams . . . 'you can safely judge that this is the onset of the Egyptian scab.'

Then a very ugly eruption of scabs appears on the face and over the whole body, accompanied by intense pains in the joints. The tibias are painful 'and their membranes also become the site of intense suffering . . . hard tumours form there . . . the forehead and head also hurt because of the nodules and ganglions formed by this large tumour.' The balls of the feet and the palms of the hands become excessively hot . . . the forehead becomes very hot and turns a deep red colour.

The variety of forms of what were later called the syphilides is once more noted: 'fiery cysts which produce a terrible burning sensation' on the face, wrists and hands, 'burning scabs' and 'countless little spots that are yellow, or sometimes red, and prurient', 'scabs which are large, rough, chapped and lead-coloured', or else 'whitish and very moist'.[30]

Early recommendations

All of the numerous writers who dealt with the new disease in the years immediately following its appearance in Europe emphasize the role of the sexual act in infection. The first recommendations given by doctors were therefore based primarily on common sense: 'I declare the sickness to be contagious,' writes Gilino of Ferrara in 1497, 'which is why I recommend once more that you should avoid any form of intimate contact with women who are infected with this dangerous malady, for I have seen many of those who are infected with it experience the greatest suffering.'[31] Also in

1497, the famous professor Widman of Tubingen advises that in order to keep oneself safe from contagion, one should take the utmost care not to perform the sexual act with a woman afflicted with the *pustulae*, or even with a healthy woman who might have had intercourse with an infected man in the recent past. Experience proves, continues Widman, that anyone who follows on after a man recently affected with *pustulae* is himself infected. Consequently, one should beware of prostitutes for the time being.[32]

A minority, including Scanaroli of Modena,[33] deny infection by coitus, and maintain that the illness can break out in the sexual organs *de novo*. To support his views, Scanaroli offers as proof the fact that he has observed the French sickness in virgins and in elderly men who were no longer sexually active. This doctor, for all that he was only an obscure pupil of Leoniceno, certainly had some supporters amongst those Bolognese families where daughters who were marriageable and therefore given out to be virgins had awakened one sad morning with the first signs of the French sickness.

However, although according to Torella the sovereign remedy consists in avoiding contact with those who are infected as one avoids contact with lepers, flight alone will not help, for the contagion is everywhere.[34] And there are those – and they are legion – unable to forgo copulation. Villalobos advises: 'when we wish to consummate the act of Venus and Mars we should ensure that Saturn, who is an unlucky companion, is absent.'[35]

Fortunately, the advice is often more practical, as, for example, when Almenar recommends the man and the woman to perform a meticulous toilet of the genital organs after the sexual act with hot water or white wine, using their nightshirts or a clean cloth, and above all to avoid using towels belonging to prostitutes because they are contaminated. If, however, a 'blemish' (*nocumentum*) appears on the penis, continues Almenar, one must make lotions with a decoction of simples (mostly plants) in wine, and then sprinkle oneself with a powder containing, amongst other things, litharge, gold and white lead.

As for Torella, he advocates some very curious procedures; if the penis is ulcerated and infected (it is always the male sex for which the doctor feels pity, the woman being strictly confined to the role of contaminator, whose chancre, moreover, is difficult to discover), you must immediately wash it thoroughly with soft soap, or apply to it a cock or a pigeon plucked and flayed alive, or else a live frog cut in two.[36]

Nevertheless, the tendency was to avoid giving advice regarding individual prophylaxis on the grounds that it was not wise to encourage sexual excesses by guaranteeing those who performed them impunity from venereal disease. As for those who were already contaminated, ought one to work against the will of God, who had punished them by the very means in which they had sinned?

First measures

The case was somewhat different as regards collective measures. These were concerned less with treating those afflicted with the 'great pox' than with protecting those not already infected. We have already seen how the Hôtel-Dieu in Paris was besieged by pox-sufferers from the autumn of 1496 onwards. But people reacted to these invalids in just the same way they reacted to lepers, fear of being infected getting the upper hand over the desire to be charitable and give them treatment. This explains the decree issued by the *parlement* of Paris on 6 March 1496[37] 'being a ruling on the matter of sufferers from the Great Pox', whose preamble makes it clear that the intention is to 'deal with the dangers arising from keeping company with, and being in communication with, persons suffering from a certain contagious sickness called the Great Pox, of whom there are now a great number in this City of Paris'.[38]

The parliamentary decree stipulates that pox-sufferers from outside the city must present themselves within twenty-four hours at the gates of Saint-Jacques and Saint-Denis, where their names will be taken, and each of them will be given four Parisian sous. Under pain of hanging, they must then leave the city, and not return until they are cured. As for Parisians stricken with the pox, they too are given twenty-four hours within which, under pain of hanging, they are to confine themselves to their homes or present themselves at specially prepared premises at Saint-Germain-des-Prés, 'at which place they will be provided with victuals and other necessities of life for the duration of the aforementioned sickness'. This marked the beginning of a systematic policy of refusing pox-sufferers entry to the Hôtel-Dieu, motivated by fear of contagion, both physical and moral.

In Paris, the few homeless syphilitics who could be caught were driven out of the city, and a few dozen destitute sufferers were put in two barns belonging to the abbey of Saint-Germain.[39] The proximity of this place to the leper colony is a clear sign of the terror which the pox-stricken inspired in the population at large and the city authorities, and certain chronicles of the time remark, perhaps in jest, that the few lepers who continued to occupy the

Saint-Germain sickhouse complained about having such dangerous neighbours.

However, it soon became clear that, despite the threats of hanging, these measures had little effect. Great numbers of pox-sufferers continued to flock to the Hôtel-Dieu, causing great agitation amongst canons of the chapter, who demanded a meeting with the Provost and city authorities of Paris 'to debate with them the matter of those afflicted with what the vulgar call the Neapolitan sickness, who flood in ever greater numbers to the aforesaid Hôtel-Dieu de Paris, so much so that the whole establishment is infected'.[40]

On 25 June 1498 the Provost of Paris issued an order reaffirming the instructions in the parliamentary decree, this time under pain of being cast into the river. The threats were not in fact carried out, and pox-sufferers continued to besiege the Hôtel-Dieu, and the most poverty-stricken of them even went so far as to beg at the gates of the palace of Tournelles, under the eyes of the king himself.

As usual, it was money that was lacking. As the bishop of Paris observed to the *parlement*, charitable donations and the income from fines levied on 'those with the Neapolitan sickness' were simply inadequate. It must be added that the introduction of the practice of whipping newcomers to the new premises (nothing more than a few barns) was hardly calculated to attract customers, even if no-one would have dreamed of denying that the pox was a direct result of licentiousness, and that its victims were suffering for their sins.

The decree of the *parlement* of Paris was renewed regularly until the beginning of the sixteenth century, ceaselessly demanding that 'persons afflicted with venereal maladies' should be put 'out of the city, like lepers'. But there is evident disillusionment: 'the malady in question has become so common that this decree is no longer observed.'[41]

Further writings (1502–1514)

After 1500, medical treatises on the *morbus gallicus* (a term which tended to stick in learned circles) became more numerous, a sure sign that the fear and interest of doctors had been aroused by this disease which had conquered Europe in less than five years.

Speculations on the aetiology of the disease varied *ad infinitum*, but everyone agreed that it involved the introduction of a poison into the body. 'It is a morbid condition,' wrote Cataneus (1504), 'originating in a total infection of the substance of the blood, linked with a poison contained in the *menstrues*.'[42]

Furthermore, everyone emphasized the grave nature of the disease and the suffering it caused. When a lesion appears on the penis following coitus, it is no laughing matter, warns Benedictus (1508), as if the idea of laughing would have occurred to the victim. In fact, he continues, it may result in the complete loss of the penis and testicles, as happened to a printer in Venice. But, this decidedly humourless author adds, there is no need to be ashamed, for good doctors, like good confessors, do not divulge the secrets which are entrusted to them.[43]

Destruction of the uvula, the nasal cartilage and the trachea is clearly understood to be a symptom of the French disease (by Cataneus in 1504 and Maynardus in 1506).[44] The *pustulae* are described in even greater detail, and first attempts at classifying them appear (Benivenius, 1507).[45]

The clearest and most complete description of the disease is undoubtedly that given by Juan de Vigo, who devotes two chapters of his *Surgical Practice*, published in 1514, to what he too calls 'the French sickness'.[46] He gives a careful account of the order in which the symptoms occur. To begin with, *pustulae* appear on the male and female genitals; they are of a livid, black or whitish colour, and are surrounded by an induration ('*cum callositate eas circumdante*'). Shortly after the first lesions have healed, hard *pustulae*, sometimes protuberant and sometimes verruca-like, break out over almost the entire body. The patient experiences intense pains in his limbs and joints. A year or more later, purulent tumours appear, along with bone-like callosities which are so painful at night that they make the sufferer scream. This is almost always followed by the destruction of the bones, and the limbs affected remain permanently twisted or stunted.

In spite of their differences, all the works which appeared before 1514 agree on the principal characteristics of the new disease: its contagiousness and ability to spread quickly, something which had initially shocked some contemporaries into classifying it as a plague; the fact that it was transmitted venereally, even though its extreme contagiousness meant that contamination through other means was fairly frequent; its multiplicity of cutaneous manifestations, and the intensity of the pains in the head and bones (the sensation that the bones are 'broken and twisted') to which it gives rise; and, finally, the fact that it is frequently fatal.

Most authors mention the primary chancre and its induration. And they all agree that it is followed by a reddish rash whose superficial resemblance to smallpox ['*la variole*'] is undoubtedly responsible for the origin of the term 'pox' ('*la vérole*').[47] In a few days the entire surface of the body is covered in small protuberant nodules, from which a fetid sanies exudes. Sometimes there were also thick scabs of a greenish-black hue which led contemporaries to report that the appearance of sufferers disfigured in this way was more repugnant than that of lepers. According to several authors, however, the eruptions could take milder forms.

After a brief respite, during which the horribly painful symptoms of the disease and the sufferer's physical weakness and spiritual depression testify to the extent to which the body had been penetrated by the disease, large rounded tumours start to appear at random in muscles or bones, eating away cavities within them. At first they are hard, but they soften into a whitish and viscous substance (hence the term gumma, used from this time onwards); they ulcerate the body extensively, exposing the bones and eating away at the nose, the lips, the palate, the larynx and the genitals.

The history of the gallant Ulrich von Hutten

Ulrich von Hutten was born in 1488 in a gloomy chateau in Franconia. It was intended that he should pursue an ecclesiastical career, because of his frail and delicate constitution, but the young Ulrich, a spirited lad, fled at the age of sixteen for a life of adventure. This did not prevent him from pursuing his studies and being made a Master of Arts in 1506. He wandered across Europe, writing poems and political essays, sometimes defending widows and orphans, but more often flirting with the ladies. It was at this sport that he caught the pox.

Following the example of Grunpeck, his compatriot, Hutten describes his illness in a work which soon met with considerable success, both because of its close concern with treatment and because of the sincerity of Hutten's views. 'Providence,' writes Hutten,

has seen fit to order things so that nowadays we see maladies unknown to our forefathers springing up around us. It was in the year of Our Lord 1493, or thereabouts, that this pestilential sickness broke out. This happened, not in France, but in the Kingdom of Naples; it was called the French sickness because before it became rampant elsewhere it appeared in the French army which fought in Italy under King Charles. The French, rejecting this denomination as ignominious and defamatory, designated the affliction the Neapolitan sickness. However, in this modest work I shall follow the usage which has prevailed generally, and call it the French sickness; this is most definitely not because I bear any grudge against a most renowned nation which is, perhaps, the most civilized and hospitable now in existence, but simply because I fear that the majority of my readers will not understand me if I call the malady by a different name.[48]

As a devout and militant Lutheran, Hutten begins by settling his scores with the Church, poking fun at priests who proclaim from the pulpit that the scourge has been sent by God to punish mankind for its depravity. Why shouldn't new diseases develop by entirely natural means? For Hutten, though, doctors are no better. They have fled from the presence of sufferers because

when it (the disease) first appeared it caused a far more loathsome stench than it does now, as if the sickness involved were a different type altogether. The ulcers and sores were like acorns in size and shape, and produced a loathsome secretion, making such a stink that it was thought that anyone who smelled it would be infected by the aforementioned sickness. The colour of the spots was something between green and black, and their appearance caused more anguish to the patients than the pain they experienced, albeit that they felt as if they were standing amidst flames.

Hutten adds that the disease spread more rapidly, and with greater virulence, amongst the Germans than elsewhere, on account of their intemperate habits. Astrologers had predicted that the scourge would last for seven years only. They were mistaken. However, the sickness has undoubtedly become weaker; the stench it causes is no longer so bad, and the ulcers are less obvious and less hard. But the 'venom' still persists, insinuating its way into the body, where it gives rise to a variety of complaints.

The sickness begins with sexual contact. Consequently children, old folk, and those whose behaviour is more restrained are less affected by it. Doctors debate the origin of the sickness endlessly, but the only fact on which they can agree is that it has appeared in their own time. They kept their own counsel during the first two years, unwilling to commit themselves.

Hutten's observations on the various stages of the disease tally with those of doctors of the period. Some of what he says, however, is unprecedented:

There persist, within the private parts of women, lesions which remain remarkably virulent for a long time; they are particularly dangerous because they are less evident to the eye of the man who wishes to cohabit with women in complete safety. And it is for this reason that the condition is so pernicious, for these lesions make it impossible to avoid the sickness, because the bodies of women of this sort are sometimes so badly infected.

The worthy gentleman soon returns to the subject of his own illness, deploring, like Grunpeck, the ineffectiveness and cowardice of doctors: they have fled from contact with sufferers, leaving surgeons to take their place. The latter, in their ignorance, have resorted to caustics in order to burn out the ulcers. Some of them were using salves, of which, amongst other things, mercury was an obligatory constituent. Patients were given frictions one or more times each day and shut up in a steamroom in which a very high temperature was constantly maintained. The treatment lasted between twenty and thirty days. The patient following this regimen would begin to weaken. His mouth and throat would become ulcerated, and swell prodigiously. His gums would tumefy and his teeth would loosen and drop out. A revolting saliva would stream continually from his mouth. Many sufferers preferred death to this barbarous procedure, which cured barely one in a hundred.

You may judge for yourself, remarks Hutten, the distress which I have experienced, having undergone this treatment eleven times. 'In great danger and in very unpleasant circumstances I have already struggled with this malady for nine years, and I have eagerly tried other remedies which looked as if they might work against this curse'. But, continues the gallant gentleman,

the saddest thing is that those who treated us in this fashion have themselves got no medical expertise. I have seen one healer cause three unfortunate artisans to perish in a steamroom whose temperature was raised on his recommendation. These patients, convinced that their cure would be quicker and more certain the higher the temperature they could bear, were stifled quite unaware of the nature of their unhappy end. I have seen others, whose swollen throats no longer allowed them to spit out or vomit up the purulent mucus, struggle in the grip of a most appalling agony and be suffocated by the corrupt fluids.

Ulrich von Hutten died in 1524 at the age of thirty-five, though it is not known for certain whether it was of the pox. He had been deeply affected by his own experience of the disease and, perhaps even more, by the sight of others with it. The Reformist religion which he had espoused early on was a great comfort to him. A short time before his death he wrote: 'Fate will cease pursuing me. My one consolation is that my courage is equal to my misfortunes.'

Gaiac versus mercury

Whilst Hutten was suffering so badly that one of his friends advised suicide he had, as he puts it, 'the boldness to resort to the services of gaiac'.[49] His boldness was a relative matter, of course, as becomes clear when one learns that doctors had tried to remove a gumma which had developed above his right heel by using caustics and a red-hot iron, and even more so when one reflects on the mercurial treatments he describes. But just what is this gaiac cure?

Wood of the gaiac, a tree imported from Hispaniola,[50] is reduced to a powder, infused, and a decoction is made; this is then simmered. The patient is put in a warm room with a close atmosphere. His intake of food is gradually reduced until he is on a strict diet, and mild purgatives are administered to him. Each day he is required to drink a large dose of decoction of gaiac, after he has made himself begin to sweat by wrapping himself in blankets. After thirty days of what is undoubtedly a debilitating regimen 'the illness has been rooted out'.

During his misfortunes, then, Hutten had the good luck to come across gaiac. This, at least, is what he says, affirming that he was healed in this manner, though the cure was prolonged well beyond thirty days. 'All the doctors considered my case to be a hopeless one, but thanks to the divine properties of gaiac I promptly recovered.' This proves, he says, that even in the most frightful illnesses one must never give up hope.

Hutten was one of the first to champion gaiac, two years after this wood had first been imported from America. Moreover, his work (of 1519) is, as the title indicates, a testimonial in favour of the precious tree. In fact the immediate vogue for gaiac, whose laxative and sudorific (sweat-inducing) properties must be acknowledged, is explained by the gathering reaction against the abuse of mercury.

When syphilis first appeared, doctors were so completely bewildered that Grunpeck said that they had been 'obliged to make a dishonourable pact with the enemy to allow him a lustrum (we shall be returning to this detail) in which he can, without let or hindrance, tyrannize, overwhelm, petrify with terror, and crush wretched mankind.'[51] In these closing years of the fifteenth century, we see the canons of Notre-Dame de Paris ordering public processions with the reliquaries of Saint Marcel and Saint Geneviève to ward off 'this dangerous and contagious sickness, against which doctors and physicians can offer no remedy'.[52]

Then, with great rapidity, doctors followed the lead of the empirics and charlatans, who, even before 1500, prescribed the mercurial treatments discredited by Galen but often used in Arab medicine for the cure of dermatoses and even leprosy – diseases which, for contemporaries, closely resembled the great pox. From that time onwards, every medical treatise devoted a good deal of space to the therapeutic uses of mercury. In 1500, Pintor,[53] who had at first resorted to blood-letting, sung the praises of mercury-based ointments used as frictions, although he does indicate that there are serious drawbacks.

Almenar, in 1502,[54] sets out his ideas on treatment at length. Almenar was the first to stress the idea that the disease, despite its diverse cutaneous manifestations, had a unique individual character, and that diathetic considerations are crucial to the treatment of it. He advocates good hygiene, laxatives, sudorifics and mercurial frictions, which are, according to him, the best remedy for the French sickness. However, he considers the use of mercury to promote salivation to be harmful, though his colleagues were soon to make it a mainstay of their therapy.

It would be tedious to list all those who, in the very first years of the sixteenth century, recommend the use of mercury in the form of an ointment (Maynardus in 1506) or a friction (Benedictus in 1505 and Cataneus in 1504; the latter also recommends patients to ligate the base of the penis to prevent the pox venom spreading elsewhere in the body). Juan de Vigo (1514) is more eclectic. He recommends, in the first instance, dieting, bloodletting, purging and the use of internal medicines. But in cases in which this proves to be ineffective one must switch to ointments, frictions administered in front of a fire, and, more especially, to mercurial plasters, for which he gives the formulae.[55] Thanks to them, he says, the pains cease completely, the tubercules disappear, and the indurations and the ulcers clear up. One must keep a careful eye on the salivation and the ulcerations caused by the mercury, but not allow them to stop too quickly, for the displaced matter will continue to be evacuated from the body.

However, many authors before Hutten mentioned the drawbacks of mercurial therapy. The first, Benedetto (1497), was well aware of the complications resulting from the excessive use of mercury – shaking and paralysis, the loosening and loss of the teeth, and so on. Torella, who had argued in favour of the use of mercury in his first work, turned against it in his second, accusing it of having caused the deaths of illustrious sufferers, and in particular of great prelates like Jean Borgia and the Cardinal of Segovia. But the most vehement opponent is Villalobos (1498), who regards the defenders of mercury as 'prize idiots'. He preferred lenitive medicines, purges, clysters, baths and bloodletting in both arms to 'render the thick humour fluid'. Though he was opposed to the use of mercury in frictions, he does recommend its use in an ointment for the bubas, but only as one part in six. Moreover, he was apparently the first to advocate the use of arsenic in the treatment of syphilis.[56]

Undoubtedly the application of increasingly strong doses of mercury to the entirety of the patient's body in an overheated steamroom over a period of twenty to thirty days resulted in dangerous intoxication of the patient due to mercury vapours entering the respiratory tract. As for mercurial salivation, the few doctors who recognized it as a problem did not know how to stop it. (Gilino, in 1497, suggested applying a red-hot iron to the skull

of the patient in order to act on the brain, the organ controlling the
pituitary, the humour responsible for saliva.)[57]

One can understand why gaiac, in spite of the debilitating
regimen of treatment it involved, was heralded by doctors, and
above all by patients, as a miraculous alternative to the formidable
mercury. However, the battle between mercury and gaiac had only
just begun.

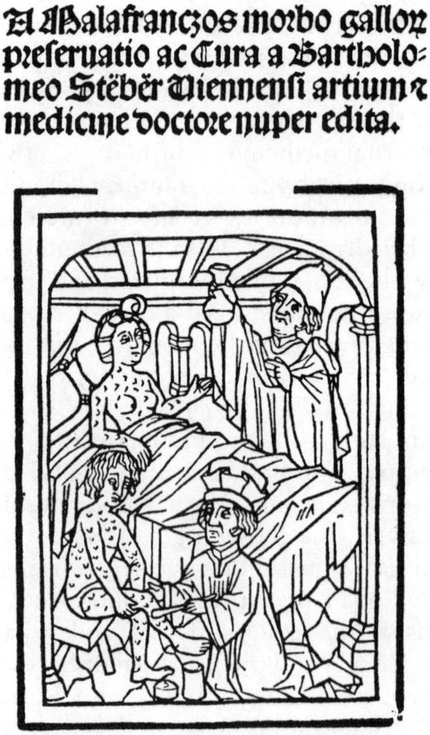

A Malafranczos morbo gallor
preferuatio ac Cura a Bartholo-
meo Steber Uiennensi artium τ
medicine doctore nuper edita.

PLATE 2 This woodcut is the first medical illustration of the pox. It shows a couple
covered in pustules. One doctor examines the woman's urine whilst another uses a spatula
to apply a (mercurial?) ointment to the legs of the husband. (B. Steber, *A mala franzos
morbo gallorum, praeservatio ac cura* . . ., Vienna, 1498; private collection)

2

A Much-disputed Origin

The first explanations

The violence with which the disease had just scourged Europe stimulated a variety of theories as to its origin. There were a number of eclectic ideas: that it was the result of the intercourse of a leprous knight and a courtesan, or of the coupling of men and monkeys, or of the vengeful Spaniards mixing lepers' blood with Greek wine, or of the Neapolitans treacherously poisoning wells at the time of the French invasion, and so on. More consonant with the venereal, and therefore impious, character of the new disease is the traditional explanation of God's anger. Ambroise Paré, in the wake of many others, was to invoke 'God's wrath, which allowed this malady to descend upon the human race, in order to curb its lasciviousness and inordinate concupiscence'.[1]

The Moors, who were driven out of Spain in 1492, were also accused. It was certainly the case that at the time when they had taken refuge in Italy, and in Rome and Naples in particular, a 'plague' had broken out and caused thousands of the inhabitants to perish. This, added to the reputation these outlaws had for lascivious behaviour, was largely responsible for the fact that the spread of the new disease was attributed to them. Likewise, the Beggards, the mystic-erotic sect which had roamed Europe since the time of the Black Death, were sometimes accused.

Furthermore, the venereal character of the epidemic, which undoubtedly made the disease a unique one, was not always perceived. Many saw it as no more than a new plague. Others considered it to be a new form of leprosy – a view which many doctors denied, however.

But it was undoubtedly the astrological explanation which received the most support in the years immediately following the appearance of the pox. Astrologers taught that the relative positions of certain stars could cause epidemics, amongst other phenomena. Thus the conjunction of Saturn (an unlucky planet) and Jupiter in the sign of the Scorpion and the house of Mars (also unlucky) on 25 November 1484 was generally considered to be the indisputable, albeit somewhat remote, cause of the epidemic.

Apart from a few enlightened spirits who, like Pico della Mirandola, were already trying to undermine the foundations of astrology, the influence of the stars was invoked by almost everyone (Grunpeck, Hutten, Almenar, Villalobos, etc.). Dürer himself expressed it in an image. In 1496 he illustrated a medical poem about epidemics by Theodoricus Ulsen. The woodcut shows a pox-stricken knight, covered from head to foot in sinister pustules. Above his head stretches the zodiac, and on it is inscribed the awful date: 1484.

Made in America

All the authors contemporary with the appearance of the pox do at least agree that the disease was a new one. 'There appeared a new malady, spread by carnal contact, called the French sickness, and unknown to the doctors of antiquity', wrote Alexander Benedictus in 1497. Juan de Vigo, for his part, wrote that 'in the month of December, 1494, a malady of a hitherto unknown nature appeared in almost every part of Italy.' Why, then, did it not occur to them that this new disease had come from the New World, which was discovered at the very time that the epidemic broke out, just as leprosy had been brought back from the Crusades?

We have to wait a few decades before we see this explanation being clearly articulated. It first appeared from the pen of Oviedo. Gonzalo Fernandez de Oviedo y Valdes was born into a family of the upper nobility of Madrid in 1478. Beginning his career as a page to the infant Don Juan, son of Ferdinand the Catholic, he was at the siege of Grenada in 1492, and then distinguished himself in the war waged by Naples against the French. The King rewarded him in 1513 by appointing him superintendent of the gold and silver mines of the New World, where he was to spend more than ten years. On his return to Europe he published his *Summary Account of the Natural History of the Indes*,[2] and, ten years later, the *Natural and General History of the Indes . . .*,[3] stressing the value of his eye-witness accounts. ('Moreover, I speak of none of these four matters on the basis of hearsay, but because I myself have seen them; I write of each at a distance, but this is all to the good; they have become firmly inscribed in my memory.')

Oviedo was at the Court when Ferdinand and Isabella received and fêted Christopher Columbus after his first voyage to America. He saw Columbus enter Barcelona 'with the first Indians and samples of the riches and knowledge of this western empire'. He made direct contact with Columbus's companions, recording their testimonies on his tablets, and then collecting, once again in person, those of the natives and the conquerors from across the ocean.

For Oviedo, then, the case was beyond doubt. He expressed himself solemnly to the King of Spain as follows:

Your majesty may take it as certain that this malady (the bubas) comes from the Indes, where it is very common amongst the Indians, but not so dangerous in those lands as it is in our own . . . The first time this sickness was seen in Spain was after Admiral Don Christopher Columbus had discovered the Indes and returned from those lands. Some Christians amongst those who went with him and took part in that discovery, and the many more who made the second trip, brought back this scourge, and from them it was passed on to others. And when, in the year 1495, by order of the catholic monarchs of everlasting memory, your grandparents Don Fernando and Doña Isabel, the great captain Don Gonzalo Hernandez de Cordoba entered Italy with an army to assist King Don Fernando the Younger of Naples (Ferdinand II) against King Charles of France, this disease was introduced into Italy by some of these Spaniards, this being the first occasion on which it had been seen in Italy. And because it was at this time that the French arrived with the aforementioned Charles, the Italians called this malady the French sickness, and the French called it the Neapolitan sickness because they had never seen it before the time of that war. From there it spread throughout Christendom, and to Africa, by means of some women or men infected with the disease, for there is no way in which it is spread more readily than by intercourse between men and women, as has been shown many times.[4]

Another testimony is that of Diaz de Isla, a contemporary of Oviedo. Diaz de Isla was a renowned doctor who was practising in Barcelona at the time the bubas appeared, and who then moved to Seville before settling in Lisbon, where he worked as a surgeon in the All Saints hospital. In 1539 he published a treatise on the pox, which he calls 'serpentine sickness'. In the first chapter he writes:

It has pleased divine justice to send us unknown maladies, such as this serpentine sickness, which have never before been seen, experienced or described in medical texts. It appeared and was noticed in Spain, in the year of Our Lord one thousand four hundred and ninety-three, in the city of Barcelona; this city became infected, and following it all known and accessible lands. This sickness owes its origin and birth from time immemorial to the island which is now called Hispaniola, as is widely and clearly understood. And since this island was discovered by admiral

Don Christopher Columbus, who had relations and congress with the inhabitants of this island during his stay, and since this sickness is naturally contagious, it spread with ease, and soon appeared in the fleet itself. The Spaniards had never before encountered this sickness, so when they felt the pains and other symptoms of the said malady they attributed them to the tiring effects of being at sea and to other causes, each to his own opinion. At the time at which admiral Don Christopher Columbus returned to Spain, the Catholic kings were in the city of Barcelona. And since they asked him for his account of his voyage and discoveries, the said malady soon began to infect the city, and to spread, as we have subsequently had many occasions to observe; and because it caused unprecedented and most terrible sufferings, those who witnessed it protected themselves by undertaking great fasts, by making vows and by alms-giving so that Our Lord would keep them from falling prey to such a sickness. In the following year, one thousand four hundred and ninety-four, the most Christian King Charles of France, who then reigned, gathered together many Spaniards stricken with this infection, and soon the army began to be infected with the said malady . . . Just as we now talk of bubas, pains, apostemes and ulcers, so the Indians of the island of Hispaniola described this sickness in ancient times as guaynaras, hipas, taybas and iças. I myself name it the serpentine sickness of the island of Hispaniola, so as not to break with the universal custom according to which each names it according to the country from which it seems to him to originate . . . . And as far as the name morbo serpentino is concerned, in point of hideousness there is no better object of comparison than the serpent. For just as that animal is hideous, fearsome and terrible, in like wise is the malady hideous, fearsome and terrible. It is a grave malady which ulcerates and corrupts the flesh, breaks and destroys the bones, and cuts and shrinks the tendons, and for all these reasons I give it this name.[5]

Elsewhere, Diaz de Isla emphasizes that he has personal experience in these matters, having treated sailors who took part in Columbus' first trip, and having also treated diseases involving the bubas in Barcelona before King Charles entered Naples. Although Diaz de Isla wrote more than forty years after the dreadful pestilence made its appearance in Europe, he is to be valued as a witness rather than as a theoretician.

Some years later, in 1498, Bartolomé de las Casas, who was ordained at the late age of thirty-six, and who was to spend most of his life defending the oppressed Indians, began a long stay on Hispaniola, where he started his *General History of the Indies*,[6] in which he too tackles the question of the bubas. He writes as follows:

There were two things on this island which were initially very unpleasant for the Spaniards, two things which are there to this day. One is the sickness of the bubas, which in Italy is called the French sickness; it is well-known that this sickness came from this island. Either this happened when, at the time that admiral Don Christopher Columbus returned with the news of the discovery of the Indies, there came those first Indians whom I saw as soon as they arrived in Seville,[7] and it was they who brought the bubas into Spain by infecting the air, or in some other way; or perhaps it happened when some Spaniards came back with the bubas on their first return to Castille, which would have been sometime between 1494 and 1496. And because at that time King Charles of France, nicknamed El Cabezudo (the big-head) was in Italy with a large army in order to conquer Naples and this contagious sickness appeared in his army, the Italians concluded that the soldiers had transmitted the disease to them, and therefore from that time onwards they called it the 'mal frances'. I, for my part, took the trouble to enquire several times from the Indians of this island if the sickness had been there for a long time, and they replied in the affirmative . . . . It is also well-known that all those incontinent Spaniards who did not observe the virtue of chastity on this island were infected with the bubas, and that not a single one in a hundred escaped, except in the case when their partner (*la oltra pacte*) had never had the bubas.

The tradition of the 'American' origin of the pox was thus firmly established at the beginning of the sixteenth century by three authors who are unanimous in insisting that they are relating what they have seen, not what they have heard tell. From this time onwards, doctors and writers who turn their attention to the subject repeat the theory *ad infinitum*. In 1564, for example, Gabrielo Falloppio, in his treatise on the French sickness,[8] observes ironically that Christopher Columbus has discovered a continent, untold islands, uncouth savages, and treasures of gold and silver, but that the precious metals conceal a thorn. In fact, he continues, the soldiers who returned to Europe were laden more with sickness than with gold, and they passed the curse on to others who took up military service with the Italian expeditions at the time of the siege of Naples (at which, he adds, his father was present).

According to a rather more tentative hypothesis which Thomas Sydenham ('the English Hippocrates') was to champion in the seventeenth century, syphilis had been brought to America from Africa by the slave trade, and was then transmitted via the Spaniards of the New World to Europe. But the transportation of slaves from Africa to America dates from 1503, whereas syphilis broke out in Europe in 1495.

The dispute

However, opposition to the thesis that the *bubas* was imported from America was very quick to declare itself. Even before 1500, the debate had already begun between those who considered that the venereal sickness had existed since time immemorial[9] and those who, even though they did not yet suspect that it came from America, believed that it was an entirely new disease.[10] (However, official texts from the reign of Francis I refer to 'the sickness from America'.) But it was not until the seventeenth century that the dispute as to the origin of syphilis, a dispute which still continues today, began in earnest.

At first the opponents of the American theory relied for their support on ancient texts, beginning with the Bible. They cited the books of Moses (Leviticus), and, more particularly, the account of Job's illness, in which the description of ulcers accompanied by pains in the bones at night seemed to them to be indicative of the pox. The works of Hippocrates, Celsus and Galen were also scrutinized. Scholars claimed to have identified the pox in the Babylonian poem of Gilgamesh, in the Eber papyrus, and in the ulceration of the genitals described by Paul of Aegina, Pliny the Younger, and so many others. What is the 'country sickness' Horace refers to? What is the ficus which, according to Juvenal and Martial, makes doctors smile, and results from debauchery, particularly pederasty? And don't the Arab doctors also describe a plethora of lesions on the genitals and the anus – ulcers, chancres, warts, verrucae and rhagades?

All, however, understand the venereal diseases (in particular the three principal ones, which are gonorrhea, chancroid and syphilis) as one and the same ailment. So, for example, Gui Patin, dean of the Paris Faculty of Medicine at the beginning of the reign of Louis XIV, asserts that Job, David and Solomon were afflicted with the 'venereal sickness'. He believes that Hippocrates described it, and also mentions Herodotus, Xenophon, Catullus and Juvenal; he likens the Indian leprosy and Horace's *morbus campanus* to the venereal sickness, and concludes that, in any case, 'the great pox was very familiar in Europe before Charles VIII set out to conquer the Kingdom of Naples.'[11] Admittedly Gui Patin never misses a chance to make a medical blunder (except when he is busy speaking ill of his contemporaries). However, the undeniable presence of venereal diseases in the ancient world proves nothing; it was only because the unicist theory of venereal disease was so unquestioningly accepted that this fact was held to be significant.

In the eighteenth century, however, Jean Astruc restored the credibility of the American theory in an erudite, polished and enormously successful treatise on the venereal sickness.[12] In it he refutes the various arguments for the antiquity of the pox. He concludes as follows:

Thus we can bring forward, as a final proof, the authority of all the doctors who lived at the time that the Pox first appeared, all of whom agree that this Sickness was brought to Europe for the first time at the end of the fifteenth century; that it has no connection with any other illness formerly known; that from the Kingdom of Naples, where first it attacked the Neapolitans and the French, it spread in all directions, by contagion, into the other countries of Europe; and, finally, that it had been brought to Naples by the Spanish soldiers who had served under Christopher Columbus in America.

From then on, the theory of the American origin of the pox seems to have become firmly established, and is supported by the most eminent writers. Montesquieu, for example, writes as follows:

two centuries ago, a sickness unknown to our forefathers made its way here from the New World, attacking humanity at the very source of life and pleasure. The majority of the greatest families in the south of Europe perished from a sickness which came to be too common to be shameful, and was instead simply tragic. It was thirst for gold which perpetuated this disease; people were continually going to America, each time bringing back new seeds'.[13]

In *L'homme aux quarante écus*, Voltaire has his hero ask 'When do you think this curse began in Europe?'. The surgeon replies:

In the year 1494 or thereabouts, when Christopher Columbus returned from his first voyage, amongst innocents who knew neither greed nor war. This age-old disease afflicted these simple and honest nations, just as leprosy reigned amongst the Arabs and the Jews, and the plague amongst the Egyptians. The first fruit gathered by the Spaniards from their conquest of the New World was the pox; it spread more swiftly than Mexican silver, which did not circulate in Europe until long afterwards. The reason is that in every town there were fine public establishments called b——, set up by royal order to preserve the honour of ladies. The Spaniards carried the venom into these privileged establishments whence princes and bishops withdrew the girls they required. It was said that at Constance there were seven hundred and eighteen girls available to serve the council which so devoutly burned John Hus and Jerome of Prague. This single detail gives an idea of the rapidity with which the disease spread through each country.[14]

Nonetheless, the opponents of the American theory were not won over. Less than fifteen years after Astruc's treatise, the Spaniard Sanchez set about proving, in an anonymous work,[15] that the disease was born in Italy because of an alteration in the elements, and was consequently not of American origin. Inverting the argument that the Indian origin of gaiac proves that the disease is from the same source since Nature always provides the remedy side-by-side with the disease, Sanchez explains that it is the Indian origin of gaiac which has caused the belief that the disease came from the New World.

There is room for a compromise between these two mutually exclusive theories, although this compromise has had few supporters.

In 1711 Charles Musitano explained that the pox had existed since ancient times, but that it was not until 1494 that it acquired 'this fermentative virulence by means of which a malady not previously capable of being communicated from an infected body to a healthy one by contagion became communicable in this manner, just like scabies and leprosy'.[16] An even more eclectic theory is that of the Dane Hensler. He explains that the disease was endemic to Hispaniola and that it had passed from America to Spain, but that it had always existed in Europe, where it appeared sporadically.[17]

The 'anti-americanist' camp rallied in the nineteenth century. The Indian origin is, wrote Dr Devergie in 1826, 'a ridiculous story, invented out of spite, spread in a spirit of prejudice and dishonesty, and made creditable by the passage of time, like so many other errors.'[18] And, of course, after Rousseau it was difficult to admit that the Indian peoples, being so morally unimpeachable, could have been the agents of the venereal sickness.

The search for textual evidence became an even more popular pastime.[19] The Ancients were scrutinized once more, and also the doctors of the Middle Ages like Guillaume de Salicet, Lanfranc and many others who, in the thirteenth and fourteenth centuries, spoke of buboes, abscesses and ulcers affecting the private parts. In short, by the end of the nineteenth century the American theory had lost its former standing, and only occasionally found support amongst doctors.

Historic bones

The dispute between 'americanists' and 'anti-americanists' came to a head in Germany at the beginning of the twentieth century. The two major protagonists were Iwan Bloch and Karl Sudhoff. Bloch, using documents which seemed to him to be incontestable, describes the successive stages of the epidemic whose origin, he has no doubt, is the island of Hispaniola. At the same time he sets about dispelling the existing arguments for the presence of syphilis in the Ancient World before the discovery of America.[20] Sudhoff is the great opponent of the 'americanist' theory. In his very numerous works[21] he maintains that it is highly plausible that syphilis was circulating in Europe from the beginning of the Middle Ages, and he makes the important observation that from the twelfth century onwards doctors recommend the use of mercury for a whole range of diseases whose various names mask the identity of the pox.

Sudhoff's school was certainly not lacking in arguments against '*die Fiktion der Amerikanister*'; it ceaselessly brought to light new references, ever more numerous in the years leading up to the 1490s. The dating of some texts, however, is questionable. For example, Maximilian's edict against blasphemers mentions '*die pösen plattern*' (*die bösen Blattern*) on 7 August 1495, although by that date the pox had not yet crossed the Rhine. However, other historians of medicine have pointed out that the mention of the *bösen Blattern* was an interpolation made in the course of the year 1496.[22]

The opponents of the American theory were often reproached, not without reason, for translating the texts they appealed to rather too freely. The result was that they abandoned textual research in favour of an enthusiastic study of necropoli. If indisputable syphilitic lesions could be found on the bones or teeth of a burial predating the discovery of the Americas then the American theory would be destroyed once and for all.

The first systematic research on osseous syphilis in the Stone Age was undertaken in 1877 by J. Parrot, a doctor at the Hôpital des Enfants Assistés in Paris. But it was in the first decades of the twentieth century that exhumation really became all the rage. Central Russian skeletons from two thousand years before Christ, Neolithic skeletons from Upper Egypt, and skulls and bones from all the anthropological museums of the globe were minutely inspected in their hundreds, even thousands. Even the noses on busts of Socrates were grist to the mill of those who upheld the antiquity of syphilis.[23]

With the enthusiasm with which they had once argued over passages in the Bible, scholars now became passionately interested in the shape of suspect humeri and ulnae. Sometimes an indisputable exostosis of the tibia would seem to herald the triumph of the 'anti-americanists', but then the antiquity of the skeleton would be called into question. As for the rare cases in which the reports give more positive support to the 'anti-americanists', they are so few that they can in no way be regarded as significant. Thus, for example, in 1930 Lorenz Michaëlis of Breslau, who examined bone fragments polished by a special process at several degrees of magnification, claimed to have found lesions characteristic of osseous syphilis on two (!) subjects buried in Europe before the discovery of America.[24]

Moreover, research on pre-Columbian skeletons is hardly more convincing. Thousands of analyses and reports end with nothing more than vague conclusions of the type 'apparent syphilitic necrosis'.[25] However, more recent studies have discovered traces of syphilis, or at least of treponematosis (I shall say more about these matters when I turn to the study of syphilis in our own time), on several pre-Colombian bone specimens from Argentina, Peru, Mexico, Guatemala, the Antilles and various regions of the United States.[26] This, added to the fact that it has been impossible to discover similar scars on European bones which predate 1500, has therefore turned the tables on the opponents of the American theory.

The Spanish perspective

It would be ridiculously presumptuous of me to decide one way or the other on a debate in which neither side has genuinely triumphed.[27] Nonetheless, it is useful to review the chronology of the beginning of the syphilis epidemic in Europe, in other words to take up the Spanish perspective once again.

On 18 June 1495, a month before the battle of Fornovo, during the course of which the first cases of syphilis in Italy were to be reported, Nicolas Squillacio, a doctor of Sicilian origin, wrote from Barcelona to a certain Ambroise Rosato, a physicist and astronomer. This letter, written in Latin, has been rightly hailed as the oldest document on the history of syphilis. What does it say? It says that the centuries bring, amongst other things, new sorts of malady, all of which are so many more roads to death. The most recent came from the Narbonne region of Gaul:

The purulent pustules spread in a circle, and there is an abundance of the most virulent lupus. The signs of the sickness are these: there are itching sensations and an unpleasant pain in the joints; there is a rapidly-increasing fever; the skin is inflamed with revolting scabs, and is completely covered in swellings and tubercules which are initially of a livid red colour, and then become blacker. After a few days a sanguine humour oozes out; this is followed by excrescences which look like tiny sponges which have been squeezed dry; the sickness does not last more than a year, although the skin remains covered in scars which show the areas it affected. It most often begins with the private parts, before spreading to the whole of the body. The disease infects neighbouring regions largely by means of contact between men and women: this is how it recently invaded innocent Spain. I first came to fear it when we landed at Barcelona, a flourishing Spanish city: I came across numerous inhabitants infected with the sickness whom doctors were treating with frictions; I came into contact with them throughout this journey; they maintain this new epidemic has come from mighty France . . . . You who know the causes of all sicknesses, who can see the storms in a threatening sky as if from an observatory; I exhort you to provide some new remedy to remove this plague from the Italian people. Nothing could be more serious than this curse, this barbarian poison. Best wishes from Barcelona.[28]

This interesting account may be interpreted as evidence in favour of either of the two sides. Although the date firmly places the first appearance of syphilis in Spain, and in particular in Barcelona (during the first months of 1495, or perhaps before?), it is meridional France rather than the New World which is held to be the origin of the disease. Of course, the French are Squillacio's enemies, but he would undoubtedly have mentioned the view that syphilis was of American origin if it had been the prevailing one. But this was clearly not the case.

Other accounts corroborate the anteriority of syphilis in Spain. Thus, for example, the Genoese Bartolomeo Senarega, an ambassador to Charles VIII in 1494, also mentions the arrival of a new and hitherto unknown disease which 'began to appear two years before the arrival of Charles in Italy. It had overrun the two kingdoms of Spain, La Bétique, Lusitania and Cantabria, before reaching us.'[29]

It also seems that it was from Spain that syphilis spread into the Netherlands and Flanders, perhaps by means of the fleet of twenty sails which carried the Infanta Joan of Aragon to her unhappy marriage to Philip the Fair in the summer of 1496. In any case, several chronicles explicitly link this event with the appearance of the pox, and one specifically observes 'that several Spaniards were ill with a sickness which was going around at the time; this sickness, known as the Neapolitan sickness, made people look like lepers.'[30] Was it for this reason that people in Ghent and Leyden came to speak of *spaansche pokken*?

Whatever the case, it seems certain that Spanish soldiers, who were present on both sides in all the 'theatres of operation' of the period, and who were keen customers of the foreign prostitutes who followed the troops closely, were the first agents by which syphilis was disseminated in Europe. Of course, this does not explain how they caught it . . .

Could Christopher Columbus have introduced the *bubas* into Spain from the New World? We must look more closely at the timing of his trips. Christopher Columbus returned to Spain, to Seville, for the first time on 31 March 1493. On 20 April he made a triumphal entry into Barcelona, where the enchanted sovereigns could gaze upon six Indians and sundry parrots which had been brought back. It seems impossible that such a small contingent could have been capable of propagating the epidemic. As for the members of the crew, there is no mention of any of them having brought back such a disease. The second expedition did not return until June 1496, and thus could not have triggered off an epidemic which had broken out more than a year before. But this is to reckon without two intermediate convoys, both under the command of Antonio de Torres, which brought twenty-six Indians of both sexes back to Spain in the course of 1494, and around three hundred in the early Spring of 1495.

The use to which the conquistadores put the Indian women is beyond doubt. From the moment their discoveries began, the Spaniards proved to be greedy for more than just gold, taking women by force and carrying others off as slaves. Columbus himself encouraged the capture of Indians with their wives, writing in his diary that 'the males will withstand captivity in Spain better if they have wives from their own country with them' (though this did not prevent two hundred of them dying of cold in the second convoy led by Antonio de Torres).[31]

It is therefore quite possible that several of these Indian slave women had ended up as prostitutes in Naples by the time that Charles VIII entered the city. Certain authors record this, albeit somewhat after the event: 'At the which (the siege of Naples) there were a large number of Indian women who had been brought there from the Indies by Spanish soldiers . . . and this was the reason why the soldiers (of whom there were as many French, German and Spanish ones wandering around as Italians) who mixed with these shameless and unchaste Indian women and behaved lewdly with them were struck down with this deplorable sickness.'[32]

This hypothesis, appealing though it may be, is not proven, for it remains to be demonstrated that the captured Indians had syphilis. The opponents of the American theory find it easy enough, today as in earlier times, to express astonishment that no contemporary, from the time of Christopher Columbus and his companions onwards, mentioned the existence of the new disease. Likewise, not one of the first authors to describe the pox at the time it appeared (Torella, Pintor, Almenar, Villalobos, etc.) makes the slightest allusion to an Indian origin. For that we have to wait for the writings of Oviedo and Ruy Diaz de Isla some thirty years later. The idea was not at first compelling, then – though of course that proves nothing.

However, there is no reason why the New World, which was ravaged by smallpox, measles and diptheria imported from Europe (all of which erupted with the same force as did syphilis in Europe), should have had nothing to give us in return. Was it perfectly isolated as far as infectious diseases were concerned, as is frequently asserted by those who pursue the infant study of historical epidemiology? The New World may still pass for an island, but it is, after all, a whole continent . . .

The poet's perspective

In an area of such uncertainty there remains a place for the poet's imagination. Oscar Panizza was born in Bavaria in 1853, son of an implacably Catholic Italian father and an equally implacably Protestant mother. It is not entirely surprising, then, that Panizza published, in parallel with some serious medical studies, antireligious poems which soon earned him the hostility of both Church and State. But no-one could have anticipated the flood of hatred which was precipitated by the appearance in 1895 of *The Council of Love, a celestial tragedy*, written, as Panizza explains, 'in the form of a medieval mystery, but in modern colours'.[33] The play was immediately withdrawn from sale, and earned its author a year in prison, a term which he served in full.

The exiled *poète maudit* Panizza, who had been a doctor in a mental asylum in Munich from 1882 to 1884, himself experienced the first effects of madness. Retrospective diagnosis is a dangerous game, but it is difficult not to wonder if what was involved was general paralysis. In fact, in his autobiography dating from 1904[34] Panizza confesses that he contracted syphilis as a student and that 'although it was treated according to the rules of the art it is still apparent today in the form of a gumma on the right tibia, and resists the strongest doses of potassium iodide.' In the early 1900s, after a lecture in 1891 on 'Genius and madness', Panizza began to develop a persecution complex which led to his being confined to a mental hospital.

It is syphilis which is the theme of *The Council of Love*, and it is not the least of Panizza's merits that he mocks at the cause of his own suffering at a time when most people were absolutely terrified of the disease. And how he mocks at it! The play which cost its author a year in prison is a tremendous jubilatory and blasphemous farce which offers its own explanation of the epidemic of syphilis which broke out in Europe in 1495. It is dedicated to Ulrich von Hutten, who provides, in epigraph, the theme of this 'celestial tragedy': 'It pleased God to send us in these times maladies which, as we are well aware, were unknown to our ancestors. Those entrusted with the Holy Scriptures said that the pox was the result of divine wrath.'

The scene is paradise, in the spring of 1495. A completely senile God the Father reigns, flanked by hypocritical and wicked angels, a feeble and depressive Jesus, and a Virgin Mary who, in contrast, is very emancipated, even something of a harlot. The only decent fellow there is the devil . . . . We can begin to understand the reaction of the authorities of the period, in a Bavaria entirely subject to the authority of the Church!

A winged messenger arrives in Heaven to inform God that dreadful things are happening in Naples: 'the city, besieged by the King of the French, is given over to the most ignoble vices. Bare-breasted women, full of lust, are running around the streets; the men are burning with animal passion. Vice is breeding vice . . . .

GOD THE FATHER (*Having heard the tale with increasing amazement, musters all his strength, rises from his throne, and, unable to master his anger, extends a vengeful fist.*): I shall exterminate them!
(*All throw themselves to the ground and hide their faces.*)

THE CHERUBIM (*beseechingly*): Don't do that, dearest, most Holy Father! You wouldn't have a human race left!

Instead of exterminating the human race there is to be an exemplary punishment. But what? The devil, an expert in nastiness, is summoned by Mary, who announces to him: 'we have decided on a well-chosen vengeance in the style of the Flood.' Mary has the idea of a poison 'which can check man's obscenity'.

THE DEVIL: So – we should – put – this – thorn, this poison – hmm! in (*lifting a finger as if to make himself better understood*) in the thing itself, in the . . . hmm! (*giving a little cough, and looking aggressive*) . . . in the . . . conjunction?

MARY: (*very much a woman of the world*) Delightful, oh it's delightful!

THE DEVIL: So that the man may infect the woman, or the woman the man, or each infect the other, which would be the most desirable case – and all without their knowing, lost as they would be in their ecstasy, in the delusive dream of a supreme happiness! Thus, babbling like infants, they would be paddling in the ghastly culture medium!

MARY: Glorious! Charming! Diabolical! But . . . how? (*God the Father and Jesus are still looking on wide-eyed.*)

THE DEVIL: Ah, I'll look after that, Ma'am! (*He paces up and down for a few moments, stopping several times to reflect.*) So, it must be enticing, this 'thing' – otherwise they won't rise to the bait, of course!

Mary said that it should have a feminine character
– perfect! Women know their own sex better
than anyone. But there must also be poison in it,
because that is what the punishment consists in –
and above all they mustn't discover it! They
must swallow it like a syrup! very well! You see
it's not difficult, one must stay within the limits
of despair, and madness. Now, they want to see
men twist and break, to empty their souls like
they do their stomachs! Very well! Nevertheless,
the soul must not be entirely destroyed, it must
remain capable of 'redemption', as they say –
fine! I can easily do them this favour, both of
them. They didn't say anything about the body,
did they? Perfect! As if the two could be
separated! When I have infected the very fibres
of my fellow's body and he is on his way to the
five hundred devils – oh, excuse me! – when he is
done for, will they still want to redeem his soul?
The soul which is already making its way to me?
Holy mercy! Well – we shall see!

We should have guessed: the Devil is a monist. So there he is,
rubbing his hands and telling us that it is his turn to do some
creating. He is going to introduce the poison into a creature of
exceptional beauty, whom he will father. But a mother must be
chosen . . .

Whom should I choose to bear my glorious
creature? . . . Beautiful, seductive, sensual –
poisonous! Capable of inflaming the brain and
the veins! Innocent, clumsy, and ravenous!
Uncomplicated! A blackened soul, and naive to
boot!.

There follows an identity parade of all the beautiful and famous
women (of whom, it turns out, there are few) in Hell. Which one
to choose? Helen of Sparta, Phryne of Athens, Héloïse and even
Agrippina are, after all, simply the victims of a sincere love. After a
good deal of investigation, Salome is chosen because she had the
only man she loved beheaded.

The devil drags her into his chamber and of their union 'the
Woman' is conceived (it should be noted in passing that on the rare
occasions when anyone addresses him, Jesus is called 'the Man').
She is amazingly beautiful and explosively sensual.

THE DEVIL: The poison within her veins is so strong that anyone who touches her will have eyes like marbles a fortnight later! His very thoughts will coagulate. He will gasp for hope like a desiccated carp. Six weeks afterwards he will look at his body and wonder: Is this me? His hair and his eyelashes will fall out, and his teeth too; his jaws and his joints will become rickety. After three months his skin will be as full of holes as a sieve, and he will go window-shopping to see if he can't buy himself a new one! Despair will not only fill his heart but run out of his nose in the form of a foul-smelling impetigo. His friends will scrutinize each other, and whoever is at the first stage will make fun of whoever is at the third or fourth. At the end of a year his nose will fall into his soup; he will go and buy himself a rubber one! Then he will change his address and his job; he will become sympathetic and sentimental, he won't hurt a fly; he will start to moralize, play with insects in the sunshine, and envy the lot of young trees in the springtime. If he is a Protestant he will become a Catholic, and vice versa. After two or three years his liver and his other organs will be like lead weights in his body; he will think of light foods. Then one of his eyes will start to smart. Three months later it will close. After five or six years his body will begin to tremble and burn like a firework; he will still be able to walk, and will look anxiously to see if his feet are still attached to his body. A little later he will prefer to stay in bed because the warmth will do him good. One fine day, after eight years, he will lift a bone out from his own skeleton, sniff at it and throw it into a corner in horror. He will become pious, very pious, ever more pious, he will love leather-bound books that have gilt edges and are stamped with a cross. Ten years later, his skeleton rotting, he will be confined to bed, gaping, his mouth open towards the ceiling, asking himself why things are as they are, and finally he will die . . . . Then his soul will be yours!

The last act takes place in the palace of Pope Alexander VI in Rome, represented as a whores' paradise. It is clearly the Pope who is giving the lead, but the atmosphere of a straightforward orgy is transformed into a frenzy of rutting by the arrival of 'the Woman', who accomplishes the first stage of her destructive mission there. As is only right and proper, the Pope is the first to be served, but we can rest assured that there will be plenty for everyone, according to the Devil who, in the early morning, awaits his creature who is a little tired from this first night:

THE DEVIL: (*imperiously*). And now, to the cardinals! And then to the archbishops! And after that to the legates – first the legates of the Italian states, then to those of foreign countries! Then to the chamberlain! Then to the Pope's nephews! Then to the bishops! And then we'll do the rounds of all the convents! And finally the rest of the human rabble! At the double! And try to respect the Hierarchy!

Curtain

3

The Great Pox (Sixteenth Century)

Cruising speed

Whatever its origin, the disease was new to Europe, as is attested by all who witnessed it, and as the drastic nature of the epidemic in the years after its appearance proves. But this virulence, which resulted in many fatalities, clearly became less pronounced from the beginning of the sixteenth century onwards.

Johannes Benedictus remarks on this in 1508. Ulrich von Hutten indicates that the period during which the French disease was most virulent lasted no more than seven years. As for Grunpeck, he says that for five years doctors were obliged to make a pact with the disease, which could do whatever it wanted in complete freedom. Fracastor says:

Although this pestilential sickness is at present (1546) still fully active it is no longer the same as it was at first. For twenty years or so the 'pustulae' have been less numerous; on the other hand, the gummas of the following stage are more common, whereas the opposite was found to be the case at first . . . . Nearly six years ago the sickness once more changed dramatically. 'Pustulae' are now only to be found on a very small number of patients, and the pains are negligible or very slight. The gummas are very common, however, and everyone is struck by the loss of the hair, and body hair in general, which turns the patients into laughing stocks: some have no beards, others no eyebrows, others have bald heads.

Fracastor, to whom we shall be referring again, concludes that 'the sickness is in decline, and very soon it will no longer be transmissible even by contagion, for the virus is getting weaker day by day.'

There were even some who, inspired by this observation, announced the imminent end of the sinister disease, and were rash enough to lay down precise expiry-dates. The pox will become weaker and disappear after having tortured the human race for eighty years, announces Brassavoli. Pintor had settled on 1500 as the date of its disappearance, Maynardus on 1584 . . . .

Other doctors were optimistic without being so peremptory. Falloppio declares that the pox has become so weak that by his time (1564) it was easy to be rid of it. Likewise Ambroise Paré writes in the middle of the sixteenth century that 'the pox as it is at present is much less cruel and much easier to cure than at the time it first appeared; it is clearly becoming milder with every passing day . . . to such an extent that it looks as if it will disappear in due course.'[1] Paré adds mischievously that doctors, who are not in the profession for the love of it, attribute this alleviation to the excellence of their remedies.

The observations of the doctors are echoed by the chroniclers. 'It is a dangerous malady,' writes Jean de Bordigné in 1529, 'which at first was no less to be feared than leprosy; however, with the passage of time its fury has been mitigated to some extent, and it is now neither powerful nor contagious . . .'.[2] 'This sickness,' writes another chronicler, 'which until recently was unknown in our hemisphere . . . was for a few years so terrible that it should rightly be described as a very cruel plague . . . . People of all ages and of both sexes died from it, and a large number of those who were attacked by it were left deformed or mutilated, and suffered almost continual torments . . . . It is true that after several years the poison lost its malignancy.'[3]

It seems, then, that after having spread like lightning in the years 1510–20 the pox kept to a 'cruising speed', foreshadowing the insidious and discreet character it was subsequently to adopt. On the other hand, the epidemic gained in extent what it had lost in intensity, reaching the Mediterranean coast of Africa, the Seychelles, India, China and Japan. It is probable that India had been affected from the beginning of the sixteenth century, by means of both the land route (via Asia Minor and Syria) and the sea route, perhaps since Vasco da Gama's voyage which left Lisbon on 8 July 1497 and arrived in Calcutta, on the west coast of India, on 17 May 1498. The disease at that time went under the evocative name of 'phiranga' (disease of the Franks). The epidemic reached the Malay Archipelago, then Canton (under the name of Canton rash), which brought the epidemic to China. It moved speedily from China to Japan, perhaps 'thanks to' Chinese pirates. The first reference to the disease in Japan occurs in a medical treatise in 1512 where it is described as 'Chinese ulcer': 'in this ninth year of Eishô's era, there are many oozing ulcers and from time to time one comes across pustules or ulcers like upturned flowers' (Takeda Shôkei).[4] There are numerous descriptions of syphilis in Chinese medical works of the same period, in which the disease is often referred to, as it was soon after in Japan, by the evocative term 'plum-tree poison' or 'plum-tree ulcer' – the term 'ulcer' alone being sufficient to evoke syphilis.

The change in the rhythm of the disease did not deceive such shrewd doctors as Fernel, who in 1579 was prepared to concede that the disease looked less awful, though the pains remained atrocious. He adds: 'unless God in his clemency destroys this scourge, or men moderate their unbridled lust, the venereal sickness will never die out and will, I believe, always be the companion of the human race'.

Unlike Westerners, the Japanese did not consider syphilis to be the wages of sin, but a natural calamity like any other disease. 'In our country,' remarks the Portuguese Jesuit Luis Frois in 1585, 'we consider it to be a foul and shameful thing to contract a venereal disease. In Japan, men and women consider it to be an everyday occurrence, and are not ashamed of it.'[5]

As for the terror that the pox had evoked when it appeared, it had by no means disappeared, as Erasmus attests:

if I were asked which amongst all the diseases kills the most people I would reply that it is this sickness which has raged with impunity for several years . . . . What other contagion has ever spread so quickly to all the countries of Europe, Asia and Africa? What contagion takes such a hold of the entire body, is so resistant to the art of medicine, infects the sufferer so easily, and tortures him so cruelly? . . . . It alone combines all that is dreadful in the other contagions: pains, infection, danger of death, and painful and repugnant treatment which, moreover, does not lead to complete recovery?'[6]

Fracastor, the father of 'syphilis'

Jerome Fracastor (Girolamo Fracastoro) was born in Verona in 1483. He was a fellow student of Copernicus at Padua University, where he studied both philosophy and medicine; he later became doctor to the Fathers of the Council of Trent. He wrote numerous works, and died, respected and famous, in 1553 in his country residence near Verona. It was one work in particular which made him famous: *Syphilis sive morbus gallicus* . . ., which appeared in 1530[7] and enjoyed an immense success, going through a hundred or so different editions in the sixteenth century. This long poem in Latin, which is of undeniable literary merit, and which some have compared to Virgil's *Georgics*, tells the story of the shepherd Syphilus, who offended the Sun by overturning his altars and replacing them with altars to King Alcithoüs, whose flocks he tended. To punish him, the Sun God sent him the venereal disease which the inhabitants of the surrounding countryside named syphilis in memory of the first person to suffer from it. Thus the name syphilis was born, though it was practically abandoned until the end of the eighteenth century, doctors and public alike preferring to use the word 'pox'.

Fracastor's poetic imagination and elegance in no way detract from his precision as a doctor.[8] As for the ideas expressed in *Syphilis*, there is nothing new. Fracastor mentions the theory that the disease originates in the Americas without sanctioning it, for he attributes it to a harmful conjunction of the stars. The treatment he recommends is that of his predecessors, such as the therapy with mercury and gaiac.

On the other hand, the treatise on contagious diseases which he published fifteen years later[9] contains newer ideas. As we have already seen, he points out modifications in the disease; most importantly, though, he has an inspired intuition about the agent of the contagion, picturing the disease as being caused by the multiplication and spread within the body of 'tiny invisible living things' (*'particulas vero minimas et insensibiles'*).

What is the pox?

As far as 'modernists' are concerned ('modern', in the medical sense, meaning nineteenth century) there has been a theoretical Renaissance in medicine, and they scarcely distinguish between the sixteenth, seventeenth and eighteenth centuries and the Middle Ages, dominated by the Hippocratic–Galenic theory of the humours. Nonetheless, there was a change in the subject-matter of medicine from the sixteenth century onwards. There were local changes, such as the birth of anatomy and physiology (Vesalius) or the discovery of the circulation of the blood (Harvey); there were also structural changes, such as the beginning of medical research which parallelled the era of the great doctors. In this context, the pox was, in the sixteenth century, the object of medical attention whose importance has too often been underestimated.

From the very beginning attempts were made to define the new disease. In France, Jacques de Béthencourt was, in 1527, the first to deal with the pox.[10] This doctor from Rouen was ideally placed, for the pox, known in Rouen as 'la grande gorre' was very widespread there ('Only gold can rid you of gorre de Rouen and crotte de Paris' warns a sixteenth century dictum). In accord with his time, Jacques de Béthencourt began as a follower of Hippocrates and Galen, whose writings he refers to as his medical Bible, those of the former being the Old Testament and those of the latter being the New. The antagonistic roles of the pituitary and the blood, the bile and the atrabile are all indispensable to his theories.

Beginning with the various names which had been applied to the disease up to that point he proposes that it should be named after its cause, and is the first to use the term 'venereal sickness' (*morbus venereus*). Even though Béthencourt is willing to make some concessions to divine or sidereal influences he states clearly that it is a shameful disease which results from blameworthy passions and which is born from an immoral coupling, and that it owes its 'first origin to a pestilential germ arising from the mixture of the two seeds, or of the male seed and the menses. It is possible, moreover, that the original development of this infectious germ was favoured by some particular circumstances, such as heat, rubbing, coition at an inopportune moment, venereal orgasm, contact between impure humours, the special virulence of a courtesan's menses, etc.'

His definition of the venereal sickness is far more modern: 'The venereal sickness is a diathesis originating in sexual relations and contagion; its first signs are ulcers which appear on the genital organs or on the parts of the body where the contagion has taken place; it then alters the humours, especially the pituitary and the seminal fluids, and is then marked by eruptions, tumours, ulcers and pains.'

In a work in French, *La méthode curatoire de la maladie vénérienne vulgairement appelée grosse vairolle . . .*, which he had published in 1552,[11] Thierry de Héry, the French surgeon responsible for treating pox-sufferers at the time of Francis I's expedition to Italy, defined 'the venereal sickness or great pox (as) an unnatural indisposition caused by poisonous vapours, or by touch, chiefly through the carnal act, most often beginning with ulcers on the private parts, pustules on the head and other external parts, and later concealing itself in the internal ones . . .'.

Thierry de Héry emphasises the novelty of this disease which is 'much more widespread and common than is generally supposed', and observes elsewhere that 'the pox is a single malady, not several' (thus gonorrhea, which was given the picturesque name of '*ardeur d'urine* or *pisse chaude*', was considered by Héry as a straightforward symptom of the pox). Very much a slave to the theory of the humours, he distinguishes at length between four varieties of pox: the sanguine, the bilious, the pituitary and the melancholic.

Other authors give more summary descriptions. Guillaume Rondelet, for example, writes in 1576 that 'the pox is a hydra of ills and a confusion of divers symptoms and accidents occurring together.'[12]

Writers were unanimous as to the aetiology of the disease, and particularly as regards the means of contagion. The most usual cause is impure coitus, but extra-genital means of infection are not overlooked: Brassavoli, like several of his colleagues, describes infection by deep kissing (*'oscula cum vibratione et conflictu linguarum'*).[13] But the pox can also be transmitted independently of any sexual or amorous contact. 'It must nevertheless be recognized', writes Béthencourt, 'that it may develop as a result of contact that is modest and chaste . . . . That is why ulcers are seen to appear on the mouths of suckling infants who have been infected by their wet-nurses.'

Béthencourt goes even further, affirming that the disease may be hereditary. Paracelsus says the same thing, adding that those who, like children, catch the French sickness at the moment of conception, cannot free themselves from the infection (*contagio*), and that the disease grows with the child, revealing itself sooner or later by its power of corruption. Niccolo Massa too describes numerous cases of infected children, and also gives an extensive account of the agents of contagion: inhaled air, ordinary contact, food and drink, clothing previously worn by pox-sufferers . . . . He reports treating one of his friends who was infected through having spent a single night sleeping in the sheets of a man infected with a leg ulcer caused by the French sickness.[14]

Jean Fernel (1497–1558) is the best-known of the French doctors of the sixteenth century who took up the study of the pox.[15] Fernel was not only a famous astronomer and mathematician, but one of the greatest doctors of his century. He was doctor to Diane of Poitiers and Henry II, and was known as the modern Galen. It was he who captured most clearly the virulent (in the sense of poisonous, which the word had at the time) nature of the pox:

the efficient cause of the venereal sickness is an occult and venomous quality, or rather a pernicious venom contracted by contagion and touch; although it is light and insubstantial, and beyond the grasp of our senses, it is not simple and unmixed but subsists in a humour or some other substance which serves it as a support and a vehicle; for by what other means could an incorporeal power force entry into the human body? The force and power of this venom sometimes remains concealed in us for a long period, but in time it reveals itself by many sure and infallible signs. Just as the poison of a scorpion or a rabid dog spreads imperceptibly throughout the whole body from the first part to be infected, so too does this one, for its nature and properties are like those of all contagious maladies; however, it is caught by venereal conjunction, from which it has taken its name; and because of the frequency of such coupling it has multiplied amongst men to such an extent that the evil consequences of a single person's impurity have gradually spread throughout the habitable world, to serve as a harsh scourge to despicable lecherers.

Fernel (like Béthencourt) insists that the disease puts down roots and sets in wherever contact has occurred, providing that there is some breach by way of which the venom may penetrate, for it is too weak to enter the body unassisted. In a patient treated with mercurial frictions, he notes elsewhere, the symptoms disappear, but the root of the evil is not eradicated; in time it reawakens, reappearing after a lapse of twenty, or even thirty, years. (The importance of this observation should be noted in passing.) Those who believe themselves to have been completely cured infect those with whom they cohabit, and they bear children who show signs of the sickness, a sure indication that all the while the seeds of the disease have remained within their veins, internal organs, and even in the marrow of their bones. 'The pox may well agree a truce with the patient,' writes Vidus Vidius, 'but it never signs a peace treaty.'[16]

Lastly, Fernel was the first by a long way to advance the notion of superinfection. 'Only someone who is untainted can be infected by a tainted person; a tainted person can be infected by someone who is more tainted than he, but never by one who is equally or less tainted. Those who are equally tainted may sleep together without harming one another, and yet either may injure a less tainted person.'

In sharp contrast to the very modern ideas of Jean Fernel, Gabrielo Falloppio developed theories of contagion which might appear odd if they did not bear the stamp of the theory of the humours: men with long foreskins and a covered glans can be contaminated more easily because they are more tender, and therefore receive the virus more readily. On the other hand, of those who have an exposed glans or who have been circumcised, less than two in a thousand are infected with the French sickness.[17]

Despite the pervasive influence of the theory of the humours, the clinical observations of the sixteenth century also deserve close study. In 1527 Jacques de Béthencourt gives a remarkably modern account of the symptoms of the pox, stressing its polymorphic character from the outset. 'No other ailment,' he says, 'involves so many symptoms. It is a sickness composed of many sicknesses.' The first signs ('the first ulcers of contagion') which always appear at the point where the virus has been introduced, continues Béthencourt, are followed by a contamination of the bodily humours which is revealed by various symptoms, some short-lived (eruptions and pains), others 'when the sickness is already old, when it has aged'. The latter include osseous lesions, deep and destructive ulceration, the collapse of the nose, erosion of the nasal fossae and the larynx, oedema, the characteristics of consumption and cachexia, etc. Béthencourt also remarks on late visceral localizations particularly the liver, the nerves and the brain. He also gives a very judicious account of the way in which the nature of the disease changes as it progresses: 'The further advanced the sickness is, the more it takes on a different face to that it showed at the start.' He concludes by observing that the eruptions which appear at an advanced stage seem to be devoid of all contagious power.

The fundamental characteristic of the chancre, namely its induration, is given prominence by Thierry de Héry: 'The most certain sign of the pox is the "pustulae" and ulcers, which are hard at the root . . . and ulcers on the private parts which are especially horny and hard at their roots.' As for Brassavoli, who distinguishes no less than two hundred and thirty-four forms of the pox, he is perhaps the first to mention the anal chancre.

Fernel himself distinguishes several degrees of the disease. He mentions the loss of hair (there are some who take this to be the origin of wigs) which, as we have seen, had already been mentioned by Fracastor, and which many other doctors also emphasize. Niccolo Massa wrote in 1558 that by that date hair loss, a new symptom of the venereal disease, had become common.[18] The most serious form, continues Fernel, attacks the periosteum ('the membranes which cover the bones') and the bones, causing dreadful pains which are worse at night. Eventually, worn out by suffering and lack of sleep, the body grows thin, wastes away, and life abandons it.

So it seems that the pox, despite the fact that it was relatively less virulent than it had been when it first appeared, still had some very severe symptoms. Ambroise Paré confirms this in the last third of the sixteenth century: after the 'pox virus', conveyed by the blood, had spread throughout the body from a primary chancre, patients would

lose an eye, and often both, or large portions of their eyelids, and even after they were cured the patients remained hideous to behold, on account of their scarred eyes; some lose their hearing, others their noses; others suffer from perforated palates and deterioration of the bones . . . . Some are unable to use their arms or legs, and drag themselves on wooden frames for the rest of their lives. Some suffer from permanently contracted limbs, and are left unable to do anything but speak, which in most cases involves shouting, lamenting, and cursing the hour that they were begotten.[19]

These pains are so severe 'that the sufferers say they feel as if they have been beaten with sticks'. Paré too describes a course of development which was sometimes fatal.

Chinese and Japanese medical works contain identical observations, and they describe the different stages of syphilis well before the first treatise from the West was translated (in 1774). The first period, from 1512 to around 1520, corresponds to the invasion of the treponema, and was characterized by a very marked dermotropism with severe cutaneous lesions: multiple ulcerations after sexual contact, followed by the fairly rapid appearance of gummatous lesions accompanied by sharp pains in the limbs. In subsequent descriptions, up to 1540, the cutaneous lesions seem to be less serious, and pains in the bones are less acute, but gummatous lesions sometimes affect the nose and the tibias. Mutilating gummas of the nose leading to the collapse and perforation of the nasal cartilage gave the victim a hideous appearance which struck the popular imagination just as it had done in the Western world. A little satirical poem warns young people tempted by debauchery as follows: 'From your parents' eyes / You, son, conceal yourself; / You will lose your nose.'[20] As in the West, the pox spared neither crown nor crozier; so, for example, we learn that Yûi Hideyasu, the second son of Shôgun Tokugawa Ieyasu, who had distinguished himself by his feats of arms at the great battle of Sekighara, was disfigured and dying of syphilis at the age of thirty-four, in 1607.[21]

Remedies

Of course, the doctors did not give up, but concentrated on treating the ever-increasing number of pox-victims. And they prefaced their remedies with good advice on how to avoid the disease: Massa, in 1532, enjoins those who fear the pox to abstain from coupling with a woman afflicted with the sickness (which certainly stands to reason), especially if she has just had her period. Those who have been exposed to contamination should wash their genitals with hot white wine (Almenar had already advised the same in 1502) or better still vinegar, for the male member thus fortified could withstand the unfortunate tendency to become corrupted. If someone is absolutely determined to have intercourse with an infected woman (which is sheer folly, remarks Massa), he should wash her vulva with wine or vinegar, and not linger over the act. He should then wash the male member as described above.

Likewise, a woman wishing to have intercourse with an infected man should take the same precautions.[22]

'I would count myself as having achieved nothing,' says Falloppio, 'if I had not taught you the means of protecting yourself from the French sickness when you have had intercourse with a beautiful siren infected with the pox.' To gain protection one must wash oneself after the act, then cover the glans with a piece of cloth which has macerated in a preparation of wine, shavings of gaiac, flakes of copper, precipitated mercury, gentian root, red coral, ash of ivory, burnt horn of deer (not to mention the rest). The protective must stay in place for four or five hours. One can always have some in reserve, cut to the size of the glans and neatly packed into a small bag which one should always carry on one's person, or at the bottom of that part of one's culottes known as the *brachet*. In a sense, then, Falloppio's protective is a precursor of the 'French letter', although it is not impossible that the Romans, a highly depraved people, had already adopted methods of this sort. But it is wrong to hail him as the inventor, as has sometimes been done, for as has already been remarked, this highly inventive doctor uses his piece of cloth after the sexual act, not before it. All the same, he affirms that he has tried this method on a thousand men, swearing by God Almighty that he has not met with a single failure.[23]

A recipe similar to Falloppio's was offered in Japan to the devotees of the fixed-price delights available in the pleasure district of Edo (Yoshiwara). It involved covering the ulcerated parts with a spider's web and a band of violet fabric. The spider's web was probably intended to act like gauze and prevent the band from sticking to the wound. As for the colour violet, the Japanese used as a dyestuff the skin of a root, the Shikonsô, which is also mentioned in ancient pharmacopoeiae for its anti-ulcerative properties.[24] But note that here again it was a post-coital protective, not an ante-coital one.

As for remedies proper, mercury and gaiac continued to share between them the ever-growing market of pox-victims . . . In his *Nouveau carême de pénitence et purgatoire d'expiation*,[25] Jacques de Béthencourt, whose prime concern is therapy, begins with the idea that the venereal sickness is the consequence of debauchery, and is therefore an offence against God – hence the necessity to expiate one's sins by fasting and purification. The gaiac treatment, with its forty-day fast, constitutes the 'penitential fast', whilst the mercury treatment, by introducing poison into the body, is the 'expiatory purge'.

But which of these two forms of treatment should take precedence over the other? Béthencourt presents the discussion in the form of a 'dialogue in which mercury and gaiac expound their virtues and their rival claims to heal the venereal sickness'. Mercury and gaiac plead their respective causes, and appeal to the author, who settles their dispute. 'Treatment using gaiac is truly barbarous,' he judges, 'because the diet imposed on the patients is excessively rigorous' (gaiac had mischievously argued that almost all of the patients would undoubtedly have refused to have submitted to such abstinence if it had been a matter of purifying their souls, but they accept it willingly – and what wouldn't they accept? – to purify their bodies). But what is worse, observes the judge, is that its effect is weaker and slower than that of mercury. As for the latter, it exercises a vigorous and swift healing action by separating the humours, disposing them to fluxion and then evacuating them. Moreover, it requires a diet which is less strict and less dangerous that that required by the gaiac treatment.

Béthencourt's preference for mercury was shared by a large number of doctors. Fracastor, for example, is a champion of mercury. He exhorts the patient as follows:

Do not think that it is loathsome and repulsive to smear and cover your whole body with ointment, for it dissipates the sickness, than which nothing is more hideous. However, don't apply the ointment to your head, or to the delicate region around the heart. Then apply compresses (on top of the ointment), and fix them with coarse wool. Then pile the blankets up on the bed until you come out in a sweat and your body is soaked with the impure fluids. This treatment will be painful, but however much it costs you, you must bear it. Don't despair! There will be sure signs of your imminent recovery. You will observe liquefied wastes from the sickness flowing into your mouth and being expelled.[26]

In addition to the mercurial plasters and frictions there are mercurial fumigations: first the patient is subjected to a preparatory treatment consisting of alterants (thirst-producers) and purges to 'temper the humours'. He is then placed, either naked or in a shirt, under a tent erected in a draught-free and overheated room. At his feet is a portable stove full of embers on which pinches of cinnabar (mercuric sulphide) are thrown from time to time. The patient's body is exposed to fumigation for a long spell. If he begins to faint he is made to breathe fresh air brought in from outside through a pipe. No sooner has the patient left the tent (or 'archet') than he is put in a very warm bed, where he is buried under blankets and made to sweat for an hour. After five or six sessions he may produce a profuse mercurial salivation, which is the desired effect, and diarrhoea may also result. These two effects, together with the sweating, are channels by way of which the 'pox virus' is eliminated. As Béthencourt observes, it is fortunate that the mercury treatment is less severe and less dangerous than the gaiac treatment!

Rabelais, in the prologue to *Pantagruel*, paints a colourful picture of the 'poxy and gouty wretches' who are prey to the mercury treatment: 'Oh, we have seen them so many times when they were thoroughly oiled and covered in ointment, and their faces shone like the key-plate of a charnel-house, and their teeth quivered like the keys on an organ or spinet when they are played, and they foamed at the mouth like a wild boar driven into the toils by hounds!.'[27]

Nonetheless, there were a good many doctors in favour of the mercury method. Botal recommends the expulsion of strikingly large amounts of saliva: a *chopine* (0.465 litres) daily during the first few days, a *pinte* (0.93 litre) daily after five or six days. Some, he comments frostily, wish to force the excretion of saliva as high as four litres, but this is too much.[28]

In 1535, Matthiolus was the first to dare to prescribe mercury to be taken internally, in pills of powdered red precipitate.[29] Soon untreated mercury (quicksilver) was to be an ingredient of Barberossa's notorious pills which Francis I was said to use.

Diaz de Isla, for whom mercury was 'the only means of salvation from the bubas', scoffs at the opponents of this therapy. 'The doctor', he says,

begins by drugging his patient, and he consults his books tirelessly: a purge, then another purge, then a laxative, a minorative, some pills, and that's all for today; but tomorrow, as a result of the thinning down of the humours and the elimination of superfluities the patient has a fever, and there is no shortage of doctors to diagnose it: a hectic fever, says one; a lactic fever, says another; humoural, says a third; phlegmatic, a fourth . . . . Diarrhoea occurs, and then we have further doctors vying to contradict each other: rheumatism of the liver, the stomach, the spleen . . . Meanwhile the sickness is going from bad to worse, and can only be cured at the hands of a charlatan who, on his own initiative, administers mercury.[30] He concludes by saying that he has nothing to add but that he has earned twelve thousand ducats using mercury.

As for gaiac, there are many who, like Diaz de Isla, consider it to be at best a mere adjuvant. Jean Fernel was the only sixteenth-century doctor, albeit an important one, to declare himself a convinced supporter of gaiac. But this is primarily because he was fiercely opposed to mercury which, he says, 'is not the antidote to the venereal sickness, but the invention of quacks . . . and men of honour and champions of the public good should never risk such a deceptive, uncertain and cruel course of treatment.' He then obligingly enumerates the damaging effects of the mercury treatment:

the throat becomes ulcerated; the tongue, palate and gums swell; the teeth become loose; saliva runs constantly from the mouth, unimaginably fetid, and so contagious that the lips and the interior of the mouth become ulcerated on contact with it. Because this stench chills and upsets the stomach, the patients lose their appetites and are tormented by an unquenchable thirst; they can scarcely drink, however, because each one's mouth has been transformed into one huge ulcer. Even their speech is unintelligible, and they become deaf, sometimes incurably so. A foul smell pervades the place they inhabit.

However, although the two therapeutic methods were opposed to one another in theory, they were very often found together in practice. Because recovery was uncertain, eclecticism was acceptable. Thierry de Héry, for example, won great renown for his treatment of the pox, as much from his work during the Italian campaign as from his normal practice (so much as that a late-eighteenth-century compiler relates that a monk, seeing Thierry de Héry in the church of St Denis, praying on his knees before the statue of Charles VIII, pointed out to him that the king was not a saint; 'Perhaps not,' replied our doctor, 'but I shall never be able to thank him enough for having introduced into France the sickness by which I have made my fortune'). Having condemned 'the immoderate practice of Venus' by way of prevention, Thierry de Héry prescribes mercury and gaiac indiscriminately as cures for the pox. To them he adds a 'philosophical water' which is none other than an infusion of gaiac.

Guillaume Rondelet too is a prime example of prudent eclecticism. His treatise, which is mostly concerned with treatment, prescribes, for those who have recently acquired the pox, bloodletting, laxatives and sudatives ('this sickness [which] is caused by repletion, will therefore be cured by evacuation'), and, for '*véroles vielles*', quicksilver ointments, mercurial pills, and decoctions of gaiac.

Likewise, in a curious treatise entitled *Book on the four sicknesses of the Court, which are: catarrh, gouty rheumatism, kidney stones and gall stones, and the sickness of the bubas, dedicated to the very illustrious Don Juan de Zurriga*,[31] Luis Lobera of Avila, a doctor attached to the house of Charles V, bases his treatment on mercurial frictions or fumigations, but also recommends preparations of gaiac to encourage sweating.

Finally, Ambroise Paré rebels against 'a horde of rogues, impostors and brothel-keepers who treat all patients with a single ointment, or a decoction of gaiac with or without wine, sometimes adding purgative medicines, and make countless mistakes which leave the wretched victims of the pox maimed and listless for the rest of their lives'. (Sometimes, he adds, the rash application of a mercurial balm to the genital organs necessitates a complete severance of the 'ploughshare of the field of human nature'.) He condemns the 'buccal flux' as a regrettable consequence, and advises a combination of less drastic remedies. With characteristic good sense, Paré adds that 'Venus should be avoided at all costs.'

In the sixteenth century, then, it was more often mercury *and* gaiac than mercury *or* gaiac. The latter, moreover, made a fortune for those who imported it, notably the Fuggers of Augsburg. Gaiac is sometimes called '*saint-bois*', and Italian iconography, already excessive in religious matters, lost no time in assimilating it to that other holy wood, that of the Holy Cross, which heals all ills and, failing that, makes possible eternal life. The frontispiece of another sixteenth-century Italian work[32] depicts a devil hovering over a sick person in bed, onto whose head he is pouring a full pot of pox pustules like those which already cover the victim's body; opposite him, Jesus is healing the victim by interposing gaiac.

However, gaiac, which Paracelsus attacked in 1529, was progressively replaced by several other woods and roots with sudorific properties. Niccolo Massa (1532) is the first to mention the root of China ('China smilax' or '*squine*') imported from the Portugese colony of Goa, and sarsaparilla, originating from America. A hundred years later, Japanese commercial registers record that in the year 1648 alone (the third year of the Keian era) a remarkable 83.4 tonnes of Chinese smilax was imported.[33] Sassafras wood from Florida was also used in the sixteenth century. Anxious not to neglect a single form of treatment, eclectic doctors (who were in the majority) sometimes prescribed a decoction of all of these woods and roots boiled together, which they describe as 'infusion of the four sudorific woods'.

The organization of the campaign

In the sixteenth century the pox did not gain a great deal geographically, since it had practically covered Europe in a decade; nor did it increase in intensity, since the particularly acute forms which it had taken at first had died down somewhat; there was, however, an increase in the number of cases. In *Pantagruel* (1542), Rabelais gives us Épistémon who, on his return from Hell, gives an interminable list of the famous people who are living out an eternal damnation. Amongst them, Pope Sixtus is acting as 'pox greaser' (he gives the pox-sufferers mercurial frictions). 'What, are there pox-sufferers down there?' asks Pantagruel in surprise. 'Of course' replies Épistémon 'I've never seen so many; there are more than a hundred million, for bear in mind that those who haven't had the pox in this life have got it in the next.'

Rabelais is being satirical, of course, but nonetheless the pox was very much in evidence, and was a source of disquiet to the authorities. In a wider context, the number of vagrants increased considerably during the sixteenth century, both because of the adversities of the time and because of urbanization, a real lure for those who begged for a living. There was the classic procession of rogues, the unemployed (able-bodied and otherwise), cripples, deserters, prostitutes, abandoned children, idiots and lunatics. The indigent pox-sufferers were from that time onwards of their number.

Although able-bodied vagrants and beggars had been hunted out since ancient times (Theodosius mentions it in his code as early as 382), a new way of thinking emerged in the ruling classes from the sixteenth century onwards, the aim being to reorganize charity on the basis of a rigorous distinction between good and bad, that is to say able-bodied and invalid, paupers. This explans why, following the example set by other European countries, the Bureau of Paupers was set up in Paris in 1544, modelled on that of the *Aumône Générale* in Lyons (1531). The hunting out of beggars in Paris began at about this time with, in 1557, the conversion of the Saint-Germain leper colony into a hospital (Les Petites Maisons) 'to accommodate, confine and provide frugal nourishment for the aforementioned men and women and other incorrigible paupers, invalids and cripples'. The idea of a general hospital was already in the air.

As we have seen, however, the first measures to lock away indigent pox-victims following the 1496 decree of the Paris *parlement* were rarely put into effect. In fact, as the chapter of Notre-Dame and the hospital nuns continued to lament, pox-victims from Paris and the provinces alike still flocked to the Hôtel-Dieu, which was already overflowing and which had unsegregated wards. In 1507, two surgeons delegated by the *lieutenant criminel* had been outraged by this situation in their turn:

'we have discovered several different sorts of sickness here; but above all we are of the firm opinion that the Christian names and surnames of those in the said Hôtel-Dieu who are afflicted with the Naples sickness, otherwise known as the pox, should be taken. The aforementioned sickness is contagious and dangerous to those who communicate and keep company with persons afflicted with it; and particularly here, because the multitude of sufferers who flock here each day make it necessary to bed patients with the said victims of the Naples sickness, which can and does have most unpleasant consequences. They should be put in other, separate places outside the said Hôtel-Dieu, where they may be tended and have their wounds dressed'.[34]

The Hôtel-Dieu pox-victims were even given money to enable them to return home.[35] Attempts were also made to place these universally shunned patients in various houses which were pompously designated hospitals, but these were quickly abandoned because of the ill-will of notables with little inclination to devote themselves to such a category of patients.[36] But in 1525 people were still continuing to deplore the great number of patients at the Hôtel-Dieu in Paris which obliged 'those stricken with the plague and those who are not, those who have the pox and those who do not'[37] to be bedded together. From this there developed the oft-repeated idea of following the Italian example and assigning a separate hospital to each category of patients (the wounded, those with the plague, lunatics, epileptics, pox-victims, women, small children).

Alas, lack of money meant that not one of these special hospitals was set up. Consequently, when the Petites Maisons was constructed on the site of the Saint-Germain infirmary, from 1557 onwards, it was a good opportunity to find a place for the pox-victims no-one had known what to do with for the previous half-century. In fact this establishment, intended in principle for putting away all vagrants, quickly specialized in taking lunatics and pox-victims. There were a good hundred of the latter from the end of the sixteenth century onwards. At the beginning of the nineteenth century Ricord describes the Petites Maisons as 'the Bastille of the pox-victims'.

The Grand Bureau of Paupers, for its part, organized free treatment for outpatients on condition that they could prove that they had 'caught the aforementioned sickness by ill-luck, and not through their own fault, as for example an honest woman given it by her lecherous husband, or when the unchaste woman gives it to her husband, or the wet-nurse to the child, or the child to the nurse'.[38] The barber-surgeons were then made responsible for treating the pox-victims. They formed a distinct guild of doctors from 1505 onwards, and they gave home treatment to those pox-victims who could pay.

In numerous provincial towns, by contrast, the barber-surgeons were forbidden to have pox-victims as private clients, just as innkeepers did not have the right to take in pox-victims for treatment. To compensate for this, certain towns made efforts to take collective responsibility for the pox-victims. In Strasbourg, which led the field in this respect, (and which was answerable to the Empire, moreover), a special refuge for pox-victims was set up as soon as the epidemic appeared in the city, and was replaced a few years later by a special establishment (*Blatterhaus*) where a progressive treatment based on gaiac was instituted at the city's expense.[39]

Prostitution becomes an issue

Everyone agreed that it was a scandal that no public prophylactic measures were being taken. Montaigne writes, reasonably enough, that 'we are taught how to live when life has already passed us by. A hundred schoolboys have caught the pox before they have studied Aristotle on temperance' (*Essais*, I, 26). In any case, temperance is not an easy virtue to practise, and doctors do not dare to advocate it. In its absence one should at least avoid the greatest dangers, beginning with prostitutes . . . .

The danger represented by prostitutes as far as the pox was concerned was recognized very early on. By 1500, when the terrible epidemic had only been around for a few years, Torella was demanding that both civil and religious authorities should appoint matrons whose primary task would be to examine streetwalkers. If found to be infected, the latter were to be consigned to a place designated by the parish or the lord of the manor for treatment, and detained until they were fully recovered.[40]

Ruy Diaz de Isla also pointed out the dangers of prostitution. In fact he even went so far as to anticipate the modern notion of a health certificate by calling for prostitutes to be obliged to obtain certificates attesting that they had been completely cured before resuming their former activities. According to him, even serving-girls in inns should not be employed without a certificate of health – which raises the question, discussed from the beginning of the sixteenth century onwards, of what was to be done about casual prostitution.

It seems that the first attempts to monitor the health of prostitutes took place in Spain, notably in Valencia. There was nothing of the kind in France, and contemporary commentators do not even express the pious hope that something should be done. A few authors content themselves with pointing out the danger, 'particularly for the person who frequents whores', as Rondelet puts it.[41] Brassavoli of Ferrara, the distinguished doctor to kings and popes, and partisan of gaiac, cites the case of a beautiful woman of breeding with genital ulcerations. 'First she contaminated one man,' he says, 'then two, then three, then a hundred, for she was a prostitute, and a very beautiful woman besides.'

Fernel, with his characteristic perceptiveness, remarks that 'one often catches the sickness from a wench who is not yet infected, by lying with her immediately after someone who is tainted.'

A literary theme

Fortunately for posterity, doctors were not the only ones to write on the pox. As Rabelais has already illustrated, sixteenth-century literature was quick to seize on such a rich theme, with the opportunities it offered to those with a bent for moralizing or social satire . . .

So, for example, we discover in a work by Erasmus[42] a genuine, if satirical, reflection on the prevention of the pox – a problem which the doctors of the Renaissance neglected. Four centuries before Fournier, Erasmus addresses the question of syphilis and marriage. Can one break a legitimately contracted marriage? asks Petronius. Yes, replies Gabriel, if this marriage has been illegitimated by fraud, such as when the man has hidden the fact that he was 'slave to that very strict mistress, Syphilis' (Erasmus is the first to use the word as a synonym for the pox). In fact, pursues Gabriel, marriage can only take place between living people, and in this case it is a dead person that one is marrying. But, retorts Petronius, if you follow the adage 'birds of a feather flock together' you will not prevent scabby women from marrying scabby men. . .

GABRIEL: If it were up to me, in the interest of the State I would let them marry and then I would have them burned.

PETRONIUS: Then you would be behaving like Phalaris[43] and not like a Prince.

GABRIEL: Are we to say, then, that the doctor who cuts off a few fingers or burns a part of the body to prevent the whole from perishing is a Phalaris? It seems to me to be an act of pity, not one of cruelty. Would to God that it had been done when the sickness first appeared. The death of a small number would have ensured the safety of the whole world . . . .

PETRONIUS: It would be more humane to castrate them and banish them.

GABRIEL: But what would you do to women?

PETRONIUS: I would give them chastity belts.

GABRIEL: That would be a way of preventing bad birds from producing bad eggs . . . .

The dialogue turns to the subject of the means of contagion, with Gabriel pointing out that the disease is not transmitted by one means only; it can also be transmitted by a kiss, a touch, during conversation, or at a drinking-party. 'And we will undoubtedly find that all those who have this sickness will never be happy until they have transmitted their leprosy to many others. And then those who have been banished can flee, they can pass on their infection at night, or to those who are unaware of their condition; from the dead, on the other hand, we would have nothing to fear.'

PETRONIUS: I admit that your remedy is safer, but I don't know whether it accords with Christian charity.
GABRIEL: Come now, tell me, which are the most dangerous, honest-to-goodness robbers or the people we have been talking about?

There follows a comparison with the plague, which Gabriel judges to be less cruel because it kills instantly. 'But what is syphilis if not an unending death?'. The conversation continues:

PETRONIUS: It will be forbidden by law to drink from a shared cup.
GABRIEL: That law will not be well received in England.
PETRONIUS: And no sleeping two to a bed, except for husbands and wives.
GABRIEL: Agreed.
PETRONIUS: And innkeepers can't be allowed to make travellers sleep in soiled sheets.
GABRIEL: What will you do to the Germans, who scarcely wash them once a year?
PETRONIUS: All the more work for their laundresses. Moreover, the practice of greeting people with a kiss must be abolished, despite its antiquity . . .

The moralizing is more apparent in *Le triomphe de haute et puissante dame vérole* (1539), whose numerous illustrations in the form of a procession and whose explicit association of the pox with the follies of the world is reminiscent of *The Ship of Fools*. In several illustrations there are fools wearing hoods with ear-pieces pulling a handcart on which is perched the pox. Similarly, an engraving, perhaps a slightly later one, illustrating *La gorre de*

Rouen (which is also depicted in *Le triomphe*), shows a strange procession against the backdrop of the city of Rouen, surrounded by its ramparts. Dame Pox is being carried on a sledge adorned with a cupid. On the horse, a strange coachman wearing a hood with ear-pieces like donkey's ears is brandishing a whip: this is Folly, who is leading the world – in this case a deceptive world, beneath whose shiny surface there is nothing but putrefaction.

A poem in six cantos gives the history of the pox, before painting a series of moralistic tableaux in which the 'well of love' – perhaps the spring of voluptuousness, but also a poisoned spring and a deadly trap – is a recurrent leitmotif. Dragging at the end of the procession is the 'baggage', a crowd of injured people, heavily bandaged and struggling on crutches pressured around Dame Pox, who is in rags and tatters and is perched on an exhausted horse:

> Here is the baggage of this triumphal procession,
> Very poorly rigged out (as you can see).
> You'll take good care not to join it if you are wise,
> If you are keen to avoid suffering torment;
> For those whose wit is taken away
> By loathsome Venus, who makes them hers,
> Usually end up as her camp-followers,
> Prey to sickness and denied pleasure;
> So do not follow such a Goddess
> If you want to live a wholesome life.[44]

In a second edition, in 1540, an appendix entitled 'the buttoned doublet' mentions the perforation of the palate which makes the pox-victim speak like 'a cracked trumpet, or bray like a Poitou oboe', and also the collapse of the nose, which becomes 'remuselé' (pug-like), 'short and squashed like a fig.'

Poets of the sixteenth century wax eloquent on the subject of the pox. In 1512, Jean Drouyn warns in a ballad that the pox is no respecter of social status[45] and that it is advisable to be cautious before 'starting the job':

> Foolish sweethearts, Poxy ones, Bald pates,
> Watch yourselves and mend your ways,
> Beware of holes, for they are dangerous.
> You Gentlemen, Bourgeois and Advocates
> Who squander your Crowns, Salus and Ducats,
> On feasting, frolics and making merry,
> Take heed of the perils of love-making
> And change your ways accordingly;
> For it was to haunt dubious places that
> The Great Pox was created.

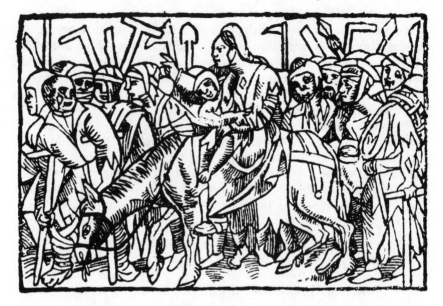

PLATE 3 In Lyons in 1539 the moralizing poem '*Le triomphe de haute et puissante dame Vérole*' was published. Here is the procession of wretched victims of the 'Queen of the Spring of Love'. (Private collection)

Be very prudent in your love-making,
And when the time for the feast comes
Make sure you see clearly.
You can cast care aside, take your fill of pleasure
And never tire of enjoying yourself
By acquiring a reputation for the highest virtue.
Avoid blotchy folk
And don't despise those who are loyal partners;
For to keep a man's lance out of any old hole
The Great Pox was created.

Stick to sweethearts, who are not to be lightly dismissed.
But make sure you don't start the job
Without a candle; don't be afraid to
Take a good look, both high and low,
And then you may frolic to your heart's content.
Be adventurous, but,
As wiseacres are wont to say,
Be learned in the school of life;
For by subtle and wily Lombards
The great Pox was created.

ENVOI

Remember, Prince, that Job was virtuous,
And even if he was blotchy and scabby,
We beg him to preserve and comfort us.
For to chastise luxurious men of the world,
The Great Pox was created.[46]

In 1525, Jean Le Maire also dedicated a poem to the pox which spares 'neither crown nor crozier':

But eventually, when the poison had matured,
They developed large, scabby spots,
So terribly hideous, ugly and enormous,
That such deformed faces had never before been seen, . . .
Few of them recovered, many died,
For this most cruel torment reigned
Throughout the world.[47]

There was also a *Pox-sufferers' Paternoster*,[48] which was in fact somewhat irreligious, and even a sonnet advising Venus' sweethearts and other slaves of Cupid be beware of 'lecherous females',

For fear of being damaged by some subtle poison,
which often sticks more firmly than glue and pitch.

And, at the opposite pole to the glorification of the female body in the *Les Blasons* of the same period, we have Mathurin Régnier's *Ode sur une vieille maquerelle*, which addresses that

Errant spirit, idolatrous soul,
Pox-ridden body covered in plaster
Blindfolded by lust,
Great barlequined nymph,
Who broke the length of her spine
On the floor of the brothel.[49]

The Spaniards too gave a place of honour to the pox in their poems, and more particularly in their novels of manners. At a very early stage the pox passed from prostitutes and private soldiers to the army officers, that is to say the noblemen. The latter introduced it to the Court, which was very much given to philandering.[50] The pox took such a hold there that some claimed that one could not pass for a gentleman unless one had had it. One writer even maintains that chancres are the 'exclusive property and privilege of gentlewomen and gentlemen'.[51] A case of 'laughter is the best medicine', perhaps . . .

It is certainly no mere chance that one of the first novels in the Spanish language, *La Lozana Andaluza* (The Andalusian

Noblewoman),[52] had pox as its theme. It focuses on a respectable girl who has been driven to prostitution by necessity and is disfigured by the 'bubas'; she simultaneously spreads the disease (through her professional activities) and treats it, for it is not for nothing that she is called the Andalusian noblewoman.

Cervantes also describes the pox in his *Novelas ejemplares*; in 'The Deceitful Marriage' he portrays a young man who has caught the pox from his young bride, and who leaves hospital sorely tested by the forty sudorific baths which he has been subjected to. But it is to the pitiless satirist and incurable pessimist Francisco de Quevedo, who in fact wrote somewhat later (at the beginning of the seventeenth century), that we owe the most gruesome description of the effects of the ravages of the pox on woman. What could be more beautiful than a beautiful woman? Yet what remains of her after the pox and 'an age in hospital'? Her voice is rasping and nasal. The smile which once inflamed lovers opens to reveal a set of wobbly teeth. The odd hair does nothing to disguise the baldness of her pate. Nothing remains of the perfectly shaped mouth with its coral-coloured lips but a dreadful grimace. She was once decked out in flowers, but now she is decked out in spots; and where once she used beauty creams she now uses mercurial ointments.

In the following century, Baltasar Gracian[53] drew the unavoidable conclusion that syphilis (like the plague) is an instrument of death, even though its envoys appear so delightful. Another Spanish author, Christobal Mosquera of Figueroa,[54] was the first to develop (in 1569) a paradox which is quite wrongly believed to have been invented at the end of the nineteenth century: the idea that between syphilis and madness there is sometimes room for genius.[55]

Mosquera's idea is an interesting one, even though he is jesting. Why should we distress ourselves about the pox? Chancres are not contrary to nature. They are delicate, and turn men infected with them into delicate beings like themselves. There follows a parallel which is very reminiscent of Aristotle: whereas the florid, sanguine man is a glutton, a drinker and a good-for-nothing bereft of imagination, the pale, melancholic man (the man of the sort that the chancres inevitably produce) is a man fit for study who is an asset to the Republic. Mosquera continues by saying that if chancres had been discovered in Antiquity altars would have been put up to them. The same idea reappears in Lucas Hidalgo's *In Praise of the Bubas*,[56] in which there also appears the amusing syllogism that since the pox is the enemy of the flesh, and the flesh is the enemy of the soul, then the pox must be the friend of the soul.

4

From Pestilence to Disease (The Seventeenth and Eighteenth Centuries)

A change in the moral landscape

At the beginning of the seventeenth century, the wind of religious reform was blowing, and social and intellectual libertinism were on the point of being indiscriminately repressed; the curiosity value which the pox had had in the previous century was to give way, for more than a hundred years, to silence and contempt. Those few writings which dealt with the subject inevitably took up a moral standpoint which led them to condemn without appeal those who had contracted the venereal sickness through debauchery, in other words the great majority of sufferers.

In 1623, David de Planis Campy, who dedicates his work[1] to Hérouard, Louis XIII's chief physician, explains in a long preface that man, though the noblest of all the animals and God's masterpiece, forgets his origins and is not afraid to debase himself. He condemns the fact that his age has become depraved through blasphemy, drunkenness, debauchery and lewdness, and he marvels that in spite of everything 'God sustains us whilst vice prevails in this disgraceful and wretched monarchy.' There are some, he continues, principally amongst the nobility, who have the pox by the time they are sixteen.

The height of abomination was that these pleasure-seekers were more concerned about what the sickness was doing to their bodies than about what it was doing to their souls. It was at this period that people began to look with suspicion, particularly amongst the gentry, at the 'wretched effeminates eager to gratify their lusts',[2] like the people of Sodom who spread the contagion.[3]

However, there was no question of abandoning these vile folk to their miserable fate (hence the book, which is a full account of the author's views on treatment). But we have these remedies only by the grace of God: 'Have pity on Your creatures, Lord, and mercifully grant that we may faithfully describe in this book the remedies received, by Your merciful kindness, for the misfortunes, calamities and suffering that our debauched actions bring down upon us.'

At the beginning of the reign of Louis XIV, an 'illustrious and pious', but anonymous, writer (it was in fact the mother of the unfortunate superintendent Fouquet) went further. On principle, she denies medical aid to those who have contracted the venereal sickness through sin, and she addresses her collection of remedies exclusively to innocent victims – an attempt at discrimination which was obviously ineffective in practice, but which says a good deal about the severity of seventeenth-century moral thinking:

Reflecting on the nature of these vile maladies . . . it is clear that they must be understood as the just consequences of, and temporal punishments for, that wretched sin which alone sends more souls to Hell than do all the others put together. Far from giving them help, we should add to their sufferings . . . . However, because experience shows us that one can sometimes acquire them through an innocent and unforeseen contagion, as for example in the case of a pious woman with a debauched husband, or a baby breastfed by a wicked wet-nurse . . . . Christian charity, which is wonderfully patient and full of gentleness and kindness, has therefore compelled me to set down here some fairly easy and very reliable remedies . . . .[4]

(There follows a list of mercury-based preparations.)

The pox and lechery go hand-in-hand, then: 'The searing droplets of this cruel sickness fall on those who are hot with love and dirtied with lust; it is a punishment for their misdeeds and their shameful desires.'[5] And this sickness, passing from one person to another, is like a deadly worm which eats away the pith of a once sturdy tree which soon must fall to the axe.

One must therefore avoid the temptations of the flesh, the

filthy pleasures of those infernal lures who, wearing enticing masks, use their attractions to make men slaves of Satan too, and who, before dispatching their victims to the other world, usually make them suffer a million pains for their one brief pleasure, as we see in the case of pox-victims, who die of this sickness with their noses, throats, fundaments, and many other parts of their bodies – even their guts – eaten away by chancres and ulcers. We even see the flesh vanishing from their rotting bones. It is a sickness which is worse than any suffered by the beasts, which in my opinion is sent to human beings as a curse to punish them for that filthy and dishonourable act which, according to Plato, makes the souls of men, after the death of the body, like those of donkeys, which are animals symbolic of lust.[6]

An engraving dating from the end of Louis XIV's reign shows us 'the three nets of the world'.[7] People of all conditions are crowding around the entrances to three immense wicker nets, all of which lead to the hospital. The first is quarrelling, the second is the tavern, and the third is the brothel, into which a bold wench wearing a low-necked dress invites everyone to enter. But a six-line stanza warns potential customers:

> Those who are full of lust
> Carry their wealth and their health
> Into my stinking crevasse.
> But after their sudden pleasure
> They come out of the Net pickled
> And go and sweat in the Hospital.

In the eighteenth century, the tone of these writings became progressively less severe with the growth of a 'non-Christian rationalism'.[8] Encyclopaedias and medical dictionaries were no longer concerned merely with describing the disease. However, some writings were still denouncing the impolite means of transmitting the 'pox virus'. They included 'lusty kisses, those horrid libertine acts in which the participants thrust their tongues into one another's mouths',[9] and even masturbation, which from 1760 was attacked by Simon Tissot.[10] One might have thought that masturbation at least carried no risk of syphilitic contamination, but that would be to overlook the fact that the hands might have picked up the virus elsewhere. It was certainly something to think about.

Despite these rearguard actions (or avant-garde if one thinks of the nineteenth century), the tone was generally lighter, and more mocking too:

Alas too-tempting desire, why do you set traps for unfortunate mortals behind the deceptive charm of pleasures? What are you playing at in fashioning new monsters for the ruination of men? O most happy ancestors, thrice happier than we! You had not discovered in the very source of life a cause of death to treacherously threaten your days. Happy and healthy you engaged in a rightful joust with your gracious spouses, happy and healthy you withdrew. But what is it that sullies the burgeoning rose of marriage today? O pitiless centuries! Know, O Man, that whilst you, pierced by Cupid's cruel arrows, dare to expose yourself to the perils of combat in Venus' camp, a sword hangs by a fragile thread above your head: everywhere implacable syphilis [the word was beginning to be used] braids a snare around the neck of the incautious soldier.[11]

The presence of the terms 'desire' and 'pleasure', which would have been unthinkable in the previous century, in this medical thesis of 1772 is ample proof of a change in the moral landscape.

The theoretical viewpoint

All those who have studied the history of syphilis consider that the seventeenth century and the first half of the eighteenth century brought nothing new. This view was first expressed at the beginning of Louis XVI's reign by Jean Astruc, a doctor famous for his teachings and writings (more so than for his practice, said his opponents), who judges the works of his predecessors to be 'dissertations without strength, genius or art, written in haste, and which barely touch on their subject matter'.[12]

Undoubtedly the medical writings of this period lack the richness of those of the sixteenth century, and, because of the censure associated with the venereal sickness, studies are rare, at least during the course of Louis XIV's long reign. Moreover, leading figures, such as Sydenham, brought nothing new to the study of the disease. However, original thoughts are far from absent.[13]

The treatise by François Ranchin, a lecturer at the Faculty of Medicine in Montpellier, is fairly typical of late-seventeenth-century writings on the pox.[14] It contains the inevitable moral tirade ('The same sin which gave death its first entry into the world also produced sicknesses as instruments for our temporal punishment and as harbingers of our ruin . . .'), and expositions which are so dependent on the theory of the humours that they might have come straight from Molière: 'one must recognize in human maladies a necessary conjunction of two causes; namely, one which is efficient, because it acts, and another which is passive, which suffers and receives by disposition the action and effect of the first. There are two efficient causes, one external and the other internal, the latter being either antecedent or conjoined . . . .'. (All this is a preamble to saying that the external efficient cause is 'actual impure contact with a pox-ridden body'.) From this pox-ridden body, continues the author, proceeds a bad and contagious quality which is unknown to us, attached to subtle humidities or coarse vapours, which begins by infecting, by way of the capillaries or the imperceptible ducts of the pores, the noble parts of the body such as the liver; once it is established it infects the substance of the blood and the natural spirits and is transmitted to all parts by the corruption of the humours, giving rise to a multitude of bad qualities in them'.

The Chinese and Japanese were not immune to the all-powerful humoural theories either, as this remarkable passage on the buboes proves:

The buboes appear in the folds of the groin, either on the right or the left. They are caused by a stasis of humid heat in the meridians of the liver and the stomach. This stasis of humid heat is itself due to an engorgement of the sperm. Consequently the buboes may appear in a chaste man who has many unsatisfied sexual desires, in a man who practises coitus interruptus, in a prostitute who receives the engorged semen, or in a man who has commerce with her and receives her vital breath contaminated with this humid heat' (Okamoto Ippo).[15]

The same author explains that the three symptoms (buboe, chancre and the syphilides) have one and the same cause, and that their difference is attributable to the degree of severity and 'the extent to which the vital breath is poisoned'.

Ranchin, however, makes other, more original observations than those mentioned above, notably that 'if one does not root it out entirely it (the pox) burgeons and proliferates once more . . .'. He also distinguishes 'recent pox', whose symptoms are lassitude, vague pains, hot feet and hands, chancres, venereal buboes and gonorrhea (which was considered to be one of the 'manifestations of the pox'), from 'confirmed or inveterate pox', whose symptoms are hard pustules on the body and (more particularly) on the head, hard and calloused ulcers around the 'private parts', and pains and decay in the bones.

There is nothing new as regards curative treatment, which is discussed at length in most treatises (it is, after all, their main *raison d'être*): diet, purges, bloodletting, gaiac and mercury, always with the idea of 'drawing the virus' (that is to say the poison) by evacuating it. As for advice concerning individual protection, it is (predictably) very much steeped in the theory of the humours:

One should not lie for long with a fallen woman, and one should wash and dry one's member most carefully. For if one lies with such a woman for long . . . and the infected quality penetrates, there is no remedy. Some women are so easily polluted that their venom is easily communicated . . . . The second condition is that the member be erect, not soft or limp, because otherwise it drinks the infection in like a sponge, and preservatives are almost useless.

(As in the sixteenth century, the word 'preservative' must not be understood in its modern sense, but as a 'preventative' medication to be administered after a suspect coitus.)

At the very end of the seventeenth century, Gervais Uçay too gives us a picture of the pox[16] in which academic notions and certain very modern touches are jumbled up together.

Like Béthencourt in the sixteenth century, Uçay remarks that the pox is a protean disease ('There are those who have jestingly said that the pox was the Proteus of sicknesses and a combination of all the other diseases'), but he also shows himself to be genuinely forward-looking by hypothesizing a spontaneous pox which could ('if the poxy ferment were more volatile') develop directly in the blood without any initial symptoms, and even more so by being the first to point out that the pox produces in its victims not only physical ills but also 'those of the mind, which also appear to be extremely bizarre in countless different ways'.

In the first half of the eighteenth century, syphilis, which was still called 'la grosse vérolle' ['the great pox'][17] once more attracted the attention of medical theoreticians. It was at this point that the chemical theory of the pox came under attack from the parasitic theory . . .

Following on from the all-powerful theory of the humours, the chemical theory had attained the status of an official doctrine. (Ranchin and Uçay subscribed to it in the seventeenth century, just as Thierry de Héry had done in the sixteenth century.) James' medical dictionary, which Diderot translated from the English in 1747[18] defined the agent of contagion of the pox as 'an active and penetrating poison (which) consists of an extremely subtle sulphurous fluid or of an ethereal and fermentative phlogistic principle, which by its communication infects the other fluids of the human body.' Soon all the solid and fluid parts of the organism are affected by a universal corruption.

For Boerhaave, the famous professor of medicine at the University of Leyden, the agents of contagion are corpuscles so small that they can enter the body through the pores of the skin and reach the veins, where they disturb the balance of the humours – each disease having its own virus (which Boerhaave defines as a subtle poison).[19]

For Astruc, it is a venom, a fermentative or, more accurately, an acid which is corrosive (for it causes gnawing ulcerations), coagulant (as the indurations prove), and fixed (it can be transmitted only by direct contact, and not by exhalations or vapours). But, observes Astruc, in regard to this theory of the acid, it is all a relative matter. The venereal venom might really be an agent which causes a vicious disposition of the humours to degenerate.

It may be noted in passing that to rank Astruc amongst 'syphilologists of the nineteenth century' seems to be something of an overreaction. He is, in fact, far less 'modern' than his sixteenth-century predecessors. Of course, he has the virtue of insisting on the unavoidability of the primary chancre, but although he produces a complete catalogue of adenoses (then called buboes or *poulains*), he does not establish a clear correlation between the character of the adenosis and that of the first attack in the way that John Hunter did a few years later.

The parasitic theory was anticipated during the second half of the seventeenth century, but it was not until the beginning of the eighteenth century that it became a subversive doctrine. It was propounded by Andry,[20] who takes the agents of the pox to be worms of a special sort, and, most importantly, by Deidier,[21] professor of chemistry at the University of Montpellier and a galley doctor at Marseilles; Deidier denied the theory of a corrosive acid, and saw in the venereal virus 'tiny living (and how monstrous they are, he writes elsewhere) worms which produce eggs by copulating and can multiply readily, as do all insects'. As regards moral thinking, however, Deidier was in the same boat as his colleagues, describing the pox as 'the true scourge of that vile carnality, and one which should induce serious reflection amongst those rash young folk who give themselves over so easily, even wildly, to a pleasure which is so ephemeral and whose consequences are so regrettable.'

Some years later, Desault[22] expresses the same theory, adding that direct infection is best explained in this way (like infection with lice), and going so far as to affirm that trustworthy surgeons had seen worms teeming on venereal chancres.

It was in the course of his savage scoffing at the supporters of the parasitic theory that Astruc unwittingly anticipated microbiology:

Besides, I would not hesitate to refute the ideas of those who believe that the venereal virus is nothing more than a great swarm of very tiny, very agile, very lively and very fecund animals which, once they have entered the body, multiply rapidly, frequently making their way to the different parts of the body, and which sting, pierce and bite the parts where they take hold, thereby inflaming and ulcerating them, and which, in short, produce all the symptoms of the pox without affecting the humours at all . . . . If we were once to admit that the pox was produced by little animals swimming in the blood then we would have as much reason to think likewise, not only of the plague . . ., but also of smallpox, hydrophobia, scabies, sores and other contagious diseases, and this would overturn the whole of medical theory.[23]

In the second half of the eighteenth century, a third doctrine, the doctrine of sympathy, was advanced by Barthez,[24] and subsequently by Hunter,[25] who gained it a wider audience. For Barthez, the venereal virus is not transported within the organism but produces a 'morbific action', first in that part of the body where it entered and then, by sympathy, in other organs (between the genital organs and the throat, for example). For Hunter, the inflammation produced by the presence in the body of the venereal poison acts simultaneously on all parts of the body which are susceptible to irritation of this sort. This is, in a sense, the first step towards Broussais' theory of inflammation (see chapter 5). All that remained to be done was to get rid of the 'venereal virus' whose nature no-one had managed to capture, though everyone had tried to measure its effects.

The vogue for experiments involving electricity and the extra-ordinary passion for Mesmer's animal magnetism (predictably enough) led to another theory, a theory according to which the communication of the venereal virus is dependent on the laws of electricity. Thus the remarkable magnetic frictions produced by an act of copulation, a kiss, a caress, or even a mere flutter of the eyelids all opened up paths by which contagion could be effected. We can imagine the terror which such a theory would have undoubtedly caused in the easygoing eighteenth-century 'high society', had it spread that far. But this was not to be.[26]

Despite the doctrinal quarrels, definite progress in the treatment of the pox was made in the course of the eighteenth century. People continued to describe the secondary and tertiary stages of the disease as 'confirmed' or 'constitutional', or even 'universal', pox. However, Hunter had already identified two periods following on from the primary stage, which had itself been carefully described since the sixteenth century. The first stage was characterized by its external signs, the second by its effects on the tendons, the aponeuroses, and the bones. Nonetheless, each of the external manifestations had been faithfully described individually – the roseola, the inguinal symptoms, the alopecia, the adenopathies and the cutaneous or mucous syphilides of the secondary stage, and the cutaneous or osseous gummas and the neurological lesions of the tertiary stage. These observations were corroborated by the founders of anatomopathology, particularly Morgagni who, thanks to the easing of restrictions on autopsies, could demonstrate the existence of lesions of the heart, the aorta (aneurism), the brain and the nervous centres on the corpses of victims of venereal disease. (The pox has a great fondness for the head, observed Lieutaud in 1777.)[27]

Doctors seem to have been indifferent to the question of the incubation period of the pox,[28] but there was a good deal of debate on many other problems which the disease posed. One of the most interesting of these was about the notion of 'latent' (or 'larval') pox championed by Sanchez, who had become famous because of his critique of the theory that the pox was of American origin. Astruc, whose hunches were decidedly unlucky, had already mocked those of his colleagues who 'commonly' believed that the pox virus and others of its type could persist unremarked, lodged in the sulphurous parts of the blood or hidden in the innermost recesses of certain glands, places of concealment in which they waited, as if in ambush, for the chance to emerge and rot the blood and the other humours, and even the 'solid parts'.

Sanchez calls this ambuscaded pox 'chronic venereal disease'. The symptoms may disappear following medication, but the poison can remain, and can even be transmitted from father to son. The insidious disease can thus pass from generation to generation, showing itself only by chronic diseases, eye pains, or crooked shoulders or backs which make the hérédo (Sanchez does not use this word, of course, but the idea is there) look like a 'thin and fleshless fowl'. Sanchez anathemizes those who thought that the disease would continue to diminish in virulence and, like leprosy, disappear. As he sees it, 'the human species will undoubtedly never be rid of it, and one day it will be the cause of a revolution in Europe (this is in 1785) like that which happened in the fifth century when the Roman monarchy fell apart because of its weakness, luxury and moral depravity.'[29]

In short, at the end of the eighteenth century syphilis was once again a fashionable topic (and it was under the name 'syphilis' that it began to appear in dictionaries and medical works, though the latter were still few and far between).[30] Advances in publishing led to the appearance of the first medical atlases in colour in which the symptoms of venereal diseases figured prominently,[31] and nearly 2,000 publications on the subject had already appeared.[32]

Anatomical collections came into vogue. Amongst them were those of the Hunter brothers, William and John. William was a surgeon and professor of anatomy at the Royal Academy of the Arts, and wrote a treatise on anatomy (*'Anatomy of the gravid uterus'*, 1774). John, known for his treatise on venereal disease, was the father of experimental pathology in England, and was responsible for the opening of a museum of anatomy in London in which the cutaneous manifestations of syphilis figured prominently. Ferrus, a French psychiatrist who made a study visit to England at the beginning of the nineteenth century, admired the collection of anatomical items which William Hunter had assembled in Glasgow. Ferrus' only regret was that this magnificent collection had been situated next to souvenirs from Waterloo. Rather than recall 'distressing and disastrous combat', it would be better to foster 'that commendable spirit of emulation which exists between our two peoples and which leads them to vie with each other in the cultivation of the sciences which benefit humanity'.

One venereal disease or several?

The end of the eighteenth century saw the culmination of the great debate between those who believed in the unicity of venereal disease and those who did not. Since the sixteenth century, venereal disease had most often been regarded as a unique disease caused by a 'venereal virus', also unique. According to this view, gonorrhea was simply one of the manifestations of syphilis, just like the chancre. 'Gonorrhea and the chancre are the effects of the same poison', says Hunter.

But why do we often find the one without the other? The unicists were not disconcerted by this question; they maintained that the same morbific substance could equally well produce either a chancre or gonorrhea, in just the same way as the intensity of these symptoms can vary considerably from one patient to another. Moreover, continues Hunter, the existence of one of these two 'irritations' has the effect of forestalling the development of the other. (Here we still have the notion of sympathy, but this time operating *a contrario*.)

According to a more subtle theory, a development from gonorrhea to the pox represents a worsening of the disease. If the former is not properly treated, the venereal virus will flow back into the blood because its 'usual exit' is blocked.[33]

Balfour was the first to pose a serious threat to the unicist theory. In a thesis which he submitted in Edinburgh in 1767 he claimed that there were two different diseases produced by two different poisons.[34] Despite vehement opposition (notably from the French) the dualist theory established itself in what might be called the 'Edinburgh school', with Duncan in 1778 and, more importantly, Bell in 1797. Bell relied on the accounts of self-inoculations performed by medical students which demonstrated that gonorrhea produces gonorrhea and the syphilitic chancre produces syphilitic chancres. Bell describes one of these astonishing experiments as follows:

Then the first of these young people introduced into his urethra, at a depth of three lines or so, some matter from a chancre with which he had charged a stylet. Not a single symptom of gonorrhea appeared; but after five or six days he observed, at the place at which he had injected the matter, a chancre which was inflamed and painful. This chancre was followed by a bubo, which eventually suppurated, even though mercury was immediately applied to it; the resulting ulcer was painful and took a long time to heal; finally the patient developed ulcers in his throat, and he could only be cured by taking a large quantity of mercury and being strictly confined to his room for thirteen weeks.

Bell adds: 'I certainly could not have hoped for better evidence of the difference between the virus of gonorrhea and that of syphilis.'[35] Those of the opposite camp appealed to identical experiments. According to his epigones, Hunter injected himself with gonorrheal pus, which was said to have produced chancres.

Other doctors adopted a more eclectic position. Swediaur, for example, maintained that 'a prostitute afflicted with a syphilitic disease in the genital organs gave one man the clap, another chancres, and a third both at once.'[36] For Swediaur there were no less than seven varieties of gonorrhea, only one of which was produced by the syphilitic virus.

Mercury is king

Those who advocated sudorifics or enervating diets became less and less numerous in the seventeenth and eighteenth centuries, and

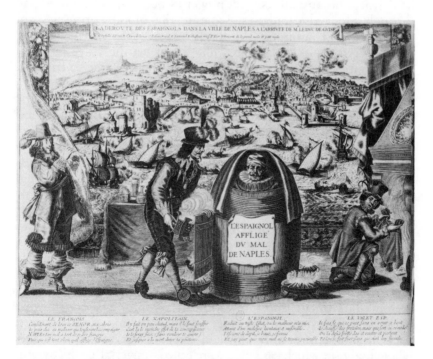

PLATE 4 Here the dreadful mercurial therapy of 'sweating one's pox' in an archet is used as a pretext for political satire following the revolt of Naples against Spanish domination in 1647 – a perfect opportunity to restore to the pox its original name (the Neapolitan sickness) and to cast the Spaniard in the role of pox-victim. (Bibliothèque Nationale, Paris)

were to be found predominantly amongst the opponents of mercury. It was certainly easy for the latter to justify their position, for they needed only to point to the accidental complications of mercury treatment, which included fatal intoxication. A few detractors of mercury even went so far as to attribute a good number of the symptoms of the pox to its use.

But although Boerhaave and his pupils were still prescribing a mixture of medications at the beginning of the eighteenth century, there was virtual unanimity in favour of mercury, which was considered to be the only specific remedy for the pox. 'Mercury,' wrote Hunter, 'is the great specific remedy for the pox and the chancre, and there is no other on which we can count to the same extent.'

The mercury treatment was as acceptable to the iatromechanists as to the iatrochemists. The former, who reduced vital phenomena and treatment to purely physical forces and actions, believed that quicksilver injected into the circulatory system in very small globules travelled through it faster than the blood itself, because of its density; because of its great power of penetration it would pass through blocked capillaries, separate the blood corpuscles and grind up and atomize the particles of the virus which it encountered on its course, expelling them via the saliva (Astruc). For the iatrochemists, whose theories gradually came to triumph, mercury, 'in the form of an oxide or of a salt, acts on the syphilitic virus more by a sort of attraction or chemical affinity; whenever it encounters the virus it promptly unites with it, neutralizes it, and forms with it a compound which has none of the qualities which either of the two substances had before they united' (Swediaur).

Even Deidier, a supporter of the iatromechanists, saw mercury as the only remedy, one which, 'by reducing itself to very small molecules is capable of penetrating the very tissue of these worms and their eggs, and can, because its great mass flows with the fluids, split their vessels, for much the same reason that it separates particles of gold, with which it mixes easily.'

Opinions differed, however, as to how the mercury should be administered. Ointments (in Italy, in the seventeenth century, there were curious anti-venereal underpants coated inside with a mercurial ointment) and fumigations fell from the favour they had enjoyed in the sixteenth century, giving way more and more to frictions, sometimes only of the ulcerated parts, sometimes of the whole body (in which case they were called 'universal'). Chicoyneau, first doctor to Louis XV at the beginning of his reign, recommended another method of mercurial friction known as 'friction by extinction', in which the frequency of the sessions was reduced as soon as salivation occurred. The medical world, in fact, continued to be divided between opponents and proponents of 'buccal fluxion'. Ptyalism, the dogma of the sixteenth century, was supported by the majority (Sydenham, Boerhaave, Astruc), but its opponents were growing in number. Some, like Desault, thought the production of diarrhoea to be preferable, because of the need to evacuate the venereal poison. But, observes Boerhaave, 'one can appreciate that this might be somewhat inconvenient for the people at Court.'

At the end of the eighteenth century, the internal administration of mercury, which for a long time had seemed too dangerous, gradually took over from external methods, taking the form of anti-venereal enemas and, more commonly, oral administration of mercury in gum form or as calomel (mercurous chloride). A new arrival, the corrosive sublimate (mercuric chloride) provoked lively debate before winning the day thanks to Van Swieten, a pupil of Boerhaave and first doctor to Marie-Thérèse of Austria. (The importance of the Dutch medical school in the seventeenth and eighteenth centuries should be noted in passing.)

Thus was born Van Swieten's liquor, destined to become famous. It was prepared in the form of grains of sublimate which were to be dissolved in a solution of water and alcohol. The success of this new means of administering mercury rested on a clearly decisive advantage: patients could treat themselves. De Horne, one of the most important specialists on venereal disease at the beginning of the reign of Louis XVI, writes that 'using corrosive sublimate one can treat, in secret, even in the very bosom of the family, a young man who has mistakenly erred or a husband whose misfortune will make him wiser and more careful, and with it one can bring about that return to duty which the public relevation of their licentiousness sometimes causes men to abandon irrevocably.'[37] This discretion, however, was also to pave the way for charlatans.

It is interesting to look in detail at the way in which a patient was treated. Take, for example, the case of Rosalie, a twenty-one-year-old native of Normandy, treated simultaneously for virulent gonorrhea and a chancre on the uvula.[38] She was bled and purged, then made to take increasingly large doses of corrosive sublimate every day. When the chancre had gradually healed over and the gonorrhea had gone she left hospital, but she returned a few months later 'having resumed her former habits' (of prostitution). She was suffering from a recent attack of virulent gonorrhea, an extensive chancre on the fourchette and 'crustaceous and suppurating pustules spread abundantly across her left shoulder and face'. She was given no less than 148 anti-venereal enemas (all mercury-based) and 17 *gros*[39] of mercury ointment in frictions, 'which was as successful as one could have hoped'.

In other cases, the number of stools and the quantities of saliva (in quarts and pints) produced by patients who had 'embarked on the remedies' were carefully recorded. Baths were sometimes used in conjunction with mercury treatments. It was thought that they facilitated the distribution of the mercury by directing its action towards the skin.

The symptoms of mercury poisoning (cutaneous eruptions, ulceration, neurological effects) were usually attributed to syphilis itself – something which further increased symptomatological confusion. However, faith in the mercury treatment did have its limits, and many doctors recognized that mercury had no effect on the later manifestations of the pox. As for its supposed efficacy in the primary and secondary stages, no account was taken of the fact, of which no-one was aware at the time, that the chancre heals spontaneously after a few weeks and that the disorders of the skin and the mucous membranes also eventually vanish, even in the absence of treatment, to make way for the serological phase of the disease. I shall be returning to the question of mercury's inefficacy, or rather its relative inefficacy, in due course.

There were only a very few forms of medication from which mercury was deliberately excluded. One such was arsenic, which was recommended for both internal and external use by Planis-Campy[40] in the seventeenth century, and had already been suggested by Villalobos, four centuries before the heyday of the arsenicals. In the eighteenth century, antimony or lead were sometimes administered internally. However, compared to mercury, these treatments were not employed to any significant degree, and they are mentioned here only for the record. Also for the record, it is worth mentioning Domenicus de Marchettis (1664), who trepanned his patients to put an end to the excruciating headaches brought on by the pox.

Empirics and charlatans

Few diseases favoured empirics and charlatans as much as did the pox. The accounts of Grunpeck and Hutten clearly show that almost as soon as the pox appeared charlatans quickly acquired influence over its victims, filling the gap left by the bewildered doctors. In the face of this new and terrifying disease they had one major advantage over the doctors: their audacity. Indeed there was often very little which they were not willing to try, and Torella,

like his colleagues, poured scorn on them for this: 'since they
know nothing they are as confident as can be, and promise
miracles; to hear them you would think they were going to bring
the dead back to life, but your hopes would soon be dashed, for
their patients suddenly and unexpectedly die; these bandits,
murderers and poisoners kill their victims pitilessly . . .'.[41]

The disapproving doctors were powerless against the charlatans
who, after all, had introduced them to the use of mercury. After
all, the barber-surgeons – and even the doctors themselves – who
promised the poor pox-victims a rapid recovery thanks to some
secret remedy or other, were they not simply legalized charlatans?
Many of them set themselves up in Paris, first around Saint-
Germain-des-Prés, where the first hospice for pox-victims (for
what it was worth) had been established.

Around 1500, one of them had some handbills printed letting it
be known in the neighbourhood that he was very expert and
experienced and that with God's help he healed all illnesses
resulting from the 'curable variety of the great pox' (note the
qualification!).[42] He also boasts that he has potions which can cure
several other embarrassing illnesses without harming his patients
and without 'rubbing with ointments or making the patient sweat'.
But tastes differ, and the surgeon adds that he will rub with
ointments and make sweat those who so wish.

Two centuries later, the tribe of empirics and charlatans had
multiplied prodigiously, capitalizing on the struggle for power
between the doctors (whose job it was to diagnose the pox) and the
surgeons (who had the duty of providing the treatment for it, in
particular the mercurial frictions). The charlatans simultaneously
filled the role of both doctor and surgeon, and they also brought
with them new forms of treatment (and therefore new hope) and a
discretion which was very desirable where a disease as shameful as
the pox was concerned.

Mercier, in his *Tableau de Paris*,[43] paints a lively comparison of
the empiric and the doctor:

A white-faced doctor with a piping voice and an indecisive gaze feebly takes your
pulse and proffers a few elegant but empty-sounding phrases. He seems to want
to play for time with the new disease . . . the empiric, by contrast, speaks boldly
and looks decisive; he gets his patient moving, claps him on the shoulder, fires his
imagination . . . . The doctor is cold, whereas the empiric is warm and energetic
and tells you in a firm and convincing voice: take this and get better . . . .

As for the charlatans (who differ from the empirics only in that
they are bigger swindlers), Mercier says that from that time on
they were the only ones to perform the indispensable function of

talking to the people – a remark pregnant with meaning for the future, bearing in mind that these lines were written on the eve of the Revolution.

The doctors themselves unwittingly aided the charlatans, by publicizing their own remedies in an extravagant fashion. This, for example, is how De Horne, the great scourge of charlatans, describes Dr Bellet's mercurial syrup, which appeared on the market in 1768: 'Of all the remedies invented and advertised for the cure of the pox there has been none with such an air of pomp and sumptuousness as M. Bellet's mercurial syrup . . . the word syrup alone seduced the imagination – it seemed as if it contained nothing that was not sweet or pleasant . . . it was believed that the most difficult and desirable goal of curing people safely and pleasantly had at last been attained.'

This new need to combine the useful and the agreeable, or at any rate less disagreeable, gave rise at the end of the seventeenth century to Belloste's pills, which were still on the Codex in 1884! But it was in the second half of the eighteenth century that the new remedies really began to multiply, with Jourdan de Pellerin's solar balm and astral water, Bru's mercurial tonic biscuits, Marbeck's health water, 'apothicaire', etc.

Everyone produced certificates boasting of the excellence of their own particular remedy. The recipes, of course, were kept secret, but most contained mercury in very small quantities. Everyone attacked their competitors, of course, accusing them all of being charlatans. They lampooned one another mercilessly. (During the reign of Louis XV a certain Dibon produced so many diatribes to advertise his wares and to reply to his detractors, Astruc in particular, that the satires of the period speak of 'dibonnades'.) Public authorities often gave permission for new remedies to be tried out on patients in military hospitals or prisons. A pamphlet would immediately be printed to report the results of these experiments; the experiments were invariably reported as being successful, and the remedy in question would thus be advertised as having received official endorsement.

The medical profession had set this bad example, but the empirics and charlatans were not to be outdone. Amongst them we must mention Le Fébure, the baron of Saint-Ildephont, who invented an 'aphrodisiac chocolate' containing some sublimate. Armed with this infallible remedy he proposed nothing less than to cure all the venereal victims in the kingdom, providing he was given exclusive rights and paid a set fee of twenty-four livres a head. In one of the many treatises he published on his method[44] he stresses the advantages of being 'one's own doctor'. (James' medical dictionary of 1747 remarks that by treating oneself at home one is spared 'the shame of a suspicious treat from society'.) One could cure oneself

right under the noses of the Athenians. A husband can take his chocolate in the presence of his wife without her suspecting a thing: indeed, she herself can take it without realizing that she is swallowing an anti-venereal remedy; by this innocent means, then, peace and concord can be maintained in the household. A father can take it in the midst of his family, a son or a daughter can take it in front of their parents . . . . A traveller can carry his chocolate with him, and need no longer load himself down with embarrassing bottles and phials.

What a far cry from the seventeenth century! The baron of Saint-Ildephont was, it should be noted, a doctor of medicine, 'professor of venereal diseases and in the art of accouchement'. In 1775 he had posters put up all over Versailles, where he practised, announcing the opening of a free dispensary to treat needy folk afflicted with the venereal disease. However, potential clients had to purchase in advance a phial of 'anti-venereal liquor', no doubt at an exorbitant price.

According to Astruc, there was also a certain Boile who, in 1726, exhibited under a microscope the pernicious animalcules responsible for the pox and, what was even more remarkable, other tiny creatures which could destroy them, like hunting dogs tracking down game. One drop of the remedy containing these salutary predators and immediately the pox animalcules would disappear before the very eyes of the astonished spectators, who were soon jostling one another to buy this miracle at a very high price. It was later discovered that an ingenious optical trick had enabled the charlatan to switch between a slide on which infusoria were moving about and a slide which was totally empty.

But all of these charlatans were mere amateurs compared to the prodigiously successful Keyser. Jean Keyser was the inventor of anti-venereal dragées, whose composition, based on mercury dissolved in vinegar, was kept a secret. In 1755 the enterprising Keyser obtained permission to test his dragées at Bicêtre, but they proved to be without effect; in 1759, however, he tested them on twenty syphilitics in a military hospital, and this time success was duly recorded. As a result of his lobbying and intriguing he was assigned the monopoly in the supply of his dragées to all the armies of the kingdom, and was given privileges and a very comfortable pension by the King. The doctors ('that treacherous company', as Mercier calls them) let loose a torrent of avenging diatribes against him.[45] Keyser defended himself, and had no difficulty in showing that his dragées could not be as ineffective as was being claimed since there were numerous counterfeits in circulation, devised by surgeons of the highest renown.[46] Until the Revolution, 'Keyser's dragées' were the sole anti-syphilitic remedy used in the military hospitals, prisons and beggars' prisons of France, and made an immense fortune for their inventor, and subsequently for his widow.

Other charlatans in the second half of the eighteenth century played on the public's justifiable distaste for mercury, offering medicines which were free from this dangerous metal. The prodigious growth in publishing which characterized the period made advertising easier, and we find, for example, a certain M. Nicole selling his anti-venereal pamphlets in the public parks, notably in the Tuileries gardens. In London at the same time an anonymous charlatan's work entitled '*A reasoned scheme and infallible means of arresting the progress, preventing the circulation and destroying the very root of venereal maladies throughout the entire kingdom*' was selling like hot cakes.

Amongst many other examples of remedies which were all the more miraculous for not containing mercury we might mention Count de Milly's 'safety water', another 'admirable water which cures without mercury' offered by M. Marie-Duclos ('correspondents are requested to supply a franked letter if they wish for a reply'), Vergery de Velnos' 'new vegetable anti-venereal remedy' and, finally, Laugier's 'Hippocrene water' and 'nectar of Cypris' (the 1785 pamphlet which sings the praises of these medications for the *Carte de Tendre* is a whole programme in itself, for it is entitled *New discovery for humanity, or Essay on the disease of Cythera*).

The summit of the genre was undoubtedly attained by Laffecteur's anti-syphilitic nectar, launched in 1779.[47] It was guaranteed mercury-free; its actual composition was kept secret, but it seems to have been a mixture of honey and a decoction of marsh reeds, aniseed (or cumin) and, as its active ingredient, sarsaparilla. Surprisingly enough, the results of a trial conducted on the venereal patients at Bicêtre which was authorized by the lieutenant-general of police were officially recognized as positive by a medical commission. Swediaur later affirmed that Laffecteur's nectar contained mercury, as proved by the fact that patients who used it salivated. Indeed it is possible that Laffecteur cunningly used a mercury-based nectar to gain the commission's approval so as to increase the sales of the mercury-free version. Whatever the case, it was a complete success, for Laffecteur became the official supplier to the Navy (a market Keyser had not tried to tap), though the high cost of his nectar restricted it to use at sea, mercury frictions being considered to be dangerous there. And, unlike the other remedies which proliferated in the eighteenth century, Laffecteur's *rob* continued its career in the century that followed.

From time to time the medical profession tried to exert some control over this thriving industry. In Lille in 1774, for example, a certain Fournier who sold an anti-venereal 'health water' was ordered to sell his wares only to those who had a doctor's prescription or, at the very least, had been advised to use it by a surgeon (surgeons and doctors had joined forces in the face of a common peril). The Lille magistrates eventually rejected this, upholding the empiric's subtle objection that rules of this kind might discourage patients who, desperate to keep their disease secret, were worried about becoming involved with official medicine!

At times the Faculty of Medicine took a hard line, as in 1776 when Dr Cézan was struck off the register of the Medical Council because his anti-syphilitic manual was judged to be 'more worthy of a low charlatan than a doctor'. Four years previously, a struggle had begun between the Faculty and Guilbert de Préval, renowned amongst the public for his 'fondant anti-syphilitic water' (as with other secret remedies, its composition was revealed by a jealous competitor: a solution of sublimate mixed with slaked lime). Struck off the list for charlatanism, Préval took the Faculty of Medicine to the Paris *parlement* in 1776, and won his case. But the Faculty refused to obey the order to reinstate him, which caused a great deal of fuss, during which satirists and student demonstrators took Guilbert de Préval's part.

However, official reprisals were rare, and left those outside the medical profession free to pursue their activities with impunity. Such persons were legion: 'now even medical students, herbalists, apothecaries' boys, monks, blacksmiths, matrons, seamstresses, clothesmenders, cobblers etc. etc. make it their business to treat these diseases, to the great detriment of the species and of society.'[48]

The only weapon left to the medical profession with which to combat empirics and charlatans was scorn. Fabre, following on from Astruc's and De Horne's indictments, wondered why 'the treatment of these diseases has almost always been abandoned to the greasy and ignorant charlatans'.[49] A disdainful silence was the order of the day ('I shall speak no more of these fellows, who would be better off on the stage'), but a plausible explanation of the success of the charlatans was offered nonetheless:

It is not surprising that men without talents who need to make a living and subsequently become ambitious of making a fortune should adopt a veil of mystery so as to impose on the public given that the disease is such that no-one dare complain aloud of having been the victim of lies and impudence. But sufferers would have been more distrustful of these dangerous frauds had they not been deceived by misused privileges, authentic Master's certificates.

In England, Dr Leake's Pills were all the rage at the end of the eighteenth century and the beginning of the nineteenth. As with Keyser's dragées, the small amount of mercury which they contained was quite out of proportion with their extraordinary popularity, as numerous satirical engravings of the period testify. Only a few of these can be mentioned here. In one of Richard Newton's engravings, for example, we see a young peasant holding a prospectus for Leake's Pills and exclaiming: 'What am I going to tell my father and mother when I go back home. My sister Anne, the Methodist, will say I have thrown myself into the Devil's burning furnace and I shall put the whole village in a commotion. What an unpleasant new-year's present.' There is also the anonymous engraving of 1784, 'The Devonshire method to restore a lost member', one of the many caricatures that were sympathetic to Pitt. It depicts the Duchess of Devonshire holding Fox by the hand (he was the leader of the Whig party, an opponent of Pitt's, and was having difficulty with his Parliamentary seat even though the Duchess, famous for her beauty and wit, actively supported his candidacy). This is all used as an excuse for some absolutely dreadful puns. The Duchess, handing a purse to an apothecary, announces: 'His Tail restore, you shall have more.' The apothecary replies: 'My famous Pills cure many Ills.' Fox, with his hand on his brow in a gesture of despair, has a paper under his feet on which we can read 'Dr Leake's anti-venereal Drops.' The woman behind him, whose hat is decorated with a fox's tail, the emblem of Fox's partisans, says 'Oh, poor Fox will lose his tail.'

Political satire was also directed against Britain's 'eternal' enemy, France. In 1799, for example, Gillray cruelly mocked the defeat of the French generals in Egypt in 'French Generals retiring, on account of their health; with Lepaux presiding in the Directorial Dispensary.' In the centre is La Révellière-Lépeaux, a member of the Directory, twisted and hunch-backed, examining a urinal and receiving the generals who are going to have to return to France for health reasons. On the table there is an open book entitled 'The Neapolitan Sickness' and a box of Leake's Pills.

The presence of prostitutes in many other caricatures testifies to the importance of their role in venereal contamination. Gillray's 'A sale of English beauties in the East Indies' (1786) merits a mention. In it, a batch of pretty whores recently unloaded in a port in the

Indies is soon to be put up for sale by an auctioneer. In the foreground stands an impressive row of barrels on each of which is written 'Leake's Pills'. With the disease, the cure . . . Another coloured engraving of Gillray's is 'The whore's last shift' (1779).[50] In a sordid room with peeling walls a naked prostitute is washing her last shift in a chipped chamberpot standing on a bench seat. Her elaborate hairdo decorated with pearls and ribbons contrasts with her laddered stockings. The inevitable prospectus for 'Leake's Pills' lies on the ground, but what the artist was concerned to show here was the miserable condition of the London prostitute, the 'Gin Palace' whore who had to conceal her poverty and, more importantly, her disease, in order to entice her clients. The theme is inexhaustible, but we should, of course, mention Rowlandson (for example, his 'An Old Member, on his road to the House of Commons' of 1802), and also Woodward; there were innumerable others.

Libertinism and the pox

At the end of Louis XIV's reign, when Mme de Maintenon had arrived on the scene, the Duc de Vendôme offended the Court. The Duke, grandson of César de Bourbon, the bastard son of Henri IV and Gabrielle d'Estrées, had been the most outstanding general in the troublesome war for the Spanish succession, and as a result had entered the favour of the King, who shut his eyes once and for all to the Duke's excesses. The Duc de Vendôme was in fact ruddy of face, filthy and coarse, and he flaunted his libertinism and homosexuality. Saint-Simon, who detested him, was indignant that the King had 'such an odd and pronounced weakness for him'.

The Duc de Vendôme's very active homosexuality had earned him the pox, and he constantly postponed having treatment for it, even though the King pressed him to do so. Finally he made up his mind to 'put himself into the hands of the surgeons who had already failed him once before'. To the great displeasure of Saint-Simon, who recounts this episode, he publicly took leave of the King to go and 'sweat out his pox'.

The King told him that he was delighted that he had finally decided to sort out his affairs and start looking after his health, and that he hoped that the treatment would be so successful that it would be safe to embrace him on his return. It is true that a race of bastards could, like the Duke, claim a certain amount of privileges; but actively to parade it when most people would have enfolded their shame in mystery was both shocking and outrageous, and demonstrated the extent to which an illegitimate birth could affect a King who was so devout, so serious, and in every way such a slave to all the rules of etiquette . . . . For three months or so he was in the ablest hands, but they failed him. When he returned to the court he had only half of his nose left, his teeth were missing and his face had changed entirely, giving him the appearance of an idiot. The King was so struck by it that he counselled his courtiers not to mimic it, for fear of upsetting M. de Vendôme.[51]

There were other courtiers who, like the Duc de Vendôme, were notorious pox-victims; one such was M. de Vaudemont, whose hands and feet, according to Saint-Simon, 'were nothing but flaccid flesh which wobbled in every direction'. These high-flying libertines were both the victims and the creators of new types of venereal disease. One example, which we do not know for sure to have been a form of the pox, was 'the crystalline',[52] which became synonymous with homosexuality in the eighteenth century, because it was frequently localized around the anus.

Whatever the case, the libertines of Louis XIV's reign could claim no right to individual prophylaxis. Uçay[53] protests that 'The libertines have for a long time been searching for a preventative remedy against the pox so as to be able to continue their debauches without danger of catching it.' The authors who promise wonders are liars who 'prostitute their consciences by promoting a remedy which encourages debauchery, for there is no doubt that an infinite number of persons of libertine inclinations would go to the brothel if they could be sure of not catching the pox, just as there are an infinite number of girls who would not keep their maidenhead if they were safe from pregnancy.' As regards this disease, which 'is the ordinary lot of those who commit the sin of fornication', the only protection acceptable to God is continence.

And when a hundred years later the Faculty took a hard line with charlatans like Cézan or Guilbert de Préval it may have been less because of their charlatanism – charlatanism was after all too widespread to be genuinely scandalous – than because these men deliberately extended their therapeutic preoccupations into the field of individual prophylaxis, in other words to sexuality, libertinism and the business of prostitution. But these were rearguard battles for, even if official medical practice was not prepared (nor would be for some while) to encourage sexual freedom in any respect, moral values had changed. Is this not best proved by the fact that the pox, and venereal diseases in general, made such notable progress?

Of course, this did not change the fact that the pox was a shameful disease. In a diary entry for December 1750, Barbier relates that Master Coffin, a senior official at Châtelet and a militant Jansenist, had been very wayward in his youth, and that it was widely known in the area that he died of the p—, for which, it was said, he has been treated either inappropriately or too late. Consequently, at the same time that he was being denied the last rites on the grounds that he was an ardent Jansenist who refused to accept the Constitution it emerged that this good Jansenist was nothing short of a victim of the p— and a debauchee who had gone through all the harlots in Paris during his lifetime. What a fine thing! It was even reputed that the disease had been in his household since his marriage began. His condition was concealed and denied as far as possible, chiefly for the honour of Jansenism. It was said to be an abscess in the chest.

Numerous writers reflect this new increase in the pox in the eighteenth century . . . . Sometimes they do so in the satirical mode, as with Voltaire when Candide recognizes a beggar as Pangloss 'all covered in pustules, his eyes lifeless, the end of his nose eaten away, his mouth skewed, his teeth black, speaking throatily, tormented by a violent cough, and spitting out a tooth with every effort.'[54] Love has reduced Pangloss to this state:

Oh my dear Candide! You knew Paquette, our august baron's pretty maid; in her arms I tasted the delights of paradise, and they have led to the torments of hell, which, as you see, have devoured me; she was infected with this thing, and perhaps she has died of it. Paquette had this present from a very learned Franciscan who had traced it right back to its source, for he had caught it from an old countess who had got it from a cavalry captain, who had it from a marquess, who had it from a page, who had got it from a Jesuit who, as a novice, had got it in a direct line from one of the companions of Christopher Columbus. As for me, I shall give it to no one, for I am dying.

Love, but also war: '[The disease] has made prodigious progress amongst us, especially in these large armies composed of honest, well-bred stipendiaries who determine the destinies of states; you can guarantee that when thirty thousand troops fight in pitched battle against an equal number, there are twenty thousand or so pox-victims on each side.' Voltaire takes the same theme up elsewhere:

The man with forty crowns was staying in a tiny canton where soldiers had not been garrisoned for 150 years. In this obscure corner of the world moral standards were as pure as the air thereabouts. No one knew that elsewhere love-making could transmit a destructive poison, that the seed of generations was being attacked, and that nature, contradicting herself, could make tenderness horrible and pleasure dreadful; people gave themselves over to love with the security of innocence. The troops arrived and everything changed.[55]

Sometimes memoirs reveal how much the pox had spread, and even become commonplace in the eighteenth century. Casanova's memoirs[56] are very instructive in this respect. The pox appears everywhere in them. Plenty of people of Casanova's acquaintance had it: the Bolognese gentleman whose limbs are paralyzed by the pox and whose sharp tongue is the only organ which the disease has left free; the abbot whose uvula has been eaten away by the pox; the Count of Vagensburg, who dies of it.

Casanova himself caught the pox for the first time in London, and really thought he would die of it. In Dresden a fresh attack once more obliged him to follow a six-week course of treatment: 'The sickness we describe as French does not curtail life, for those who know how to cure themselves of it; all it does is leave scars; but we can easily console ourselves with the thought that we have won them in pleasure, like soldiers who are delighted at the sight of their wounds, the signs of their virtue and the sources of their glory.'

In fact these successive attacks of the pox (Casanova says at one point that he is on his twentieth) seem to have been mostly gonorrhea, but this a retrospective diagnosis, and for Casanova, as for his contemporaries, the two were manifestations of a single disease. But the most interesting thing is that a disease which, in the centuries before, had provoked nothing but horror and fear had now become commonplace, for the great libertines at least. Here, for example, is the surgeon of the neighbouring village asking to speak to Casanova: 'He entered, and after having looked all around whispered in my ear that my valet had the pox. I burst out laughing for I was expecting some horror.'

Boswell lacked Casanova's audacity, and his diary, with its usurped literary reputation, reveals the extent to which this fat, pretentious sensualist worried about his health:

> I determined to have nothing to do with whores, as my health was of great consequence to me. I went to a girl with whom I had an intrigue in Edinburgh .... I waited on her and tried to obtain my former favours, but in vain. She would by no means listen. I was really unhappy and in want of women. I thought it hard to be in such a place [London] without them. I picked up a girl in the Strand; went into a court with the intention to enjoy her in amour. But she had none. I toyed with her. She wondered at my size, and said if ever I took a girl's maidenhead, I would make her squeak. I gave her a shilling, and had command enough of myself to go without touching her. I afterwards trembled at the danger I had escaped.[57]

A month later Boswell, a provincial in London at the beginning of George III's reign, still wanted a woman. But his actions were still guided by fear, all the greater since he had once had a serious attack of 'the disgusting disease' (although it was most likely to have been gonorrhea). Moreover, Boswell was miserly, and doctors in London were expensive, as he remarks. Nevertheless, a few years later he had an accident:

I gave a supper to two or three of my acquaintance, having before I left Scotland laid a guinea that I should not catch the venereal disorder for three years, which bet I had most certainly lost and now was paying. We drank a great deal, till I was so much intoxicated that instead of going home I went to a low house in one of the alleys in Edinburgh where I knew a common girl lodged, and like a brute as I was I lay all night with her . . . next morning I was like a man ordered for ignominious execution. But by noon I was worse, for I discovered that some infection had reached me. Was this not dreadful? I had an assignation in the evening with my charmer. How lucky it was that I knew my misfortune in time. I might have polluted her sweet body. Bless me! What a risk! But how could I tell her my shocking story?[58]

Here again the disease is made to seem relatively commonplace, for the woman he was courting forgave him immediately and Boswell, for his part, quickly encouraged her to overlook his misadventure. And, once again, the pox in the eighteenth century seemed to have been more gonorrhea than syphilis – an anachronism, of course, given that at the time, and for some time afterwards, the 'venereal virus' was considered to be an indivisible unity.

Prostitutes, of course, played an important role, for it was they who democratized the pox. The libertine literature of the end of the eighteenth century provides numerous testimonies. For example, the authoress of *La Cauchoise, ou Mémoires d'une courtisane célèbre*[59] caught the pox from a client who, after having made ample use of her, clearly had no intention of paying her. To get her revenge she announced that she had given him the pox. Then we are quits, he replied. 'What did he mean? . . . had the rogue given me the pox? Had he ruined me thus?' A surgeon was called, and he gave her a tisane and took payment in kind – from behind, claiming that he had avoided getting the pox by this means. The whore, allowing herself the benefit of the doubt, bestowed her favours the following evening on a generous young cavalier. Some time later he returned to see her. She was very frightened that there might be a scandal but he reassured her: 'You have given me a form of the pox, a mild form it is true, but I well and truly deserved it. Whether I caught it from you or someone else was all the same to me.' The cavalier had come to arrange an appointment for some young people: 'Just you give them what you gave me: they are rascals on whom I wished to be revenged.'

There were also at this time an abundance of poems which strove to turn the disease into a joke. An example is this *Ode to the pox*:

> O pox! O cruel plague!
> How dreadful are its ravages!
> How many cunts it has devastated
> How many fuckers it has made miserable!

It is the disease of opulence,
The French disease par excellence,
The common ill in every land,
The disease of prudes, coquettes,
Duchesses and maids,
Porters and marquises.[60]

Others, on the other hand, are alarmist, especially those written after the Revolution:

Amorous people, unwise people,
Don't you tremble with horror to see
The young girl leaving her village
To offer her honour for sale here . . .
You let a fickle swarm of girls
Attracted by voluptuousness
To lose the best years of their lives,
And the treasure of health.

Why this barbaric slowness?
More haste, O doctors,
And give the monsters of Ténare
All these poisons of the human blood . . .
If you touch them, may the pox,
By the great gods! overwhelm you with ills . . .
Must this frivolous pleasure
Lead us to nothing but the tomb?[61]

And since wise words had failed to check the pox, preventative measures were required. This, at least, is what John Hunter wrote in 1787: 'Since we must not only seek to cure patients in general, but to stop people becoming infected, it would be appropriate to examine at this point, as fully as we can, how this might be done. This disease, in fact, is one whose spread can be effectively prevented by taking certain measures either before or immediately afterwards.'[62]

The idea is certainly a revolutionary one when considered in the context of the morality of the age, but Hunter and his colleagues provided barely any practical advice. Just as in the sixteenth century, we find the classic *ante* and *post coitum* ablutions, and the scarcely newer idea of coating the genitals in a greasy substance to prevent 'the venereal matter from coming into contact with those parts'. As for anti-venereal waters, everyone declared them to be ineffective because of their low mercury content. In short, concludes de Horne, 'we still know of no genuine form of prevention.'

And yet the means of protection did exist, a fact deplored by the few doctors who deigned to mention them in passing. For men, there was the condom,[63] which was probably invented in England at the beginning of the eighteenth century. Turner[64] mentions debauchees who for some time had used bags made from very fine, seamless membranes (the sheep's caecum) in the form of a sheath. Casanova, as one might have expected, made great use of these 'frock coats from England' which were soon to be more widely known as English caps. Clients would be allowed 'an English garment' to 'put the soul at rest' by prostitutes. If the quality seemed to them to be too ordinary, they were then offered some at three francs apiece, which were sold only by the dozen. Casanova took a set, having been fitted with several samples by a maidservant of fifteen.

The brothels were supplied with enormous quantities of these accessories which, already, practical jokers were filling with air or water under the noses of passers-by. But, just like the sponge which prostitutes inserted in their vaginas,[65] they were most often regarded – quite justifiably – as contraceptives. That was where, one might say, the shoe pinched, for though the morality of the time was henceforth ready to accept the idea of *ante coitum* protection, the idea of contraception could under no circumstances be tolerated. And, in this case, it was difficult to have the one without the other.

In any case, prostitutes were still at the centre of the debate. Succeeding lieutenant generals of police in Paris in the eighteenth century took a close interest in prostitutes, but they were more interested in using them as informers (they were popularly known as 'snoopers' at the time) than in worrying about their crucial role in propagating venereal diseases. However, the question was already being raised by certain authors, as for example in *La Cacomonade*,[66] a satirical term which designated the pox. The anonymous author pokes fun at the Faculty for having initially wanted to confine mercury to barometers, and after he has pronounced himself to be a supporter of the American origin of the disease (described as 'the princess of America'), he gets to the most original aspect of his work: advice on how to prevent the *cacomonade*. It must be tracked down like contraband merchandise by setting up special offices at the points of entry to towns, staffed with specially qualified women inspectors.

They would be neither the three graces nor the twelve muses. We could have forty of them, as in the Académie Française, or sixty as in the Ferme Générale. Only those who were the most expert, the best-trained in shop practices, the most familiar with fraudulent practices and consequently the most suited to discover it in spite of the skill of the smugglers, would be appointed.

The victims who were thus discovered would be stamped 'like prohibited merchandise', then sent, at the expense of the state, to a special hospital.

A few years later, Restif de La Bretonne, in a work which was famous in his lifetime *Le Pornographe, ou idées d'un honnête homme sur un projet de règlement pour les prostitutées . . .*[67] put forward the idea that prostitution should be made a public institution. Since prostitution is 'an unfortunate but absolute necessity in the large towns', prostitutes should be restricted to regulated establishments (Restif's proposed regulations consist of no less than forty-five articles). This is the simplest way of rooting out the venereal virus . . . .

> The greatest care will be taken to protect the prostitutes from the horrible disease which makes an establishment of this sort so desirable: we will choose prostitutes who are no longer young, and whose taste for pleasure is disappearing, those who have always been the most dutiful and who are the most intelligent, to visit the men who present themselves. They will deny them entrance to the Corridor indicated on their ticket until they are satisfied that they are in a state of perfect health. They will also inspect other prostitutes every day, when they are getting up.

From the prison to the hospital

The policy of locking up beggars which had begun in the sixteenth century became more entrenched in the seventeenth. Thus, in 1656 a general hospital was set up in Paris, consisting principally of two establishments which were soon to become famous: Bicêtre, for men, and the Salpêtrière, for women. (The provinces were invited to do likewise, but financial difficulties soon put paid to the possibility of extending such provision to the whole kingdom). At first, the pox-victims were explicitly excluded from the general hospital;[68] pox-victims likewise continued to be excluded from the Hôtel-Dieu, which refused to do any more than pay for such of them as had contracted the disease innocently to be treated elsewhere.[69] But in the years which followed, the necessity of accepting pregnant pox victims was the first step towards the admission of pox-victims of both sexes at Bicêtre from 1690 onwards.

Much has been written on Bicêtre, which was considered from the eighteenth century onwards to be the epitome of prison horror: 'It is a terrible ulcer on the body politic,' wrote Mercier,

a wide, deep, oozing ulcer from which one cannot help averting one's eyes . . . .
The name Bicêtre conjures up an indescribable feeling of repugnance, horror and
scorn since it has become the receptacle for everything that is most squalid and
vile in society, and its inmates are almost all libertines of one sort or another,
rogues, informers, swindlers, robbers, counterfeiters, pederasts, etc.

In 1788 Mirabeau painted an equally gloomy picture of Bicêtre:

We had the courage to present ourselves at Bicêtre; I say courage, although for my
part I ought not to give myself much credit; in fact when I made my mind up to
go I was ignorant of all the horrors of that odious dwelling-place. I knew, as
everyone does, that Bicêtre was both a hospital and a prison; but I did not know
that the hospital had been constructed to engender disease, and the prison to give
birth to crimes. Within the precincts of the hospital, which we visited first, are
confined those persons infected with the venereal disease. They are piled up on
top of one another like a cargo of Negroes in an African ship. Each ward contains
two rows of beds; but it is common to see the floorspace between them crammed
with patients. Sometimes this is due to the complete lack of space, sometimes
to the fact that a poor, weak, emaciated patient, half-eaten by this most terrible
of diseases, actually prefers the hardness of the floor to the infected and filthy
bed. . . .[70]

Even allowing for the exaggeration of the satirical tracts, it is
clear that the fate of venereal victims sent to Bicêtre was hardly an
enviable one. In the second half of the eighteenth century a
hundred or so patients were treated for five weeks at a time. This
number scarcely varied up until the time of the Revolution, and the
restrictions on intake led to frightful waiting lists. 'The applicants
are so numerous,' writes Mercier, 'that a few libertines and several
women prostitutes have put their names down even before falling
sick. What have you moralists got to say to that?'

However, those patients who were deemed 'unworthy of
compassion', according to the expression of the administrators of
the general hospital – mostly those who were sent there on the
orders of the lieutenant general of police – lived, or rather survived,
in appalling conditions. In Saint-Eustache, men were literally piled
up in miniscule dormitories which were so saturated with
mercurial vapours that the specific symptoms appeared even before
the treatment had begun. As far as women were concerned, the
facilities at La Miséricorde were a little less deplorable. As regards
the treatment, its name alone is evocative: 'les grand remèdes'.
There was no question of regulating the administration of mercury
or of the countless secret remedies tested. All sorts of wild
experiments were allowed, and although fatal cases of the pox had
become rare in the eighteenth century, people frequently died of
their treatment at Bicêtre.

Elsewhere, the general hospitals tended to conform to the line taken by the Hôtel-Dieu by refusing admission to venereal victims. The same applied to the religious workhouses, where it was believed that nothing could be done for libertines who had reached such an advanced stage. But there were many indigent victims of the venereal disease, especially prostitutes, in the beggars' prisons which were set up after the royal declaration of 3 August 1764. It was at this point that an administration of *intendants* began to take over, introducing the first health records for venereal victims; these showed the days on which each received treatment, and even how many Keyser's dragées were administered. There was a rigorous distinction between those who were there because of their licentiousness, for whom imprisonment and punishment were as important as the treatment, and those victims who required nothing but a cure.

Often prostitutes with venereal diseases were sent there at the express wish of the military authorities, which were anxious to 'use the most appropriate means to protect (His Majesty's) soldiers from a contagion which attacks the very springs of life, and which degrades the human species.' For the first time a proper campaign of prophylaxis for the armed forces was drawn up:[71] prostitutes who frequented the garrisons or followed the regiments were to be tracked down, recidivist soldiers with the disease were to be punished . . . . But, although the systematic medical visits of the army surgeons bear witness to the extension of the disease, attempts to create military hospitals exclusively for victims of venereal disease still encountered much resistance, especially from the nuns, who exercised a tight control on anything which even slightly resembled a hospital.

However, despite growing financial difficulties, the reign of Louis XVI saw reforms in medical care and in the hospitals, following on from and parallel to the philanthropic movement which was developing throughout western Europe at the time. In the 1780s there were numerous inspections and enquiries (Howard, Colombier, Tenon, La Rochefoucauld) which exposed shortcomings, and measures were introduced on behalf of the sick, the insane, and prisoners, particularly through the efforts of minister Necker.

The question of the victims of venereal disease was therefore aired once more, and it was all the more pressing because there were very few of the fifty or so large and small hospitals in Paris at the end of the eighteenth century which took this category of patients (even though from that time onwards they were at least acknowledged): Bicêtre, the Petites Maisons[72] and, exclusively for soldiers, the Les Invalides hospital and the military hospital of the French and Swiss Guards. The latter was little used in consequence of an unfortunate order in 1778 which decreed that any soldier receiving treatment three times for venereal disease would have to serve two extra years over and above the twelve he had enlisted for. Of course, the soldiers did not change their behaviour, they simply concealed the sad consequences.

Small establishments were set up for civilian victims, often as charitable initiatives. And on 10 November 1776, something previously unheard of happened: the parish priest of Saint-Étienne-du-Mont was heard reading from the pulpit a notice from Lenoir, the lieutenant general of police, informing the congregation that these health establishments would take pox-sufferers of both sexes on presentation of certificates from their curé and a surgeon.[73] But these establishments soon had to close through lack of money, and after an edifying visit in 1784 by minister Breteuil to Bicêtre it was finally decided to set up a proper hospital devoted exclusively to venereal diseases in the Capuchin convent in the Saint-Jacques district. This institution complemented the Vaugirard hospice, created in 1780 'for new-born children afflicted with the venereal disease. . . .'

Saving the race

A paradoxical aspect of the Malthusianism which developed in the eighteenth century was the refusal to let new-born babies die[74] and the birth of a populationist doctrine of the theoreticians of power (contraception as harmful to the state) which was objectively akin to that of the Church (to waste the seed is both sinful and a murder by default). In this context, the pox was soon accused of destroying not only 'the present race' but also 'that yet to be born'.[75] Here we have the idea, which we have met with already in Sanchez, of the pox being the cause of the 'decline of the French temperament'.[76] 'To marry when one has such diseases,' writes Raulin in 1768, 'is to cheat one's fatherland by bringing into the world children who cannot serve it, and to deceive and distress oneself by inoculating one's family with the seeds of a premature death, a sword of Damocles which threatens all those born into the family in question for several generations.'[77]

Numerous writings examined the medical aspects of this grave topic, with regard both to the obstetric consequences (with a notable contribution by the Swede Nil Roseen de Rosenstein in 1764) and the problem of hereditary pox, a question on which agreement was still a long way off. Van Swieten believed that a healthy foetus could be infected during delivery if there were venereal ulcers on the mother's genital organs, whereas Fabre believed that the venereal virus could be communicated at the moment of conception. Swediaur, reliable as ever, gives a comprehensive overview of the possibilities: hereditary syphilis (he was one of the first to use the term) communicated by means of the father's semen or as a result of being in the womb; congenital syphilis, more common and contracted at birth; and, finally, syphilis transmitted by the nipples of a wet-nurse or the kisses of a pox-infected mouth (from this period onwards, many cases of accidental infection were recorded). This gave Swediaur the opportunity to denounce the women of the cities of Europe who preferred their own comfort and pleasure to the responsibility of feeding their children themselves and therefore abandoned them to hired wet-nurses who were frequently infected.

One of the first emergency measures was taken in 1780 by the lieutenant general of police, who gave Colombier, the inspector general of hospitals (the post had just been created), the job of opening a hospice in Vaugirard in which syphilitic children would be breastfed by their mothers or by wet-nurses who were already infected. At the time this new hospice was considered to be a model establishment, since wet-nurses and pregnant women had beds to themselves, each child had its own cot, and standards of cleanliness were scrupulously observed. The use of mercury to treat women who were breastfeeding was not abolished, but it was at least very much reduced. It was, however, anticipated that their milk would contain a small amount of mercury and would therefore act as an antidote for the babies, who received no direct treatment. Fifteen months after the Vaugirard hospice opened, Colombier addressed a report to the King in which he congratulated himself on having saved more than one-third of the newborn babies suffering from the venereal disease. That two-thirds continued to die does not seem excessive if one remembers that in former times the mortality rate had been as high as 90 per cent. Moreover, as Mercier pointed out, fewer were saved at the Enfants-Trouvés hospital, even though it admitted only babies who were free from the pox.

Faced with the desolate picture painted by the doctors of the Vaugirard hospice[78] – women with the pox having series of abortions, decrepit children who survived looking like little old men, the eruptions which covered their bodies – the public authorities eventually became aware of the urgency of the problem, a problem which affected the whole kingdom and not just the capital. Of course there were also plagues, epizootic epidemics, famines caused by bad harvests, the problem of abandoned children, and a hundred other calamities to contend with. But in the crucial decades of 1770 and 1780, the administrative infrastructure of the *intendants* made possible a health care investment in the provinces. These *intendants*, steeped in the Enlightenment, were eighteenth-century 'technocrats', the effective, docile and intelligent tools of a henceforth well-organized centralized monarchy who had the power and the means (notably the wide circulation of the printed word) to bring about the necessary reforms.

It thus came about that the problem of the pox generated a multiplicity of instructions on the treatment of venereal diseases in the provinces,[79] and memoranda on the need to use cow's milk in place of the milk of wet nurses. The practice of sending children, particularly abandoned children, from the cities to the provinces to be suckled, was often considered to be one of the causes of the spread of the venereal disease.[80] In short, from this time onwards, anathema gave way to education.

5

The Nineteenth-century Impasse

The Revolution and the pox

In 1789, a certain Mittié, a professor at the Faculty of Medicine, assailed the Constituent Assembly, and subsequently the Legislative Assembly, with memoranda and petitions, and had soon launched a full-scale attack on the inadequacy of the material provisions for combatting venereal disease:

Bicêtre, the Vaugirard hospice, the civil hospitals and the beggars' prisons of the Kingdom, which received the unfortunate victims, were unable to cope with all of those who presented themselves, and even the help which they did give was of questionable value! The treatment was long, cruel, short-sighted, difficult, complicated, inconsistent, unpleasant, costly, inadequate, and sometimes fatal.[1]

Even allowing for the settling of scores between the Faculty and the powerful Royal Society of Medicine, radical criticisms and demands for reform were undeniably in the wind. There were full-scale attacks on the inefficacy of the treatments ('it is astonishing that the experience of three centuries has been unable to shed any light on its cure!'), and especially on mercury. Behind all this, however, lies an admission of general disarray: 'Even today there is not a single man of science in the kingdom, nor yet in Europe, who knows how to treat this disease, what he is doing, why he is doing it, what he is using or what the effects will be . . . .'[2]

The question of the victims of venereal disease figured large amongst the very many debated by the Mendicancy Committee:

It must not be forgotten that in the account of the state of the hospitals of Paris which we gave to the Assembly we brought to its attention the fact that each year only 600 patients of both sexes afflicted with this disease received free treatment, which was given only at Bicêtre, whereas more than 2,000 persons applied for it, and a further five or six times that number did not even make an application because they had not the least hope of being accepted for the treatment, horrifying and inadequate though it was.[3]

The Mendicancy Committee concluded by demanding that two hospitals for the victims of venereal disease should be set up in Paris. As for the situation in the provinces, they postponed examining it until more auspicious times.

However, not only was no new hospital for sufferers from venereal disease created in Paris, but it was not until 1792 that victims began to be systematically referred to the establishment which had been instituted in 1785 but which had opened late because of lack of money. Male and female venereal victims from Bicêtre and also pregnant sufferers and milkless mothers with the disease from the Vaugirard hospice were transferred there. The increase in the number of admissions, which rose from 1,600 in 1792 to 3,000 in 1810, gives a clear indication of how important this establishment became, particularly from the time of the Consulate onwards.

Henceforth in the Hôpital des Vénériens, as in all those founded during the Revolution and the Empire, as much as possible was done to run it as a therapeutic establishment rather than simply as a refuge for paupers, which is what it had been under the *Ancien Régime*. The various departments (men, women, pregnant and nursing women) conformed to principles of hygiene which were rigorously adhered to from then on: good ventilation and drainage, bathrooms, inner courtyards and corridors to allow freedom of movement. Infirmaries, which catered for the same districts, treated non-venereal diseases, which were legion amongst the poor. And, finally, the staff was augmented to a certain extent by the creation of medical teams which included, in addition to doctor and surgeon (the distinction between whom survived for some time after),[4] new characters such as the chief pharmacist and the student treating patients whilst pursuing his clinical training.

Cullerier, chief surgeon since 1792, had particular responsibility for the men's and women's departments; he suppressed the 'grands remèdes' without entirely abandoning mercury. He published a good deal whilst he was closely involved in the activities of the hospital service and in teaching, and he was one of the prototypes of the great clinicians of the nineteenth century, even though his theoretical oeuvre contributed nothing to knowledge of the disease. He also instituted a free outpatient service, which became a regular feature from the year VIII onwards.

Bertin, who was appointed chief doctor in 1799, was given responsibility for the care of the wet-nurses and children, who were the object of special concern. In a report which he wrote 'in the light of observation and experience' he depicted the Hôpital des Vénériens as

an establishment in which those mothers of indigent families, or women who have been abandoned by their husbands, who have fallen victim to the most dreadful of scourges, can find healthy and sustaining food, and where they and their children can recover; an establishment to care for wet-nurses of pure and simple morals who, though they lived in the country, were not safe from the grim consequences of the corruption of the towns; an establishment in which the child abandoned by those to whom it owes both its existence and the poison so apt for its destruction can still smile at another mother . . . in which the corrupt woman, at first almost astonished by her own maternal feelings, can find a beneficial diversion in the performance of these functions.[5]

Aside from this fine flight of oratory, what were the results? It seems that if what was now increasingly being described as 'syphilis' rather than 'the pox' was not actually being cured then at least fewer patients were being killed – if we can believe a report from the General Council of Hospices which gives the figure of one death in every forty-seven cases. However, if we consider only the figures given by Bertin himself, who was hardly likely to have been pessimistic, infant mortality remained highly significant, with 617 deaths out of 1,024 admissions between the years IX and 1809 (a span of ten years).

In any case, syphilis undoubtedly continued to make progress. It extended its geographical spread to Canada, taking virulent forms which recall the outbreak of the scourge in Europe at the end of the fifteenth century, and it spread to all social classes during the wars of the Revolution and the Empire . . . This is reflected in a satirical engraving of 1816, '*Les adieux au Palais-Royal ou les Suites du Premier Pas*'. It depicts officers in the allied armies who are preparing to quit French soil turning their backs on the Palais-Royal, which was famous for its prostitutes, whilst a doctor hands them prescriptions and medications for the venereal diseases they have contracted. (Amongst the remedies there is prominently figured a bottle of 'Rob Boyveau-Laffecteur', which is clearly continuing the fruitful commercial career on which it had embarked at the end of the *Ancien Régime*.) The height of irony was that one of the buildings requisitioned by the Prussian troops when they occupied Paris in 1814 had been the Hôpital des Vénériens.

Ricord and the birth of symptomatology

According to the 1821 *Dictionnaire des sciences médicales*,[6] syphilis is a 'contagious disease which can be caught in so many ways, and which manifests itself in forms that are so varied and numerous, that it defies philosophical definition'. 'A bizarre appelation,' adds the 1836 *Dictionnaire de médicine et de chirurgie pratiques*,[7] 'synonymous with venereal disease, which is neither more exact nor more meaningful, and which has for a long time been used to refer to a group of affections which are very diverse as regards their origins, causes and natures, and which people persist in grouping together as if they were one and the same.' Cullerier, the co-author of these articles, denounces the 'syphilomaniacs' who 'blame on syphilis any pathological affection which does not respond to normal treatment' (scrofula, cancer, phthisis, asthma, rheumatism, etc.). Once again we have the question of the unicity of the venereal diseases . . .

During the same period, Broussais added to the confusion by founding the physiologist school, according to which the inflammation of the tissues was the sole cause of all maladies (including insanity). Syphilis was thereby reduced to a phlegmasia, and the venereal virus was either dismissed as non-existent or reduced to the level of a mere irritant. Jourdan,[8] one of the supporters of this ephemeral but powerful doctrine, even went some way towards denying the existence of contagion, relying on the apparently irrefutable argument that there must ultimately have been a point, albeit the birth of the first man, at which syphilis broke out spontaneously!

For his part, Cullerier, whom the 'physiologists' tried in vain to rally to their cause, advanced the theory of a primitive syphilis (characterized by the chancre) and a constitutional syphilis (characterized by the syphilides and subsequently by the later manifestations which had been remarked on at all periods), the idea being that the former could progress as far as a cure without the latter even appearing. This same doctor was amongst the first to specify the length of the incubation period, estimating that it was between three and five days until the initial chancre appeared. Elsewhere he notes that syphilis is less common in women, even allowing for the fact that chancres situated in the depths of the vagina or on the cervix can go unnoticed. He maintains that this is because women 'generally behave more moderately'.

At last came Ricord, as historians of medicine traditionally say. And, it is tempting to add, he arrived at just the right moment. A

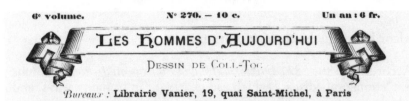

6º volume.   Nº 270. — 10 c.   Un an : 6 fr.

LES HOMMES D'AUJOURD'HUI

DESSIN DE COLL-TOC

Bureaux : Librairie Vanier, 19, quai Saint-Michel, à Paris

DOCTEUR RICORD

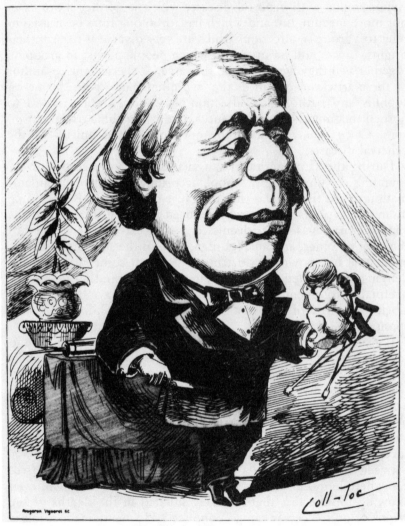

PLATE 5 Philippe Ricord (1800–1889) was, if not the first, then certainly the greatest, and at any rate the most famous specialist on syphilis of the first half of the nineteenth century. (Bibliothèque Municipale de Caen)

student of Dupuytren, he joined the Hôpital des Vénériens as a surgeon to wet-nurses in 1831, following on from a period of training complicated by an initial lack of funds and an immoderate penchant for irony, neither of which was calculated to promote a great hospital career. He quickly became famous for his brilliant lectures, to which flocked students and doctors from France and abroad, and he soon had a classy private clientele queuing up at his private residence in the Rue de Tournon. He was born a brilliant socialite and a true savant. He remained at the Hôpital des Vénériens (which was renamed the Hôpital du Midi in 1836 when a new hospital was founded in Lourcine for female venereal patients) for three years before devoting himself exclusively to his ever-growing private clientele. A doctor to Napoleon III, he was laden with honours and died in 1889 at the age of 89. In 1893 the Hôpital du Midi was renamed the Hôpital Ricord, and was subsequently incorporated into the Hôpital Cochin in 1903.

Ricord's clinical observation was rigorous. He was, for example, one of the first to make systematic use of the speculum. His prime achievement was to distinguish syphilis from venereal papillomae, balanoposthitis and, above all, from gonorrhea. Already, a few years earlier, Hernandez (to whom Ricord refers) had inoculated convicts in Toulon prison with gonorrhea and concluded from the fact that they did not contract syphilis that gonorrhea and the chancre were of a different nature and did not belong to the same disease.[9] Thus syphilis came to be recognized as syphilis, gonorrhea as gonorrhea.

Ricord also established ideas which were, at the time, revolutionary: there is no such thing as a syphilis whose first manifestation is the bubo; syphilis produces constitutional effects; it affects the patient by making him resistant to a fresh dose ('you cannot catch a double dose of syphilis'); there is a strict chronology of symptoms ('there is therefore order and discipline where people have persisted in seeing nothing but confusion and unregulated chaos').[10]

He also delivered the coup de grace to the doctrines of Broussais' followers:

It is now a question of determining the specific cause, the fatal poison which produces syphilis. This poison, which we are now in the position to name, is the syphilitic virus. People need to be reminded of the fact, since efforts are being made to make them forget it, that the existence of this virus was contested and formally refuted when I began my first researches into syphilopathy. In those days many doctors could not name it thus without fearing that they would thereby compromise themselves. It was at that time that the learned Jourdan exclaimed in a bizarre fit of rage: call it what you like, but don't refer to it as a virus![11]

Those whom he wittily calls 'the athletes of the physiologist school' tried to defend themselves, denying him the 'role of reformer and chief exponent of doctrine'[12] and reproaching him both for the content and for the over-romantic form of his works; these works, however, contained certain expressions which subsequently became famous, such as 'les pléiades ganglionnaires' for the lymphatic propagation of the indurated chancres.

There are, however, shortcomings in Ricord's clinical work. He makes no reference to the incubation period; as regards treatment he falls back on mercury as a specific remedy, having condemned the antiphlogistic remedies favoured by the physiologists; he denies contagious powers to the secon   .1anifestations, and in particular to the mucous plaques, on the grounds that he was unable to induce infection using them – yet at the same period William Wallace proved that they *are* infectious by infecting healthy men with them![13] But in 1852, on the rostrum of the Academy of Medicine, Ricord upheld his earlier conclusions: 'If I am to change my mind I want more convincing evidence than this.' The works of Julius Bettinger (who published his first paper anonymously in 1855 and was thenceforth to carry for posterity the disquieting pseudonym of 'l'Anonyme du Palatinat'), and even those of Rollet,[14] failed to change Ricord's mind.

Moreover, although he recognized that the indurated chancre is infectious and makes the subject resistant to another dose of infection, and that the soft chancre is a local lesion with which the carrier can be reinfected any number of times, Ricord did not conclude that the different characters of these two chancres implied that they are the product of two different diseases. It was Léon Bassereau who, in 1852, was the first to maintain that the soft chancre was different (even though it can be associated with syphilis in the mixed chancre), thereby destroying the last vestiges of the unicist theory.

The failure of syphilization

Given the remarkable precedents set by William Wallace and company, and also the extraordinary vogue (justified in this instance) for vaccination in the first decades of the nineteenth century,[15] it was virtually inevitable that there would be a search for a 'vaccine' against syphilis. Hence from 1844 onwards we find the theory of syphilization, as expounded by its promoter, Dr Auzias-Turenne, who was widely talked about in medical circles for more than ten years.

Auzias-Turenne was a contemporary and enemy of Ricord. Like Melchior Robert he was one of the last supporters of the unicist theory. He still believed in syphilitic gonorrhea, and thought that the soft chancre was the result of a mild attack of syphilis – hence the idea of injecting healthy subjects with it in order to make them immune to the more virulent form of syphilis. 'I am introducing a new concept into science,' writes Auzias-Turenne,

and consequently I must adopt a new word to express it; the word is syphilization. Its root is so well-known that no-one will have any difficulty understanding the meaning I wish to give it. It can be defined as follows: it is the state of the organism whereby this latter is no longer susceptible to developing syphilis, this being the consequence of a sort of syphilitic saturation. The suffix which I have given to the word syphilis perfectly conveys the idea of a sort of impregnation or impression which can no longer take place . . . . Repeated injections of the syphilitic virus taken from a developing chancre do not give rise to more serious chancres, as one might naturally have expected, and as syphilologists have thought until now; instead they produce artificial chancres which become increasingly smaller, up until the point at which the last injections have no effects whatsoever.[16]

What were the implications of this postulate? The syphilitic treated by syphilization would be cured and would thenceforth neither contract nor transmit any sort of syphilitic affection. Whores in particular would be singled out for syphilization, and those who frequented prostitutes would from then on be able to escape contamination by going to those who had certificates of syphilization. The inventor of this radical new specific measure intended it principally for men and women who were already afflicted with syphilis, but he also went so far as to advocate, albeit tentatively, the syphilization of healthy subjects who were at risk of infection.

Syphilization, however, was an utter failure. After the demonstration of the dual nature of the chancre no-one believed in it except Auzias-Turenne, who clung to it, secretly trying out the first experiment on himself (a secret which came to light in his will: 'It might be profitable to dissect me, for I am the oldest syphilized person in the world'). Auzias-Turenne's honesty is beyond question, and he can in no sense be classified as a charlatan.[17] He was, moreover, an outstanding clinician. 'The most remarkable symptoms of syphilis,' he wrote, 'appear on the skin. These are like the label on a vase, or better still like the signature of the pox written in large characters. Be sure that you can read them with ease.' But this is just a small part of the picture of syphilis, a mere 'fraction of the whole'. It is a question of unearthing syphilis 'in every case in which it feigns absence'.[18]

The fact remains that in 1852 the Imperial Academy of Medicine, to which the question had been referred, condemned syphilization as dangerous:

1 Neither reasoning, nor analogy, nor experiments on animals, nor observations of people who are said to have been syphilized by natural means can justify the application of syphilization to either healthy persons or sick ones.

2 Its use as a supposed preventative measure against syphilis is a monstrous act which gratuitously risks seriously damaging the health of those people who are foolish enough to undergo it.

3 As a method of treating the symptoms of syphilis in all their forms it has no basis in any positive, detailed, authenticated fact, or in any comparative statistics; indeed, the only exact and authenticated information which we have points only to the method's uncertainty, its difficulties and, above all, to its dangers and the shameful scars it leaves behind.

In the same year, a commission appointed by the prefect of police to decide on Dr Auzias-Turenne's application for authorization to syphilize syphilitic prostitutes in the infirmary of Saint-Lazare prison opposed the experiment. (Gone were the blissful days when one could experiment to one's heart's content on the human material confined in Bicêtre.) Ricord, who was a member of the commission, and who had for several years put his uncontested authority behind syphilization, abruptly abandoned Auzias-Turenne: 'I saw the birth of syphilization, and I gave it all the help I could; I gave it a public. I was soon obliged to reject it with indignation.'[19]

The bizarre practice of syphilization, the idea behind which was that one could protect oneself by an overdose of the disease, was condemned in France, but it enjoyed a certain success in Piedmont under Dr Sperino and in Norway under Dr Boeck (who went as far as to attempt to cure a leper by syphilization in 1862). No man is a prophet in his own country, and France was not syphilized. Unless, that is, we understand the word in the sense that Baudelaire gave it a decade earlier when, disappointed by the failure of the revolutions of 1848, he declared: 'When we talk seriously about revolution they are horrified; we all have the republican spirit in our veins, just as we have the pox in our bones. We have been democratized and syphilized.'

What should be done?

The nineteenth century was not simply a new century. In the aftermath of the revolutionary watershed it declared itself to be a new era of democracy, rationalism, science and progress. Amongst the tasks to be undertaken, the struggle against pauperism and the crime and disease which it brought in its wake was of particular importance given that nothing had been done in this connection during the 'Ancien Régime' (a pejorative term at the time). Whereas alcoholism, for example, offered plenty of scope for the introduction of educational, hygienic and preventative measures, syphilis, by contrast, had the effect (as was increasingly acknowledged) of discouraging practitioners and the public authorities because of the lack of an effective remedy for it. Syphilis was more elusive than other ills, and seemed to be making a mockery of the declarations of war against it.

The doctors of the period were in disarray, agreeing that 'this cruel disease can never be completely destroyed.'[20] 'Are we not forced to admit,' writes a doctor of the Empire, 'that the end of our troubles is a very long way off?'[21] Ricord blamed charlatanism for having made everyone sceptical. As for Dr Baumès, the chief surgeon at the Hôpital de Antiquaille in Lyons, he writes that 'the medical profession certainly has good reason to be weary of all these theories on the origin, cause and appearance of syphilis, the action of mercury, etc., which have seen the light of day in no less than twelve hundred treatises, pamphlets and memoirs since the fifteenth century.'[22]

Morale was equally low in medical circles in Japan, judging by what we hear from Sugita, an old and disillusioned doctor who in 1810 recorded his memories in his *Keiei Yawa* (*'Nocturnal Dialogues with my Shadow'*):

When I was young I made a point of questioning those with a reputation for treating syphilis successfully, and I learned their therapeutic methods. But when I put them into practice I never obtained the desired results . . . I collected all their theories and recipes. Every time I encountered a syphilitic I would try one of them, choosing it to suit the symptoms, but I have not found the miraculous recipe which works every time. Later I perused all the books which describe the prescriptions of the Dutch medics and I tried those too, but the outcome was no different. In the meantime I had acquired an undeserved reputation over the years and my patients grew in number day by day and month by month. Eventually I was treating more than 1,000 a year, of whom seven or eight hundred were syphilitics. Over a period of forty to fifty years I must have treated several tens of thousands. I am seventy this year, but I still have no perfect knowledge. Is it that my patients are insubordinate, or are my methods of treatment inadequate? It seems, in fact, that this disease is increasingly difficult to cure, and nothing has changed since I was young.[23]

The general public too was disillusioned. Syphilis has become 'a terrible bugbear of family life' writes Cullerier, who mentions the increasing number of 'syphilophobes'. Soon it became one of a doctor's tasks to 'boost the patient's morale', for the latter were for the most part convinced that they were afflicted with an incurable illness.

Syphilis was not in decline geographically; indeed, it had conquered new territories, notably Canada which was affected by the end of the eighteenth century. 'In Canada of late,' writes Swediaur,

we have seen a new sort of venereal disease to which the name *Mal de la baie de Saint-Paul* has been given. Within just a few years this disease has made rapid and substantial progress amongst the Canadians. Fathers transmit it to their children, and it is spread in food and drink. When it breaks out in a family it is rare for even one individual to be spared. In some cases the virus seems to enter the body by absorption, and lies dormant there for years; eventually the disease appears, and in its tertiary stage exhibits all the symptoms of the pox. The victims often drag out a miserable existence to an advanced age; they lose, in turn, their noses, eyes, the soft part of the palate, and sometimes even the lower part of the cranium. Five thousand eight hundred people were found to be infected in Canada in 1785, not counting those who did not declare that they had the disease; it was, however, still unknown amongst the Indians of the neighbourhood at that time.[24]

The severity of the symptoms, which according to Swediaur were often the result of subjects contracting syphilis by non-venereal means, is reminiscent of what happened when the pox appeared in Europe at the very end of the fifteenth century. Jutland and various places in Dalmatia were also affected between the end of the eighteenth century and the beginning of the nineteenth century. There too the majority of cases were of non-venereal origin – which brings us to the question, to which we shall return briefly in chapter 10, of the treponematoses in general.[25]

As far as treatment was concerned, no progress was being made. Mercury lost a good deal of its credibility at the beginning of the nineteenth century with the success, albeit ephemeral, of Broussais' inflammatory theory; the supporters of this theory were vigorous opponents of mercury,[26] for which they substituted an antiphlogistic treatment consisting of baths, enemas, laxatives and lenitives, the intention being to counteract the irritation of the tissues. But mercury was quick to recover its position, even though thenceforth practitioners were less enthusiastic about it, and some of them were already openly opposed to it.[27] Only a few extremists still advocated 'mercurializing' the patient, that is to say saturating him with mercury.[28] In the 1860s mercury enjoyed a revival when injections were added to the classic treatments of frictions, pills and Van Swieten's liquor. New compounds appeared at the same period: acetate, nitrate, phosphate and sulphide of mercury.

In Japan, as in China, sublimate of mercury was very popular in the eighteenth century, but its high toxicity brought it into increasing disrepute as an internal treatment. Opposition to mercury was also a consequence of the dogma according to which health is the result of a balance between Yin and Yang, antagonistic forces an excess of either of which necessarily causes a deficit of the other. Venereal infections fell into the nosological category of 'emptiness of the kidneys'; this was characterized by a loss of Yin, and consequently mercury, a Yang metal, was contraindicated. However, certain daring doctors unhesitatingly defended the prescription of mercury, even if it meant administering it to themselves after they had voluntarily infected themselves with syphilis. One doctor who did this was Funakoshi Keisuke:

Out of fear of misleading future generations I decided to spend a month frequenting five prostitutes who had recent chancres and buboes, and I contracted a chancre and buboes in my turn. I then swallowed my 'pills of longevity' until they made my mouth hurt. Despite this, I persisted in swallowing these pills, which were reputed to be toxic to fish and birds, and I quickly recovered. I then once more had commerce with ten prostitutes, and was not contaminated. This was ten years ago, and I have never been afflicted with the pox since. (Baidoku Sadan, *Table talk on syphilis*, 1843).[29]

Other forms of treatment found it difficult to compete with mercury, or even to gain acceptance in combination with it. Some mooted potassium iodide as a new specific.[30] There were also the arsenical preparations which had been pursuing the tentative career which had taken shape at the very end of the fifteenth century; and, for the record, there was the usual collection of gold, platinum, silver, antimony and iron (the latter was intended as a tonic). We must also mention homeopathy, which Dr Hoffmann advocated in the following euology in 1848: 'All of you young people for whose benefit I am speaking out, if you wish to preserve yourselves from the chronic diseases which could poison your futures, remember homeopathy as soon as the slightest symptom of syphilis appears.'[31] Opponents of homeopathy were justifiably ironic: 'Homeopathy! We would of course have been very careful not to wake up this beautiful golden-haired lady, especially for a disease with such serious consequences, for it is certainly no laughing matter.'[32]

Another method of treatment was the cauterization, or even excision, of chancres, something which took place on a large scale at the beginning of the 1870s. But this radical response (radical because it involved mutilating operations) did not prevent the appearance of the secondary symptoms. Hence, as a counterpoint to the triumphal – and rigged – statistics we find the following euphemistic assessment, typical of the style of official medical pronouncements: 'Numerous experiments whose drawbacks for the patients outweighed the benefits.'[33]

And, in despair of anything better there remained one simple method worth considering: simply to abstain from treatment and leave the body to rid itself of its enemies on its own.

Faced with what must undoubtedly be described as a therapeutic impasse, charlatanism continued the dazzling career it had begun so promisingly in the previous century, albeit that the charlatans had nothing to add to the classic recipes based on mercury. Pamphlets and advertising posters became more numerous despite nascent attempts to introduce restrictions, in particular on the sale of so-called secret remedies (Law of 2 Germinal, year II). The title of one of these pamphlets which was widely circulated in 1828 gives a fair indication of their tone: 'Venus' medicine without the doctor, for the prompt and radical treatment of syphilis or other secret diseases, including the means of recognizing them all . . ., to cure oneself of them in the greatest secrecy without interfering with one's affairs and even whilst travelling, with the aid of safe

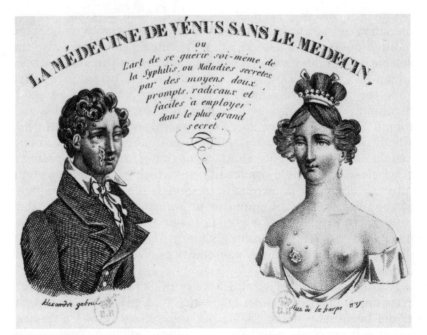

PLATE 6 This advertisement of 1828 is one example of the many quack pamphlets which from the eighteenth century onwards promised pox-victims who had been let down by conventional medicine some secret and painless cure. (Bibliothèque Nationale, Paris)

and gentle remedies which are as infallible as they are inexpensive.'
(In this instance it is pills that are being advertised.)

It is also worth mentioning a *Guide pour le traitement des maladies vénériennes à l'usage des gens du monde*[34] or, more especially, the *Vade-mecum des jeunes gens*,[35] which offers us, amongst other gems, the following:

> The European thinks he is so powerful and so civilized, but all this is mere illusion. Nineteenth-century man has managed to do away with long distances, tunnel through mountains, harness the power of fire, and yet he has not thus far managed to preserve himself against disease. As a conqueror of matter, a new Icarus, he sets out boldly heavenwards; as the threadbare king of creation he is slave to a hideous sickness which eats him away and lays him in the tomb. He is less prudent and has less instinct for his personal preservation than the savage who, sheltering under a shred of fabric, scans the dark night of the desert, defying the lion and the jaguar. Civilized man, behind the golden panelling of a palace, falls prey to a disease which the simplest of precautions would enable him to avoid.

(All this simply to recommend a certain 'lustral lotion'!)

Given the context, it is not so very surprising that Laffecteur's *rob* made a forceful return. In 1828 the brand-name Boyveau-Laffecteur was bought up by Dr Giraudeau de Saint-Gervais, whose daring advertising earned him a trial in the criminal court. However, the celebrated *rob* became ever more successful, so much so that in 1851 it was glorified in a long poem (*Syphilis, poème en deux chants*). The author, Auguste Marseille Barthélemy (1796–1867), who had been famous since the appearance of his *Némésis*, a violent satire against Louis-Philippe's ministers, had translated Fracastor before he composed *Syphilis* . . . The first canto is devoted to the 'sickness', and paints a horrifying clinical picture before denouncing syphilitic degeneracy:

> It has produced this infirm and degenerate race,
> This people of runts destined for the orthopaedist,
> It has produced these young folk who are already cadaverous,
> With narrow chests, pale foreheads and hollow eyes,
>
> ....
>
> It has produced these young flowers, these sixteen-year-old virgins,
> Precocious reservoirs of a thousand bitter ills,
> Who langorously bend on their stalks,
> A prey to swoons, vapours and dizziness.
>
> ....

The second canto is devoted entirely to condemning mercury:

But this art, too often slave to a system,
Combats the excess of the sickness with an extreme remedy,
Ardently fond of the liquid metal,
It infuses it into the body, which it kills in the attempt to save it.

Did Giraudeau de Saint-Gervais give Barthélemy a handsome bribe, or did he simply convince him of the benefits of his *rob*? Whatever the case, a canto celebrating Laffecteur's *rob* was added to the highly successful fourth edition of the poem.

Disappointing results

Under the July monarchy, just as under the Second Empire, everyone agreed that hospital provision for victims of venereal disease was deplorably inadequate. In Paris at the end of the Second Empire there were only 460 beds for women and 336 for men. In the provinces, except perhaps in Lyons, there was next to nothing, though the number of cases of syphilis continued to increase, particularly in the army. This is mainly attributable to the persistent tendency (amongst the Church, the local authorities and, indeed, the public at large) to ostracize syphilitics, a tendency which the medical profession at the end of the eighteenth century was unable to check. 'We must keep up with the times,' argues Ricord, 'and nowadays we can no longer follow the foolish prejudices of a false and petty so-called morality and regard venereal diseases as a divine punishment for libertinage, one which the wise man must respect.'

All doctors agreed that 'it is quite within the power of the state to root out this modern leprosy which we call syphilis. Preventative measures and the isolation and treatment of venereal diseases must be organized in a consistent fashion throughout France and, if possible, Europe, and not left to the whim of local authorities or to the mercies of the preventative measures of an earlier age.'[36] 'This prejudice,' says another, 'so out of step with the high-minded ideals of our age, is nonetheless a powerful one, and governs all the departmental health committees from one end of France to the other. I should say that I am not including Paris, for in this capital they have the unashamed selfishness to isolate all the foul and contagious elements in society.'[37]

Parent-Duchâtelet, whose work on prostitution[38] was to become a milestone (see chapter 9), attacks hospital administrators in particular, comparing them critically with their predecessors under the Ancien Régime:

They would have considered that they had dishonoured the establishments under their control if they had admitted a syphilitic; they would have considered that they had dishonoured themselves if they had taken the least trouble to improve the lot of those wretches. We pity the extreme short-sightedness of these good bourgeois; we excuse them because of the times in which they lived; however, let us take care not to regard them in too harsh a light, for in our own time, in many of our provinces, syphilitics of both sexes are being denied treatment, and this is the nineteenth century!

Hospital administration in England was better, if we can believe the French psychiatrist Ferrus, who made an official visit to the mental asylums there: 'In England, national and individual pride, though taken to extremes, even in matters of charity, are working wonders. This is amply proved by the number of different establishments in which the hapless sufferer may take refuge or receive cursory treatment.'[39] Following on from this qualified compliment (Ferrus' Bonapartism – he served as a military doctor in all the Napoleonic campaigns – accounts for his animosity towards England) we learn that sufferers from venereal disease had their own wards in general hospitals, and even that in certain towns there were establishments specializing in venereal diseases:

but they are exceptional in that patients are hidden from the public gaze; outsiders are rarely aware of these asylums. Only in Glasgow did we visit one of these establishments, which was very well maintained, and was directed with great zeal and intelligence by Dr Gibb. The majority of those suffering from venereal disease receive advice and medicine in charitable dispensaries. In the great London hospitals, such as St Bartholomew's and Guy's, the ablest doctors bring all their skills to bear on treating the symptoms of syphilis. This disease seemed to us not only more common but also more serious in England than in France. We attribute this circumstance to the fact that the common people never bathe, to the fact that they are ashamed to declare a sickness they regard as degrading, and, even more importantly, to the fact that the health of harlots is not monitored.[40]

A question raised for debate by the Brussels Société des Sciences Médicales in 1836 shows clearly, however, that public prophylactic measures must include more than just the admission of syphilitics to hospitals and free dispensaries (which were very slowly coming into operation, most often in hospital annexes). The question was as follows: 'What are the most appropriate health regulations for stopping the spread of venereal diseases?' (Note the term 'health regulations', which was to become the watchword of the struggle against syphilis in the nineteenth century.) Most answers to this difficult question were decidedly severe (notably close supervision, or even isolation, of prostitutes). One dissertation, perhaps more realistically, suggests that victims of venereal disease who present themselves at hospital of their own accord should receive an allowance 'at least in the beginning, so that people's very unfavourable opinion of hospitals for venereal diseases will be gradually altered'.

In the 1850 *Gazette Médical*, Dr Diday of the Hôpital de l'Antiquaille in Lyons suggests that schools, the judiciary, the civil service – in fact all state institutions and services – should be closed to anyone who could not, produce 'proof of freedom from syphilis'. 'I would,' he says, 'like to see all sorts of restrictions of this type placed on those with venereal disease; without the special certificates of health no-one would be allowed to contract marriage, buy their way into an office, inherit an estate, take a case to court, deposit savings, vote in elections, receive public relief from poverty, obtain a passport or a hunting permit etc. etc.'

But although a good deal of ink was spilled (another reformer proposes that every doctor should have the right to arrange an immediate examination of a woman implicated by the patient consulting him, whether she was a prostitute or not), barely any legislation followed in France, unlike in Belgium where, as a result of the question raised for debate in 1836, a number of regulations aimed particularly at prostitutes and military personnel were introduced. The silence of the public authorities in France provoked the indignation of many doctors. Syphilis is the worst of diseases, they repeated tirelessly.

It is not just the responsibility of statesmen, public health officials and economists to study syphilis, to combat it and to make its elimination their crowning glory; the whole of society must unite its efforts to wipe out this great destroyer, this deadly enemy of the human race, to root out this foul leprosy, which is all the more dangerous because it strikes from the shadows . . . . Humankind has allowed this evil to multiply its stealthy attacks, and to spread its poisons into the veins of every nation, every family – I was on the point of saying every individual! . . . Not one government has yet dared to bring the question of syphilis out into the open, to nail it with a public enquiry, to raise it to the height of a question of public hygiene, of social health. On the contrary, we dare not even pronounce its name. Even practitioners of the medical art themselves have been reduced to disguising the thing behind euphemistic circumlocutions; . . . I have known doctors of the highest renown who would hasten to pass pox-ridden clients on to their humbler colleagues . . . . How prudish our corrupt nations are![41]

Individual prophylactic measures made no greater advance than public ones, and even Ricord does no more than repeat the advice on hygiene *ante* and *post coitum* already given by doctors in previous centuries. There was scarcely anything but the condom which, for Ricord, as for the majority of his colleagues, was considered to be effective (though more as regards gonorrhea than syphilis), even if there were moral objections to it as a form of birth control. On this count it was condemned by Rome in 1826 as thwarting the decrees of Providence. But that did not lessen the popularity of the French letter. In 1877, Bertherand and Duchesne of Lyons made a close study of this interesting topic. Made exclusively in England by women, alternating with red balloons for children, the condom was exported in two grades, the superior for the Russians and the Austrians, the inferior for the French, Italians, Spanish and Portugese. Despite its failings, particularly in the inferior grades (a faulty umbrella which the storm can rupture or toss aside, as Ricord wittily remarks), the net result was positive. It is the least bad system and, add certain hygienists and moralists, so much the better if the condom is more likely to inspire disgust than provoke desire. The number of couplings, and consequently of cases of contamination, will thereby be reduced.

Syphilis in literature

Baudelaire, scanning the barricades of 1848 and seeing nothing in the offing, exclaimed in disillusionment and disgust 'We are democratized and syphilized.' Echoing his sentiment, the elections to the legislative Assembly of 13 May 1849 returned an antirepublican coalition of royalists and catholics who lost no time in intervening against the infant Roman republic. (Not to 'stifle Italian liberty,' explains Louis-Napoleon ingeniously, 'but, on the contrary, to guide it by preserving it from its own excesses.') The taking of Rome on 2 July 1849, its occupation by a French army and, furthermore, the reappearance of syphilis on the scene were reminiscent of Charles VIII's army's unfortunate odyssey three and a half centuries earlier.

Where one might have expected a doctor, a poet appeared on the scene, in the person of the young Théophile Gautier who had just embarked on his trip to Italy, as was the fashion. His *Lettres à la Présidente*,[42] a work which long remained in obscurity on account of its highly pornographic character, is a sex-obsessed account of his trip. But where there was sex there was the pox, especially in French-occupied Rome. The city had kept up an appearance of decency but, writes Théophile Gautier,

there is a splendid American pox here, as pure as at the time of Francis I. The entire French army has been laid up with it; boils are exploding in groins like shells, and purulent jets of clap vie with the fountains in the Piazza Navona; rhagades and papillomata like coxcombs hang in crimson festoons from the seats of sappers, sapped in their own foundations; tibias are exfoliating in extoses like ancient columns of greenery in a Roman ruin; the deltoids of the staff officers are spangled with constellations of pustules; lieutenants walking in the streets look like leopards, they are so dotted and speckled with roseola, freckles, coffee-coloured marks, warty excrescences, horny and cryptogamic verruccae and other secondary and tertiary manifestations, which appear here after a fortnight.[43]

As we can see, syphilis has become more to literature than simply the literary theme which it had been in past centuries. As Patrick Wald-Lasowski writes, in a brilliant study of the role played by syphilis in nineteenth-century French literature:[44]

So many Divinities and Demons vie with each other as to who can claim to inspire the nineteenth century, to preside over its terrors and its delights, to rule its ecstasies . . . . Alcohol, Drugs, the Muses, Oracles, Voluptuousness, Black Idols; and the 'diseases' join this procession. Phthisis appears, with her burning cheeks and her throng of pale suitors . . . . But the most important is Syphilis, who, with her greedy eye and bloody mouth, enters the scene.

And the prime role syphilis was to play was that of an instrument of vengeance. In Maupassant's novella *Le lit 29*, a handsome captain accumulates female conquests in the fine town of Rouen, in 1869. He forms closer links with Irma, the most beautiful of the kept women of the town. War breaks out and the regiment departs. The war ends and the regiment returns. The captain seeks out his Irma. She is in hospital. He hurries there. But why does he get such a cold reception from the doctor? Everything becomes clear when the captain reads on the door of the ward: 'syphilitics'. In bed 29, pale and unrecognizable, Irma explains: 'It was those Prussian bastards. They took me almost by force, and they have poisoned me.' . . . 'Didn't you go for treatment?.' A spark of fire comes into Irma's eyes: 'No, I wanted to have my revenge, even if it killed me! And I have poisoned them too, all of them, all, as many as I could. For as long as they were in Rouen I refrained from going for treatment.'

Likewise in Barbey d'Aurevilly's 'La vengeance d'une femme' (*Les Diaboliques*, 1874), set in the reign of Louis-Philippe, we follow a dandy, Robert de Tressignies, a connoisseur of women, though of a more blasé type. One day he follows a prostitute 'with superb flesh', and has a good time in bed. But during the most passionate bout of lovemaking he catches this Spanish beauty staring at a portrait. The time for confidences arrives. The man in the portrait is her husband, a Spanish grandee whom she abhors. She is the Duchess of Arcos de Sierra Leone, trapped in a loveless marriage. One day there came Don Estaban, for whom she conceived a love that was 'burning and chaste' – which did not prevent the wicked husband from having his rival strangled before his wife's eyes. The still-beating heart was torn to pieces and thrown to the dogs. From then on the Duchess thought of nothing but revenge. But the Duke was courageous and did not fear death. 'It was therefore necessary to dishonour the name of which he was so proud' (to commit 'a civilized crime', comments Barbey).

Hence the idea of abandoning herself to prostitution and dying of the pox in hospital. De Tressignies, disappointed (what he had taken for passion was nothing but the product of despair) but reassured (the Duchess has only just started out on her fatal journey), was haunted by this encounter, and took on 'the airs of Hamlet'. Later, the scandal breaks: a Spanish duchess has died at la Salpêtrière amidst fallen women. Thunderstruck, de Tressignies hurries to la Salpêtrière and is told of the Duchess' sad end (for it is definitely she) by the chaplain. 'She caught the most dreadful of diseases at this terrible game she played,' says the old priest.

In only a few months she was rotten to the bones. One of her eyes had suddenly jumped from its socket one day, and had fallen at her feet like a large coin. The other had liquefied and melted. She had died – but stoically – suffering intolerable tortures. She had still had a great deal of money and jewels, all of which she had bequeathed to patients like herself, at the establishment to which she had been admitted, and she had requested a ceremonial funeral. Except that, to punish herself for her dissolute behaviour [so said the old priest, who had not understood this woman at all], she had demanded, out of penitence and humility, that after her titles on her coffin and her tombstone it should be written that she was a REPENTED PROSTITUTE.

Syphilis in the novel need not be confined to the role of a mere instrument, albeit an instrument of vengeance; it can stand at the very heart of a novelistic composition, as in *A Rebours* by Huysmans (who may have had direct experience of syphilis himself). We should be wary of des Esseintes' hyperbolic naturalism and his decadence which is too unrestrained to be credible.[45] Here it is a matter of soul and being. In the extraordinary episode of the flowers, des Esseintes suddenly discovers the unreal, even monstrous, appearance of the rare species he has amassed:

Not one of them seemed real; fabric, paper, china and metal seemed to have been lent by man to Nature to allow her to create her monstrosities. When she had been unable to imitate human artefacts she had been reduced to copying the inner membranes of animals, borrowing the lively tints of their rotting flesh and the magnificent hideousness of their gangrenes. There is nothing but syphilis, reflected des Esseintes, his attention caught, fixed by the horriby mottled Caladiums caressed by a ray of sunlight. And he had a sudden vision of humanity ceaselessly tormented by the age-old virus. Since the beginning of the world, from father to son, all creatures passed on the immutable legacy, the eternal disease which had ravaged man's ancestors, which had even burrowed into the now-exhumed bones of ancient fossils!

It had come down, inexhaustible, through the centuries; today it still raged, concealing itself behind the symptoms of migraines, bronchitis, vapours and gout; from time to time it would surface, preferring to attack those who were poorly looked after and poorly fed . . . . And here it was again, in its original splendour, on the coloured foliage of the plants!

Obsessed by this thought, des Esseintes falls asleep, and is soon 'tossing in a dark and fantastical nightmare'. He is walking beside a woman whom he has never seen, but whom he guesses to be attached to him. Suddenly a figure on horseback appears before them, and turns around in its saddle:

His blood froze in his veins, and he was rooted to the spot in horror. The ambiguous, sexless figure was green, and its purple eyelids opened to reveal eyes of a terrible cold light blue; its mouth was surrounded by pustules; its extraordinarily thin arms, the arms of a skeleton, which were bare to the elbows and protruded from tattered sleeves, trembled feverishly; its fleshless thighs shivered in its over-wide knee-boots. Its frightful stare fixed on des Esseintes and bore into him, chilling him to the marrow . . . . Immediately he understood the meaning of the dreadful apparition. Before his eyes was the image of the great pox . . . . On the ground something stirred, and became a very pale woman, naked, wearing tightly-fitting green silk stockings. He looked at her curiously; like horsehair crimped with over-hot irons, her hair was frizzled and broken-ended; pitchers of Nepenthes hung from her ears; light the colour of cooked veal radiated from her half-open nostrils. Her eyes ecstatic, she called to him in a low voice. He did not have time to reply, for the woman was changing already; flamboyant colours appeared in her pupils; her lips took on the angry red of Anthuriums; her nipples burst forth, like two glossy pods of red pimento.

He had a sudden intuition: it's the Flower, he said to himself; . . . Then he noticed the frightful irritation on her breasts and mouth, discerned blackish-brown and copper-coloured blotches on her body; he stepped back, distraught; but the woman's eyes fascinated him, and he advanced slowly, trying to dig his heels into the ground to stop himself walking, letting himself fall, but getting up all the same to go towards her; he was almost touching her when black Amorphophallus sprang up all over her, thrusting towards her belly, which was rising and falling like a sea. He had pushed them back, feeling a boundless disgust at seeing the firm, tepid stems swarming between his fingers; then, suddenly, the loathsome plants had disappeared and two arms sought to entwine him; a dreadful anguish made his heart pound, for the eyes, the awful eyes of the woman had become a terrible cold light blue. He made a superhuman attempt to free himself from her embrace, but with an irresistible movement she held him back and clamped onto him; haggard, he saw flowering beneath her exposed thighs the savage Nidularium, which gaped in bleeding sabre-blades.

It might seem surprising that syphilis, which cuts such a brilliant figure at the turning-point of Huysman's literary career, should figure so little in the novels of Balzac and Zola. The game of retrospective diagnosis of Balzacian characters seems to be somewhat rash and unproductive.[46] In *Béatrix* (1839) it is not certain, or at any rate not explicitly stated, that it is the pox which Shontz voluntarily receives from Du Ronceret to give it to Arthur who finally gives it to Béatrix, the ultimate target of his revenge. Similarly in *La cousine Bette* (1846), Balzac's study of the archetypal poor, ugly and repressed relative who busies herself making mischief for her cousin, the pulpy Adeline, in a complex plot of the sort so dear to him. Just what is the 'terrible disease' which passes from Baron Hulot, the husband, to Valérie Marneffe, the mistress, by means of Baron Montes, the vindictive Brazilian millionaire who communicates the disease to Valérie, albeit indirectly, to punish her for not responding to his love?

There is no syphilis in the Rougon-Macquart cycle either, though there is plenty of vice and misfortune;[47] the exception, perhaps, is Maxime Saccard, though neurosyphilis (which it would be in this case) had barely begun to be discussed by Zola's contemporaries. Syphilis was as disconcerting for literature as it was for the medical profession. One might have expected to find it in studies of society like those of Balzac and Zola, but it remains elusive here; however, it looms at the very heart of the nascent symbolist movement, petrifying the writer and mirroring his own modernity to him.

And the encounter with syphilis was often more than just a figurative one. It would be rash to try to draw up a list of all those literary giants who crowned their bohemian, dandified or decadent lives with syphilis – or even of those who boasted of having done so. Nonetheless, we must still mention the key figures. First there is Flaubert, who, during a trip to the Middle East, indulged in an unrestrained frenzy of sexual activity whose (somewhat sordid) details he smugly records in his letters to Louis Bouilhet. The inevitable happened: (14 November, 1850) 'You must know, my dear Sir, that in Beirut I caught seven (sic) chancres, which reduced to two, then one. Eventually it cleared up. In two or three days the scar will have healed over. I am taking meticulous care of myself. I suspect a Moroccan woman of having given me this present, but perhaps it was a little Turk.'[48]

Roseola, sexual asthenia and alopecia followed ('One thing which is disappearing is my hair. Next time you see me I'll have a skullcap. I shall have the bald pate of a clerk or a worn-out notary, all the deuced signs of premature senility.') His teeth were to follow, after mercurial treatment ('My ivories are going.') Was this the end of Flaubert's sexual exploits? Not a bit of it: 'Ah, you old

blaggard, my false friend, so you made fun of my luckless sabre,'
he wrote to a friend, 'but I'll have you know that it is cured for the
present. A slight induration remains, but that is the hero's scar. It
just adds to its poetic quality. One can see that it has lived, that it
has weathered misfortunes. That gives it a fateful and doomed air
which cannot but please the contemplator.'[49] And Flaubert
confides that he is once again in 'a state of arousal which I would
be so bold as to describe as venereal, even libidinous' (which from
him is no small admission).

We find the same sexual frenzy and the same pride in the
'wound' in Maupassant. Much has been written about Maupassant's
syphilis and the effect of his psychopathology on his work – and
on his sexuality. Frank Harris, with whom he became friendly in
1880, and who also had a one-track mind, tells of Maupassant's
sexual vigour and boasting: 'The strange thing is that he was
prouder of his amorous exploits than of the stories he had
written.'[50] And a good deal could be said about Maupassant's wild
nights. He could have an erection at will (as he once told Harris
whilst they were out walking); he had coupled, before witnesses,
with six prostitutes in an hour; one day he had painted a false
chancre on his penis and paraded thus in front of his mistress,
whom he then raped to make her think that he had given her a dose
of the pox.'[51]

In the course of these little games, Maupassant really did catch
syphilis, though his own doctor (respecting professional confidentiality) long denied it. But the question was finally resolved in
the thirties when Maupassant's letters began to come onto the
market. One of them, addressed to his friend Robert Pinchon,
dated 2 March 1877 (Maupassant was then 27), leaves no room for
doubt:

You will never guess the astonishing discovery which my doctor has just made
about me . . . . Because my body hair had all fallen out and not grown back,
because my father was fussing over me, and because my mother's lamentations
could be heard all the way from Étretat, I took my doctor by the collar and said to
him 'Find out what's wrong with me, you blighter, or you'll get what for.' . . .
'The pox', he replied. I hadn't been expecting that, I can tell you; I was very upset,
but at length I said 'What's the remedy?' 'Mercury and potassium iodide', he
replied. I went to see another Sawbones, who made the same diagnosis, adding
that it was 'an old syphilis, dating back six or seven years.' . . . In short, for five
weeks I have been taking four centigrammes of mercury and thirty-five
centigrammes of potassium iodide a day, and I feel very well on it. Soon mercury
will be my staple diet. My hair is beginning to grow again . . . the hair on my arse
is sprouting . . . . I've got the pox! at last! the real thing! not the contemptible clap,
not the ecclesiastical crystalline, not the bourgeois coxcombs or the leguminous

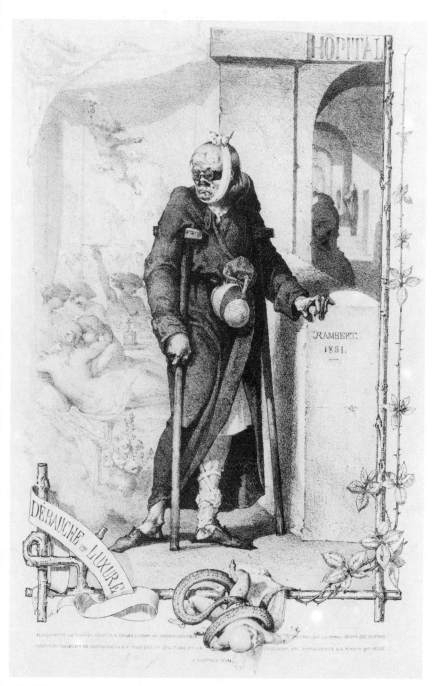

PLATE 7 In the middle of the nineteenth century Rambert executed a very fine series of engravings on moralizing themes. Here a syphilitic with his phial of mercury turns his back on luxury, prepares to enter the hospital and sees his own line being devoured by the hideous sickness. (Bibliothèque Nationale, Paris)

cauliflowers – no – no, the great pox, the one which Francis I died of. The majestic pox, pure and simple; the elegant syphilis . . . I've got the pox . . . and I am proud of it, by thunder, and to hell with the bourgeoisie. Allelujah, I've got the pox, so I don't have to worry about catching it any more, and I screw the street whores and trollops, and afterwards I say to them 'I've got the pox.' They are afraid and I just laugh.[52]

6

The Great Turning Point (around 1900)

The era of Fournier

Three-quarters of the way through the nineteenth century, research and theoretical reflection on syphilis was at something of a low ebb, and treatises did nothing but repeat the classic texts: a primary period with chancre and adenopathy; a secondary period, between the first month and the first year, in which the tissues were only superficially affected; a third period marked by late lesions much deeper and more serious than before. Amongst the tertiary symptoms, osseous syphilis was the one most remarked on: 'Of all the symptoms of tertiary syphilis, the osseous lesions are those which give us the most accurate and complete idea of the anatomical disorder caused by this disease.'[1]

The debate still raged between the proponents of congenital syphilis and the proponents of hereditary syphilis (those who regarded the sperm as the agent of contamination), whilst the question of syphilitic children placed with wet-nurses continued to confront doctors with problems of medical confidentiality (what should be said to the wet-nurse?). Moreover, these same wet-nurses continued to pose the problem of accidental infection (mostly from child to wet-nurse, but also from wet-nurse to child). Further means of accidental contamination were discussed, though some of them were somewhat dubious: syphilis in glassblowers observed in the years 1870–80 (owing to the blowing-rod being passed from mouth to mouth); vaccinal syphilis (caused by the gathering of vaccine from unsuspected syphilitics); chancre of the gum caught at the dentist's; chancre of the chin, cheek or neck due to a contaminated barber's razor; chancre of the finger in a doctor or midwife etc. But the most priceless of them all was undeniably contamination from lavatory seats, an explanation which, thanks

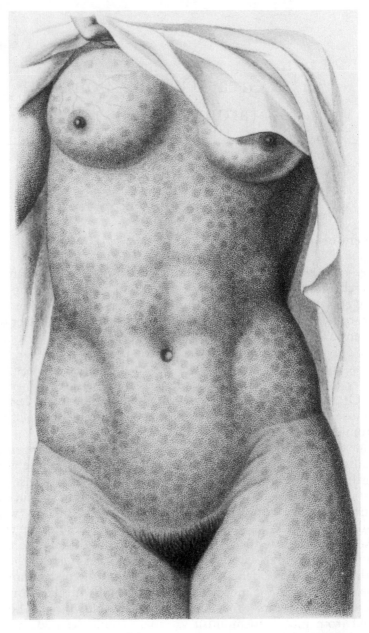

PLATES 8 and 9 Before the arrival of medical photography there were some splendid clinical illustrations, notably the magnificent watercolours in Devergie's and Ricord's atlases of syphilis. Here we have two roseolas (secondary syphilis), that of the woman beginning to diminish. (Cullerier, *Précis iconographique des maladies vénériennes*; Bibliothèque Nationale, Paris)

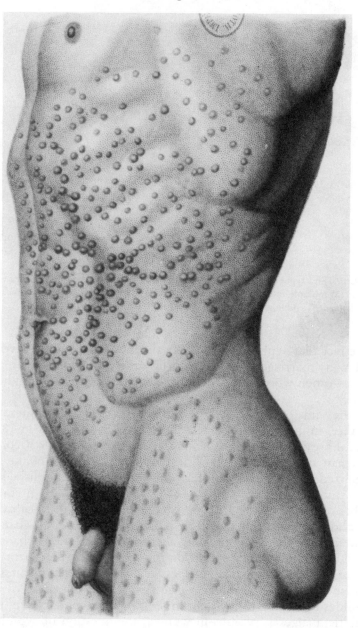

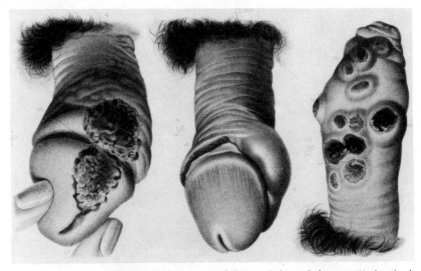

PLATE 10 Three types of chancre (primary syphilis): (1) indurated chancre; (2) cicatrized chancre; (3) multiple indurated chancres. (Cullerier, *Précis iconographique des maladies vénériennes*, 1861; Biblioghèque Nationale, paris)

to the fact that syphilis could be localized in the genitals, saved a good many marriages. (Three centuries earlier, Falloppio had made fun of women who claimed to have 'caught the pox through holy water'.)

In the midst of this stagnation, the works of a newcomer, Dr Fournier, immediately attracted attention. Born in Paris in 1832, Alfred Fournier studied medicine there, and became Dr Ricord's houseman at the Hôpital du Midi. Ater qualifying in 1860, he too specialized in the treatment of syphilis, and in 1857 published an initial study *(Recherche sur la contagion du chancre)*, the first of a number of important clinical works on topics such as the incubation of syphilis, the primary syphilitic induration, the pseudo-chancre of the tertiary stage, the cephalic chancre, the infectious chancre, the extra-genital chancres, the diagnostic role of the chancre's satellite buboes,[2] the contagiousness of the secondary manifestations (in particular the mucous plaques), the classification of the syphilides according to their chronology,[3] late secondary syphilis, syphilitic analgesia, syphilis in women, the question of syphilitic abortions etc.[4]

Most importantly, however, Fournier affirmed the syphilitic origin of tabes dorsalis in 1875,[5] thus initiating, in spite of general scepticism, a series of works which, until the revolutionary discovery – also his – of the syphilitic origin of general paralysis (see the following chapter), gave to the nervous symptoms of tertiary syphilis the prominent place they deserved.

His theoretical work, though enormous, was not done at the expense of practical activities. At the hospital he taught that one does not treat syphilis, only one or other of its stages.[6] But should it be treated? (This was in response to the *'méthode expectante'*, which was already very old and which had gained renewed impetus from repeated therapeutic failures; this was the idea that syphilis would get better by itself without being treated, perhaps even only on condition that it was not treated.) Yes, it is always worth treating it, if only to alleviate its effects, and all the more so since it is impossible to distinguish at the early stages between serious and mild forms of syphilis. (He formulates, in passing, the disturbing aphorism that 'A case of syphilis which begins well is no less likely to end badly.') Fournier cites numerous observations and statistics.

However, Fournier was obliged to recognize that there was not, as things then stood, a genuine abortive treatment for syphilis. So an effective set of prophylactic measures was required, measures which should be drawn up by doctors, not the public authorities. In 1886 this question was brought before the Academy of Medicine, which the following year appointed a commission, presided over by Ricord, to look into the means of containing the spread of venereal diseases. After lively discussions, the Academy of Medicine voted in favour of Fournier's conclusions, and Fournier thereafter emerged as the champion and mastermind of the struggle against syphilis. His programme was based on a set of administrative measures intended to monitor prostitution, to institute medical surveillance of the army and the navy, to provide hospitalization and treatment ('to hospitalize syphilis in its contagious forms is to render it harmless; therein lies safety'), and to train doctors, whose studies were to include a compulsory course in syphilology.

In 1901, Alfred Fournier founded the Société Française de Prophylaxie Sanitaire et Morale, following the first international conference for the prevention of syphilis and venereal diseases in Brussels in 1899 (the second conference was in 1902), which launched the struggle against syphilis on an international scale. At the conference he explained his ideas: syphilis is a social disease like alcoholism and tuberculosis. It must become the object of a crusade, as have the other two diseases. Society has a particular duty to defend itself against syphilis by public prophylactic measures.

Fournier also developed the idea that syphilis threatens those who do not expose themselves to it as well as those who do, and took pains to enumerate the cases of 'unmerited' contagion amongst his female patients. For these 'unmerited' cases of syphilis, and even more so for the merited ones, the hospital is, as well as a place of treatment, an instrument of prophylaxis: 'by isolating subjects afflicted with contagious manifestations who could spread the contagion. From this decidedly unusual point of view, the hospital is the safest means of neutralizing syphilis.' But there must also be outpatient clinics which are 'numerous, free, easy of access and open at hours which allow the worker to visit them without prejudice to his job or to his purse'. Here we have the idea of the community clinic.[7]

At the end of the nineteenth century, then, it was Fournier who, more than Ricord, was to succeed in bringing about significant progress in a field in which progress had up until then been irritatingly slow. It was Fournier who was to make syphilis a respectable branch of medicine (with the terms 'syphilology' and 'syphilologist' receiving official approval);[8] and, most importantly, it was he who put into operation for the first time a programme of public prophylaxis involving the creation of national organizations supported by public authorities, a programme whose effectiveness as regards the 'venereal peril' we will shortly be assessing. Even Léon Daudet, usually so cruel in the portraits he paints of the doctors of his time, heralds this new era: 'As for Professor Alfred Fournier, courteous, inscrutable and unaffected, he was the first syphilologist of his time, and probably of all time' (*Devant la douleur*).

Syphilology and syphilologists

The setting up of the first chair of dermatology and syphilology in 1879 shows, paradoxically, both the promotion of syphilis to the rank of a medical discipline and its subordination – a rich source of future ambiguities – to a branch of pathology which was, after all, only relevant to the disease's most obvious manifestations. As was only right, Dr Alfred Fournier became its first incumbent at the Hôpital Saint-Louis, which during the nineteenth century gradually became 'the Mecca of dermatology'.[9] First intended under the Ancien Régime for plague-victims, the Hôpital Saint-Louis had subsequently directed its activities towards the treatment of chronic diseases, including skin diseases. Alibert, a doctor at Saint-Louis from 1801 onwards, had founded the first specialist clinic in this latter branch of pathology, and devoted himself to classifying these diseases in his 'family tree of dermatoses'.

But instruction in the clinical treatment of syphilis did not take off until the arrival of Fournier, from Lourcine. From then on the Hôpital Saint-Louis was to become the capital of syphilology, both in France and internationally. The first international congress on dermatology and syphilology was held there in 1889, and enjoyed a great success in the medical world – a success due in no small part to the opening, for the occasion, of an extraordinary museum of dermatological waxworks.[10] In the years which followed, the hospital had no less than six departments for cutaneous or syphilitic diseases.

It was also an age of statistics, and here too Fournier played a crucial role. What, for example, was the distribution of cases of syphilis in women? In twenty-seven years, Professor Fournier was consulted by 887 syphilitic women, in forty-five of whom the disease was not of venereal origin but inherited or contracted accidentally from midwives, wet-nurses, children etc. That leaves 842 cases of syphilis of sexual origin, distributed as follows: 366 women of loose morals and 'irregular persons' of all sorts, 220 married women, and 256 women of unknown social standing. Out of the 220 married women, the only ones who interested Fournier in this instance, 164 had undoubtedly caught it from their husbands, who were examined later. 'So you see, gentlemen, the significance of such a statistic? In the case at issue, what a reply, what a crushing reply, to those who would have us believe that syphilis is the monopoly of the demi-monde!'[11]

And what was the age-profile of syphilitics? Edmond Fournier,[12] who consulted his father's medical records in 1900, first separated the hospital patients from the more bourgeois town patients (11,000 of the 20,000 looked at). But it was the resemblances rather than the differences which were striking, in particular the fact that the majority of cases occurred in young, even very young, subjects. Moreover, women clearly caught the disease at an earlier age than men (between 17 and 22 in women, peaking at 18; between 18 and 25 in men, peaking at 20). Suddenly statistical researchers became more interested in minors with the disease, most of whom were girls, and an overwhelming majority of whom were prostitutes – hence the increasingly pressing question of prostitution.

All these preoccupations led to the setting-up of medical journals devoted entirely to the study of syphilis. *La syphilis*, which appeared for the first time in 1903 under the direction of Dr Barthélemy, a doctor at Saint-Lazare and a follower of Fournier as far as public prophylaxis was concerned, sets the tone fairly explicitly: 'It seems that syphilology is making slow progress', it says in the foreword, hence the necessity to 'create a sort of stir about so many problems on which depend the fate, the health, the existence and the happiness of a great proportion of the human race . . .'. The *Annales des maladies vénériennes* were launched in 1906 to take an international perspective, whilst the *Annales de thérapeutique dermatologique et syphiligraphique*, founded in 1901, aimed to attack what had, alas, remained the most intractable part of the question, namely the fact that mercury and potassium iodide were the only known treatments for the disease.

Notwithstanding this impasse, clinical research flourished, as the numerous works of Fournier have already shown. To them we must add the re-examination of the dogma of the non-reinfection of syphilis ('You cannot catch a double dose of syphilis', Ricord had proclaimed), a view which Fournier himself favoured, the manifestations known as the secondary chancre being for him nothing but a chancriform syphilide. However, in 1884, Erik Pontoppidan had communicated to the Copenhagen conference five positive cases in which syphilitic chancres had infected carriers. In 1906 L. Queyrat verified Pontoppidan's results and, in 1909, with Marcel Pinard, succeeded in infecting subjects with the symptoms of tertiary syphilis using products of primary syphilis.[13] Thus was demonstrated the possibility of syphilitic reinfection, and also that of superinfection, in other words a second dose of syphilis grafting itself onto one which was weakened but not extinct.

Léon Daudet's novel *Les morticoles*, which appeared in 1894, confirms in its own fashion the advent of syphilology and syphilologists. In this savage sketch in which doctors are the absolute masters of an imaginary kingdom, Pridonge, a doctor who deals with shameful diseases, is high on the list of great specialists. Indeed it is he who leads the dance (both literally and figuratively, as we shall see). He lives, mingles with the nobs and gives sumptuous receptions in a fine private residence (one thinks here of Ricord) at the entrance to which is the device of a doctor pulling an arrow from Cupid's foot. Thanks to the venereal diseases, and syphilis in particular, he has become successful despite his brutality and coarseness: 'Pridonge saw his clients out with coarse laughter and shouts of "Goodbye you dirty old man! Old lecher! – Ah, what a funny old devil!" Syphilis, in all its forms, never failed to elate him.'

The height of cynical jubilation is attained at a grand supper for *morticoles* at the syphilologist's house. Medical confidentiality not being permitted between *morticoles*, everyone gets a proper dressing-down:

'Look at our friend Burnone', continued the host, full of good humour. 'He had consulted Tartègre and Wabanheim, and all manner of specialists like Purin-Calcaret, and none of them spotted anything untoward. But you can guess what he had, ladies and gentlemen! Our Burnone was pickled!' A chorus of laughter rippled around the table, and all the ladies, a little red, leaned back fanning themselves; all eyes, bright with tears of laughter, turned towards the hilarious Burnone, who also joined in. The servants were laughing at the idea of so comic a disease, and even the family portraits, the wine in the carafes, the crystal and the silverware seemed to be highly amused. Everyone pretended not to feel concerned, but the infernal Pridonge pursued his attack: 'Besides, all of you male guests, why act so innocent? I've had each of you in my surgery, very humble, very anxious, very submissive. Ah, the stories I could tell! And I might just tell them too! I like a bit of fun, I do, I love it.

Pridonge is the only one laughing now, for sure. No-one else is speaking or eating.

What's wrong? Have I gone too far? Is it my fault if I'm hale and hearty? I am always asking the fools who come to consult me, looking chaste and crestfallen: Won't you take off your mask? You're not the first one I've examined. And when he spins me some yarn or other, you should see how quickly I get back to the point: What cock and bull story is this? You caught it getting into a boat, I suppose, or doing the splits, or on a rainy day, or blowing your nose, or from a pipe? Ah, the pipe – now there's an instrument that's always good for an excuse! . . . amongst senators especially. Begging Vomédon's pardon, his venerable colleagues are as obscene as they are hypocritical. They may preside over the League of Modesty but they plague the young ladies and are the bane of my life. Not to mention that they don't pay me, the old rascals.'

His guests are vexed, but they stay on, if only from fear of being still more cruelly mocked in their absence. There follows a ball in the library – a truly allegorical ball in which the young ladies twirl before the spines of huge volumes: *The bubo*, *On the chancre*, *Secondary syphilis*. Here, marked out in advance, are the flames at which these white moths are soon to burn themselves.

In search of the little beast

During the first and second thirds of the nineteenth century the word 'virus' continued to mean poison or venom, with the additional idea that there existed a specific one which was the agent of transmission for each contagious disease. We have seen how, from the time of the Ancien Régime (and in particular with the parasitic theory), there had been a premonition of the existence of a syphilis microbe. But, as Auzias-Turenne observed in the middle of the nineteenth century, 'syphilis is a fallow field for micrographers.' And indeed microscopes were not yet sophisticated enough to allow a sufficiently extensive study of microbes. However, Donné claimed in 1837 to have discovered a spiral microbe in syphilitic lesions.

But only with the work of Pasteur, beginning in 1877, did the nature of transmissible diseases cease to be a mystery. From then on, the search for the syphilis microbe began. In 1878 Klebs claimed to have found in the chancre 'the syphilitic helicomonad, a short and very slow-moving rod'. In 1881 it was a fungus, Aufrecht's 'diplococcus'; the next year a bacterioid with a gyratory motion, or perhaps also an immobile bacillus (Martineau and Hamonic). Such a diversity, a compiler of Dechambre's dictionary sagely observes in 1884, proves that the causative agent of syphilis has not been found, for syphilis 'can only arise from a single parasite'.

The gonococcus, the pathogenic agent of gonorrhea, was discovered in 1879 by Neisser, but by 1900 not a single syphilis microbe had turned up, except perhaps for Donné's spiral, which was observed and re-observed, though in most cases it was not observed at all. However, the first step in the right direction was made when experimental research on monkeys (1903, Metchnikoff and Roux)[14] proved indubitably that monkeys could be infected with human syphilis (the first attempts at infecting animals with syphilis, always in the hope of creating a vaccine, had been performed by Klebs in the 1870s). The syphilis microbe therefore existed, fragile and still mysterious.

In February 1905, the zoologist Siegel claimed to have observed protozoons which he christened *Cytorryctes luis* in blood and syphilitic lesions. The Berlin health authorities then made the zoologist Schaudinn, the syphilologist Hoffmann and two bacteriologists responsible for verifying this. Nothing was found, but on 3 March Schaudinn observed in a sample from a syphilide 'a very small spirochaete, mobile and very difficult to study'. A few days later, Schaudinn and Hoffmann rediscovered the same spirochaete in syphilitic ganglions, chancres, syphilitic papules and the blood of the spleen some days before the appearance of roseola. There was no more doubt: the spirochaete was undeniably the syphilis microbe. After various suggestions it was baptised *Treponema* (because of its resemblance to a twisted thread) *pallidum* (because of its pale colour).

As one might have expected, the news of the discovery was greeted with scepticism in Germany, no man being a prophet in his own country. Japan, England and the USA, on the other hand, recognized Schaudinn's discovery which was confirmed in the months which followed. From then on things moved quickly. The following year the use of the ultramicroscope allowed better research to be done on the pale treponema and made it possible to verify immediately the syphilitic nature of the lesions that were examined. Also in 1906, following Bordet's clarificatory work on reactions to non-treponemic antigens at the very end of the nineteenth century, Wassermann, Neisser and Bruck applied a complement derivation or complement fixation reaction (called a haemolysis reaction) to the diagnosis of syphilis. Bordet-Wassermann's diagnostic (subsequently known as the 'BW') was born, and looked set for a bright future despite its empiric foundation and the occasional uncertainty of its results (a + or even a + + not being infallible signs of syphilis). At last, following the attempts of Levaditi in 1907, Schereschewski (1909) and, more importantly, Noguchi (1911), managed to produce, using different techniques, short-lived cultures of the treponema.

The discovery of the treponema in 1905 sparked off once again the dispute between those who believed that reinfection with syphilis was possible and those who did not, and once more raised the hope of obtaining immunity to syphilis in man by experimental means. On 8 May 1906 Metchnikoff[15] explained to the Académie de Médecine the results of research carried out at the Institut Pasteur with Dr Roux on the attenuation of syphilis. Twelve subjects were infected and then rubbed with a mercurial ointment. The microbe remained inactive, he claimed. A student was subjected to the same experiment without the slightest symptom being triggered off.[16] This news caused a great stir in the press, although the medical world remained for the most part very cautious, wisely judging that whilst they were waiting for more information there was a risk of increasing the number of syphilitics by creating a false sense of security. However, a circular dated 23 September 1907 ordered Metchnikoff's treatment with frictions (minus the infection!) to be used in the army and the navy. The vogue for this 'first strike' prophylaxis continued during the First World War (particularly amongst the Americans) and beyond.

However, there was a moral question: before the experimental induction of syphilis in animals several doctors and students had been brave enough to experiment on themselves, but did that justify experimenting on patients, or even on healthy subjects? No doubt this was discussed in the first years of the century, when the discovery of the pale treponema raised new hopes of a cure. What did Fournier have to say about this?

We should not use the lancet on a healthy subject; if the doctor wishes to study and verify a scientific fact he must chose himself as the experimental subject, not the patient who entrusts himself to his care. The practice of researchers who, in the attempt to obtain some crucial datum, have exposed their patients to indisputable risks is clearly open to criticism. There is particular cause for concern when research has been attempted without their having been informed of the nature of the disease with which they were being infected.

'606'

In 1905, in the course of their studies on sleeping sickness, Thomas and Breinl of Liverpool demonstrated that atoxyl (a sodium salt of arsenic) had a remarkable effect on the trypanosomiases, diseases whose pathogenic agent is in some respects analogous to the syphilis treponema. Many then applied atoxyl to the treatment of syphilis, thereby reviving the ancient practice of prescribing arsenic. Atoxyl was soon abandoned after accusations that it had toxic properties.

Paul Ehrlich (1854–1915) of Frankfurt had, for his part, been obsessed from the beginning of his medical studies by the difference in colouration of identical cells which he observed under the microscope; this led him to the idea of tropism, which opened the way to that of cellular receptors. Ehrlich set about applying this phenomenon for therapeutic purposes, aiming to isolate a toxin which would affect microbes but not damage the cell. This was the marvellously simple theory of the *'wünder bullet'* (magic bullet) which thus opened the way to a new era of chemotherapy. Now, the great enemy of the moment was indisputably the treponema which had just been discovered. Ehrlich, taking up once more the experiments in which the pathogenic agent was attacked with arsenicals, formulated the notion of arsenoresistance, and endeavoured to substitute trivalent arsenicals for pentavalent ones. In May 1909, in collaboration with the Japanese Hata, he had arrived at his 606th compound (one of his mottoes was *'Geduld'*: patience). It was a miracle, albeit a planned one; the magic bullet had reached its target. Twenty-four syphilitics were treated experimentally in October 1909; Salvarsan (arsphenamine), or '606', was born.

A few years later, in his 914th experiment, Ehrlich modified the formula to create '914' or Neosalvarsan (neoarsphenamine), which was easier to use. So began the era of the arsphenamines, which at last appeared to be a suitable substitute for mercury. The latter, however, was not to be ousted so easily.

In 1921, Sazerac and Levaditi discovered the treponemacidal power of bismuth.[17] This, in conjunction with the other treatments, heralded a new therapeutic era, with the early cicatrization of the chancre, the rapid disappearance of the cutaneous and mucous symptoms of secondary syphilis, the early breakdown of the gummas, and the Bordet-Wassermann test becoming negative in the blood and the cephalorachidean fluid. As far as treatment was concerned, the sole ambition of Fournier and all the syphilologists of his time was still that of establishing a *modus vivendi* between the syphilitic and his syphilis. From then on, doctors claimed to be able to scotch the disease with the arsenicals and bismuth.

But syphilis was not so easily defeated. After several years of euphoria it was perceived that neither the clinic nor the laboratory could guarantee recovery – hence the already ancient idea that it was always possible for the disease to lie dormant, and that consequently it had to be treated intermittently over an indefinite period. Thus for a long time the treponema came to have the reputation of being both fragile and yet invincible, as this staff-room song entitled *The Treponema*[18] proclaims:

I am the Spirochaete, slender and serpentine,
And here in the indurated chancre I live.
That Japanese Hata would like to drive me out
From my mucous palace where I vegetate in contentment.

Mercury and hectine lie in wait for me, I know,
And Ehrlich's 606 which has always missed me.
I don't give a damn for them! Believe me, they never
Took away my appetite for supping

On your lecherous bodies. Humans, pale humans,
You can use phenol and wash your hands all you like;
But you can't get rid of me, I'm hereditary.

I'm prince of the blood, I'll have none of your laws,
I'm a protozoon, an eternal parasite,
I've killed plenty of rogues and a few kings to boot.

The venereal peril

In an article dedicated to the venereal peril at the beginning of the century,[19] Alain Corbin clearly shows that from 1900 onwards the much-needed prophylactic measures against syphilis tended to be combined with a desire to restrict to dissuasion the sex education which was their logical consequence. 'It is not wrong to encourage one's fellow citizens to be obsessed by it when it is in a worthwhile cause,'[20] declares Dr Burlureaux straightforwardly at the Brussels conference of 1902, in reference to the sexual education of young girls. This postulate gives us an insight into the nature and aims of the activities of the Société de Prophylaxie Sanitaire et Morale which had just been created (the conjunction of the last two terms is significant in itself). Admittedly the thinking involved here is conservative in its content, but it is nonetheless revolutionary in its form, for this is the first time that anyone had dared to speak in this way of the sexuality of young ladies other than prostitutes.

At what age should sex education be given? The age at which young girls of the working classes were deflowered was debated at length by the learned society (girls of the bourgeoisie being deemed to remain virgins until the age of marriage, as Alan Corbin mischeviously points out). But the discussion soon foundered because of the unwillingness of families, and even of numerous medical practitioners, to warn young girls about anything what-soever. Thus Dr Burlureaux's pamphlet *Pour nos jeunes filles quand elles auront seize ans*[21] (For our daughters when they are sixteen) was poorly received, whereas Alfred Fournier's *Pour nos fils quand ils auront dix-sept ans*[22] (For our sons when they are seventeen), intended to be distributed in the upper forms of educational establishments, was well received even though it was still only in draft form.

What he says, however, deserves our attention. My friends, announces a doctor, paternally, you will soon be men, and grave dangers are looming on the horizon. Women interest you ('Women! Ah! the things I could tell you on that score if I were a moralist, a philosopher, a religious teacher, etc. But I am a mere doctor.'). It is only a short step between desiring a woman and possessing her, a step which is not always made with impunity. And then it's the doctor's job to take care of the casualties. Following this, the doctor, 'in no way blackening the picture', describes at length the venereal peril, and in particular syphilis, which ruins marriages and families, kills children and debases the species both physically and spiritually. And all it takes is a single contact. Beware, young men, 'feminine provocation' will assail you in all its forms, and in particular in its worst form, which is that of clandestine prostitution. How dangerous they are, these bogus little factory girls who pace up and down the boulevard pretending to put off going back to work! Is that all that public prophylaxis has found to preserve us from this hideous scourge? you may ask. 'Alas yes,' I must reply, 'that's what things have come to.' A final piece of advice, however: if an accident were to befall you all the same, the worst attitude to adopt would be silence, which renders the medical art ineffective.

In fact doctors definitely felt that this campaign to increase public awareness, not to mention public guilt, was a double-edged sword, and that there was a risk that those affected would not admit to having such a degrading disease – hence the notion of a social disease which caught hold at this time: 'There is a social disease which is so general, so deep-rooted, so terrible and so contagious that the famous specialist Professor Alfred Fournier went so far as to refer to it, along with alcoholism and tuberculosis as the "triad of contemporary plagues"; let us therefore have the courage to look it in the face and call it by its name: syphilis.'[23] The author then endeavours to demonstrate that we must combat prejudice against this shameful disease, 'the first evil we must uproot.' It is this prejudice which leads the patient to conceal his disease and not take proper care of himself. Syphilis then takes root in the body, contaminating the spouse and, more importantly, the offspring – which is the worst social danger.

So here we see young people being dissuaded from pre-marital sex and encouraged to take up sport instead. (When, on the eve of the First World War, German psychiatrists tentatively remarked on the dangers of excessive sexual continence, early marriage was suggested as a compromise solution.) The Société de Prophylaxie Sanitaire et Morale was, in fact, a long way from meeting the goals it had set itself as regards preventative education in schools. Always concerned to operate with discretion, the heads of institutions followed suit, and only a few directors of teacher-training colleges agreed to organize conferences on the subject. On the other hand, as far as prostitution was concerned, a massive preventative campaign was organized in the army.

The propaganda against the venereal peril was more successful in the street (posters were even put up in urinals), and even more so in the family, with lectures (at the Sorbonne, and even in Notre-Dame as a Lenten address),[24] articles, pamphlets and even popular novels specifically written to carry a prophylactic message. The archetype of the genre seems to have been *L'Infamant* by the appropriately-named Paul Vérola, published in 1891.[25] 'Now I am clean', exclaims Marc Favrot, the hero, contaminated since the early pages, recalling a visit to the Hôpital du Midi where his father had taken him for his edification.

An obsession tormented him at that time, blighting his past and his future. He could not rid his nostrils of the acrid and penetrating exhalation of the iodoform which had lodged there the day he had visited the Hôpital du Midi. This odour, tyrannically evocative, conjured up before his weary eyes faces half-devoured by an indescribable evil. One head in particular haunted him, a head of living death, without nose, without lips, with decomposed and greenish cheeks, a head straight out of a Dante-esque nightmare.

Marc Favrot denied his illness for a long time, but there came a day when he had to bow before the evidence. He had syphilis.

Melancholically, sighing ceaselessly, he undressed, painfully resigned, like a virgin slave who has just been designated for the master's bed – and what a master! Man has even imperiously applied his social prejudices and his passion for hierarchies to the realm of diseases! . . . Phthisis and typhoid fever are noble and aristocratic; apoplexy belongs to the rich bourgeoisie; varicose veins and boils are poor devils, outcasts to whom one sometimes gives alms. Then come the pariahs that we hunt down and chase out, the whole string of shameful diseases that no-one admits to or acknowledges, epilepsy and syphilis which turn any human being they enslave into a pariah.

This gave rise to a whole generation of popular novels devoted to the service of anti-syphilitic prophylaxis. It was no longer Syphilis in Literature, as in des Esseintes' dream, but anti-syphilitic literature. In 1900 there was *Les Mancenilles*, by André Couvreur, who intended it as a clinical study of the evolution of syphilis in Maxime Duprat, a government minister struck down at an early age by the insanity of the tertiary stage. Nothing has been left out of this novel; there is a marriage to a virgin which should have been postponed, the birth of a monstrous infant, and the doctor friend who, in the midst of all this to-do delivers anti-syphilitic messages ('Profit from your fear and avoid women').

We must also mention *Vénus*, which appeared in 1901,[26] a 'physiological' novel[27] about syphilis which is just as terrifying as its predecessors, but which stands out from them because it is much more modern in tone. It does not defend morality, continence and marriage; instead there is a defence of the pleasure which is constantly marred by the fear of pregnancy and syphilis. But the message is all the stronger for that . . . The hero, Léon Mirat, an indifferent poet living on his annuities, is, as one might expect, a great aficionado of women (particularly 'the curvaceous type') – a fact which causes his doctor friend some anxiety: 'But I assure you, old chap, many of these women are dangerous. Their plumage is deceptive; just you beware of infectious parakeets.' Mirat scoffs. The friend insists, describing the ravages wreaked in society by sexual diseases, and even admitting that his own brother, a dashing lieutenant, committed suicide on learning that he had contracted syphilis (this explains Léon Mirat's friend's medical vocation). For a moment, Mirat is shaken: 'Mirat did not answer. Instinctively he dragged his friend towards the brightly-lit and lively boulevards. But the women now appeared to him through a melancholy haze, like enemies – no longer cheerful ships decked out in flags, but hostile warships whose sides bristled with destructive weaponry.'

But Mirat, a great number of conquests later, catches syphilis all the same. Without saying that he himself has got it, he goes for information to his friend, who is searching for a vaccine at the Institut Pasteur. He gets more than he bargained for.

With this poison, anything is possible . . . it assumes the most unexpected and disconcerting forms. It almost seems to know the ridiculous shame it inspires. So it kills under a disguise. It makes its victims die of an intestinal obstruction, for example, or a nice little liver disease. You don't recover, but your honour is safe. At least the bereaved don't have to blush at the mention of the deceased . . . . So much for its caprices. But it also has its little habits. It loves to come out into the daylight. And then you get the whole gardenful of cutaneous manifestations, those burgeonings, those dreadful efflorescences, the lupus – you can find fine examples of them all at Saint-Louis, or in its museum. And, of course, it eats away your bones . . . . But above all, you see, the disease attacks the nervous system. That's its treat, its desert. It chooses its spot. It snaps the network of the nerves at whim. It can cut off communication with the outside world, suppress the five senses. And then we've got a pretty bouquet of infirmities. Or it plays with a man as if he were a puppet. By pinching the nerve at the right spot it makes him jump or dance or start; then, tired of this Punchinello, it casts him aside, legs broken. And then we have ataxia. Such a cruel game. You have heard tell, for instance, of the acute pain which strikes unendingly in the small of your back. Or perhaps it lays into the brain, the kingpin of it all. And there's your general paralysis, senility in all its glory, all its regularity'.

Imperturbably the doctor continues his account, explaining that the disease attacks the organ which, having worked the most, is the most worn out ('It takes workers in the muscles, and intellectuals in the nerves'), and that treatment is useless. The position is clear. Léon Mirat will commit suicide (being a poet, he throws himself from a mountain).

Works as pessimistic as those of Michel Corday[28] have played no small part in increasing people's fear of syphilis. As early as the beginning of the nineteenth century doctors were deploring the 'syphilomania' of certain patients,[29] but this was nothing compared to the full-blown psychosis which took hold at the beginning of the twentieth century. The effects of this 'syphilophobia' were lamented by the medical profession which had been so instrumental in creating it. 'Syphilophobes' ranged from the neurotic besieging his doctor's surgery to the potential suicide,[30] and included those who, for years on end, inflicted, far-fetched remedies on themselves (like the 'syphilophobe' who cauterized his lips, tongue, throat and

MICHEL CORDAY

VÉNUS

ou

LES DEUX RISQUES

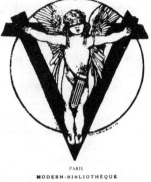

PARIS
MODERN-BIBLIOTHÈQUE
ARTHÈME FAYARD, ÉDITEUR

PLATE 11 The first edition of *Vénus*, a novel by Michel Corday, appeared in 1901. Morality, or rather, in Corday's case, the survival of the species, is cleverly defended in a very modern way. Pleasure itself is not condemned, though it is constantly threatened by the double fear of pregnancy and syphilis. (Private collection)

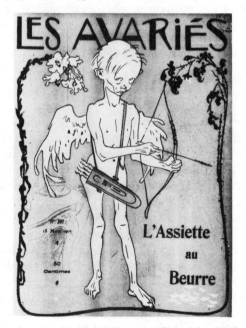

PLATE 12 Brieux's play, *Les Avariés*, which was performed for the first time in Paris in 1905 was, perhaps, the first manifesto for the campaign of anti-syphilitic prophylaxis which reached its peak between the wars. *L'Assiette au beurre* devoted an issue to *Les Avariés*, and on the cover was this cupid, apparently born syphilitic, a 'hérédo'. (Bibliothèque municipale de Caen)

nose with silver nitrate every day for twenty-six years).[31] In short, writes Alain Corbin, 'the excessive fear of the "pox", a formidable obstacle to pleasure, took over from the fear of sin; and it was this which fuelled the very wide spread of syphilophobia.'[32]

But when we look more closely we find that the general public remained, for the most part, immune to this medical and literary stir. Admittedly syphilis frightened everyone, whatever their social class. But proper medical information had by no means reached the masses. This was particularly true in Anglo-Saxon countries, where the press chose to use euphemisms such as 'rare blood disease', and it is with good reason that Prince Morrow writes that 'social sentiment holds that it is a greater violation of the proprieties of public life publicly to mention venereal disease than privately to contract it.'[33] The same author is justifiably indignant that many journals which spoke freely and at great length about prostitution were reticent about raising the spectre of its pathological consequences. When, in 1906, Edward Bok, editor of the journal *Ladies' Home*, broke the silence by publishing a series of articles on venereal diseases, he lost 75,000 subscribers, claims Morrow, who founded the American Society for Sanitary and Moral Prophylaxis (ASSMP) in 1905, a society intended to 'prevent the spread of diseases which have their origin in the social evil'.

This association, says Allan M. Brandt in '*No magic bullet . . .*'[34] began modestly in spite of its ambitious name, drawing only twenty-five doctors to its inaugural meeting, which took place in the New York Medical Academy. Nonetheless, it attracted not only doctors but social and religious leaders, and the society spread to Philadelphia, Baltimore, Detroit, Milwaukee, etc. The ASSMP, absorbed in 1910 into the American Federation for Sex Hygiene, aimed to break the conspiracy of silence in all areas, demanding in particular sex education in schools. No-one went that far, in fact, and even those doctors who were the least steeped in the Victorian morality which was then on its last legs confined their advice to men, concentrating entirely on the preservation of the line.

Syphilis and marriage

In this context, marriage became the keystone of anti-venereal prophylaxis; on the one hand it was necessary to preserve the line, and on the other it was necessary to restrict sexual relations – conjugal fidelity being, after chastity, the means of avoiding catching venereal disease. Once again, morality and medicine overlapped.

There was a flourishing genre of medical literature dedicated to the health of married couples and 'the philosophical hygiene of marriage'.[35] It is the married woman who is the greatest object of solicitude in this matter: 'The woman must submit to her husband – consequently, whereas *he* catches it when *he* wants, *she* also catches it when *he* wants! The woman is ignorant . . . particularly in matters of this sort. So she is generally unaware of where and how she might catch it, and when she has caught it she is for a long time unaware of what she has got.'[36] The woman must be told![37] But this brings us back to the question of educating young girls.

The doctor may sidestep this problem, notably by asking mothers to arrange for their daughters to receive sexual information (though only in matters of hygiene); but he cannot escape the role of mediator, or even arbiter, which is forced on him when a former syphilitic comes to his surgery and asks: Doctor, it is safe for me to marry? This thorny question was pondered by numerous syphilologists, and in particular by Alfred Fournier.[38] A Cornelian conflict arises, in which the interests of the patient and the public interest are opposed, 'for beyond this client stands a young girl, unborn children, a family, and society, and your prohibition will safeguard them all. What importance the doctor's mission assumes when he becomes the arbiter of so many common interests in this way!' (Fournier).

There was a middle way between the two extreme attitudes that a doctor might take up, namely either systematically forbidding marriage because he believed syphilis to be incurable, or just as systematically allowing it as soon as the primo-secondary symptoms had disappeared. This was to forbid marriage and sexual relations not only whilst the symptoms remained, but also after they had completely disappeared, for a surveillance period of between six months and two, or even three years, depending on the severity of the case. This, of course, was to suppose that one regarded syphilis as curable, something which Fournier for one made an absolute dogma: 'So yes, a hundred times yes, you can marry after you have had the pox, and the consequences of such a marriage can be, medically speaking, entirely happy ones.' Must one, in fact, under the pretext of doubt deprive a former syphilitic of family life and progeny, 'the two things which, after the turbulence of the first years of youthful folly, become the natural and common aspiration?' (Fournier). However, there were many doctors who, whilst allowing marriage, were much more evasive about the prospects of complete recovery.

And what was to be done if the marriage took place before the time-limit stipulated by the doctor? In that case, the patient should receive treatment, and above all not confess to his spouse that he has the disease, so as to preserve 'the peace of mind and honour of the family', says Dr Langlebert,[39] who all the same is willing to admit that this is a 'thorny point of medical ethics'. Issues of medical confidentiality became pressing when, for example, parents came to enquire about a prospective son-in-law suspected of having syphilis, or when a patient asked for a divorce on the grounds of syphilitic contamination by the spouse. It was, however, unacceptable to break medical confidentiality. In 1886, for example, a doctor was sentenced to a year in prison and ordered to pay 1,000 F in damages for having sent a bailiff with a request for payment worded as follows:

Owes M.M.—— the sum of 300 francs for visits and treatment given to his mother-in-law for a disease; for consultations, operations and treatment given to his wife, who was infected with a venereal disease given to her by her husband; for consultations with him at an agreed time, and cauterization of his troublesome chancres, venereal ulcers, rhagades and other growths; and for having treated him for, and cured him of, two serious syphilitic diseases contracted at different times during the years 1862 and 1863.

Raymond Villey, who cites this case in his *Histoire du secret médical*,[40] adds that the mere fact that a psychiatrist or venereologist undertook legal proceedings against a patient on any pretext whatsoever constituted a serious breach of medical confidentiality. (Some venereologists were so concerned about medical confidentiality that they would never be the first to greet a client in the presence of a third person, so that the client would have the option of ignoring the venereologist in order to prevent any undesirable surmises being made!)

This accounts for the difficult position in which doctors were put by patients who refused to reveal their syphilis to those, such as relations or prospective spouses, who had the right to know the truth. The doctor was faced with a fresh dilemma: he had the duty to warn, but not the right to do so without the patient's consent.[41] Certain practitioners nonetheless made subtle distinctions, requiring the syphilitic to submit with good grace to their injunctions (notably in the matter of postponing his marriage plans) or else the warnings would be given regardless. In the first case, writes Dr Diday,[42] 'his cause is mine, and he can count on my discretion.' In the second, he continues, discretion would be connivance, and it is appropriate to do one's utmost either to force the party concerned to obey or to let the truth out without betraying confidentiality – a minefield which Dr Diday did not always manage to negotiate successfully, it seems.[43]

'Les Avariés'

The serious question of syphilis in marriage was taken up in *Les Avariés*, the first play to be concerned with anti-syphilitic prophylaxis, which Eugène Brieux, already a well-known play-wright,[44] had performed at the Théâtre Antoine in November 1901, and which he explicitly dedicated to Alfred Fournier:

Sir, I ask your permission to dedicate this play to you. Most of the ideas it seeks to popularize are yours. Like you, I think that syphilis will be considerably less serious when people dare to speak openly of a disease which is neither shameful nor a punishment, and when those afflicted with it, knowing the miseries they can spread, are more aware of the duties they have towards others and towards themselves.

Before the curtain rises, the stage-manager addresses the audience as follows:

Ladies and gentlemen, the author and the director are pleased to inform you that this play is a study of the relationship between syphilis and marriage. It contains no cause for scandal, no unpleasant scenes, not a single obscene word, and it can be understood by all, if we acknowledge that women need have absolutely no need to be foolish and ignorant in order to be virtuous.

And its plot? A patient consults his doctor. There is no doubt, it is definitely the pox. 'Don't be alarmed,' says the doctor to the 'Avarié', 'at least one in seven of the men you meet in the street, in polite company, or in the theatre is or has been in your predicament.' This thought does not console the Avarié, who talks of suicide.

THE DOCTOR: Every other person who sits where you are sitting now has just the same reaction. And they are quite sincere about it. Each considers himself to be more miserable than all the others. But on reflection, when they have heard me out, they realize that this disease is a companion one can live with; as in all marriages, harmony can be achieved by making mutual concessions, that's all there is to it. Really, sir, I assure you once more, it is all very ordinary, very natural, very common. It is an accident which could happen to anyone, and one might almost depict this disease (so inappropriately called the French disease, for there is no disease more universal) by addressing those who seek venal love with the famous lines:

Behold your master . . .
That is, or was, or must be.

But the Avarié, being neither a statistician nor a stoic, is
distressed and indignant. He had taken all the right precautions,
no-one could have worried as much as he had done about what
might happen to him. He had only had two mistresses, both
carefully chosen. One was the wife of his best friend, a man well-
known for his strict morals, and she had had the fear of syphilis
drummed into her ('I told her almost all men had it, so she
wouldn't get the idea of deceiving me'); the other was a young
factory-girl who was closely supervised by her own family, and
who had even been brought back to religion thanks to the efforts
of her prudent lover. And then our man had become engaged to a
rich party. And just as he was burying his bachelor life, this stupid
accident happened, with a woman who was 'almost honest', and
who lived in a fashionable neighbourhood to boot.

There remains the question of what to do next, in other words
the question of his marriage. The doctor is both firm and
reassuring. Yes, the Avarié can marry and have children, but not
for three or four years (this long time-limit poorly conceals the
uncertainty of a complete recovery: 'Even if our remedies weaken
or almost suppress the disease, it remains a threatening unknown
quantity'). Now the Avarié hopes to get married in a month's time,
and springs the trap of medical confidentiality on his doctor:
'You're not just a doctor, you're also a confessor.' The latter
deploys all the arguments he can to sway the Avarié: 'To get
married without saying anything is to enter society failing to
disclose crucial information' (the Avarié is a lawyer). In the first
place, his wife will almost certainly be contaminated and the
doctor inflicts on the Avarié a particularly horrible description of
an unfortunate young wife whose face was eaten away by a
'phagedenic syphilide' thanks to 'a benighted idiot who had had no
scruples about embarking on marriage whilst the secondary stage
was in full spate', and who, of course, said nothing. And, most
importantly, there are the children:

THE DOCTOR: In the name of those innocents, I beseech you, it is
the future, the race I am defending! Listen to me . . . .
Syphilis is above all a killer of children. Herod
reigns in France and over the whole globe, and
begins his massacre of innocent children anew each
year. And if it is not blaspheming against the
sanctity of Life, then I would say that the luckiest
are those who have passed on. Visit the children's

hospital. We doctors know the distinctive features of the children of syphilitics. The characteristics are classic ones, and doctors can pick them out from all the rest, these little old men who seem to have had their lives already, and to bear the stigmata of all our infirmities, all our failings. Of those children with rickets, children with tiny bodies crowned with oversized heads which they cannot support, children who are hunchbacks, deformed, monstrous, those who have club feet, or hare-lips, or who limp because of congenital dislocation of the hip, a great number are the victims of fathers who got married without knowing what you know now, what I would like to be able to shout out in public! I have told you everything, without dramatizing anything.

Shaken all the same, the Avarié goes off at the end of the first act promising to defer the date of his marriage. But his good resolutions do not last, and he gets married all the same. A sickly little girl is born, and has to be sent to a wet-nurse. The fatal disease finally becomes evident, and the child has to be taken from the wet-nurse, who runs the risk of being infected. The doctor recommends proceeding with great care: 'You never know what a wet-nurse is capable of, you never know what rancour, and legitimate rancour at that, combined with the rapacity, greed and spite of the peasant might cause such folk to do . . . people for whom the bourgeois is always something of an enemy, who are savage when they get the chance to take their revenge on him for their own inferiority.' The Avarié and his mother try to pay the wet-nurse off, keeping her as ignorant of the true nature of the situation as Henriette, the wife. But the latter, entering unexpectedly, hears and understands everything. She falls to the ground, and the curtain does likewise.

The third act takes place in hospital, where we meet the first doctor once again, coming to visit Henriette's father, a Deputy known for his diatribes on health and morality. This indicates the political dimension which the author wishes to give to this last act. The Avarié's father-in-law has come to demand a medical certificate which will allow his daughter to obtain a divorce. His arguments are unyielding:

FATHER-IN-LAW: This man has inflicted the supreme insult on the woman he married, he has made her the victim of the most odious attack. He has debased her. He has, in a manner of speaking, forced her into contact with the streetwalker whose curse he has transmitted to her. He has created I know not what mysterious link between her and this woman who is used by everyone. It is the poisoned blood of this prostitute which poisons the child, and her too. This abject creature lives in us, it is in our family, he has brought it to sit at our hearth. He sullies the imagination and thoughts of my little one as he has sullied her body.'

The doctor refuses the certificate on the grounds of medical confidentiality. Moreover, he does not wish to help bring about a divorce. Marriage must be maintained, come what may; forgiveness and treatment are what is required. All hope is not yet lost, and the couple can have healthy children later providing they do not 'neglect' the disease. 'Syphilis is imperious, and doesn't want her power to be underestimated. She is harsh to those who believe her to be insignificant, and benign to those who know how dangerous she is. Like certain women, she gets angry only when she is neglected.'

The father-in-law has no time for these subtle reasonings. There is to be no question of forgiveness. But the doctor suddenly makes an artful thrust at him: 'Have you yourself never sinned?'

THE FATHER-IN-LAW: I haven't had a shameful disease!
THE DOCTOR: That's not what I'm asking you. I am asking you whether you haven't ever exposed yourself to one. You have! . . . In that case, sir, it is not virtue . . . but luck which has protected you. And this term 'shameful disease' which you have just used is one of the things which irritate me most. It is one of our misfortunes, like all our other diseases, and there is never any shame in being unfortunate – even if one has deserved it. (*Becoming excited.*) Come, come! – you must agree! I would like to know how many of those puritans, those who in their bourgeois English prudishness dare not pronounce the name of syphilis, or who look as shocked and disgusted as they can when they deign to speak of it, who treat syphilitics like criminals, have never exposed themselves to such a misadventure, how many of them have pos-

sessed only virgins. Only those who have are
entitled to speak. How many are there? Are
there even four in every thousand? Well!
apart from these four, it is only chance which
has kept the rest from becoming syphilitics.

This unanswerable argument appeases the father-in-law, and
allows the doctor to move onto politics. The Deputy and his 500
colleagues are accused of having done nothing to combat the
'savage trinity' of Tuberculosis, Alcoholism and Syphilis. To open
his eyes once and for all, the senior doctor will show him the social
effects of syphilis. In comes a factory-girl. Once her situation was
an enviable one. But her husband had the pox and died insane,
having ruined the marriage and infected his wife. Now she can no
longer get treatment, for in order to attend the dispensary she is
obliged to take time off work, and also she cannot bring herself to
wait there with the streetwalkers. Overcome by emotion, the
doctor tells her that in future she can come to his own home on
Sunday mornings, and he even gruffly obliges her to accept a small
handout.

Then there is the father of an infected schoolboy – which poses
the question of the conspiracy of silence as far as information on
venereal diseases is concerned ('Pornography is admissible; science
is not'). And lastly there is a prostitute (of the 'streetwalking'
variety), a former maid made pregnant by her master at the age of
seventeen and then dismissed by her mistress. It was her clients
who infected her, though they were fashionable folk, gentlemen
wearing decorations. ('It is rather funny really . . . They are
wearing decorations when you meet them . . . they follow you . . .
Hey presto! . . . the decorations are gone. That intrigued me . . . I
saw in the mirror, they don't seem to be doing anything, but while
they are walking along they get rid of their ribbons with a flick of
the thumb, the way you shell peas, you know what I mean?') The
day the prostitute learned that she 'was laid up' she had her
revenge: 'My blood boiled . . . I took all those who wanted it . . .
for whatever they offered me, for nothing if they offered nothing
. . . I took as many as I could . . . and the youngest and the most
handsome . . . What the hell! I only gave them what they had given
me!'

After this descent into Hell there is nothing left for the doctor to
do but show the distraught Deputy out in silence. But the message
is made clear enough in a previous scene:

THE DOCTOR: We don't need a new law, we have laws enough
already. There is no need for it. It would be enough

if people knew a little more about what syphilis is. It would soon become customary for a fiancé to include amongst all the paperwork required of him a doctor's certificate testifying that he does not have to go through a period of quarantine and that he can be received into a family without them having to fear that they are receiving the plague along with him.

Astonishing, though it might appear in an age in which the concept of the venereal peril was so strongly established, the play was banned by the censor – a fact which the medical journals were quick to criticize, expressing justifiable amazement that blatantly licentious plays could be shown with complete impunity in the little theatres and café-concerts whereas a work of public utility was censored. The *Chronique Médicale* even produced a special issue in which Professor Fournier had free reign to express his indignation at a measure which he found inept, ridiculous and above all damaging, for Brieux's play was in his opinion 'essentially elevating'. So, he concludes, if 'the novel reaches only a part of the public, the theatre reaches a greater part.'

A controversy ensued, in the course of which certain syphilologists like Dr Balzer, a doctor at the Hôpital Saint-Louis, took the liberty of expressing doubts as to the utility of such a play. Of course, Dr Barthélemy, the Secretary-general of the Société de Prophylaxie Sanitaire et Morale, was in favour of it. Clemenceau, a doctor and playwright when the fancy took him, doubted the efficacy of such a play, even though he was opposed to censorship of the theatre. In particular, he thought that it was more urgent to combat alcoholism. Sarah Bernhardt, who had not read the play, nonetheless declared *a priori* that such subjects were not displeasing to her. As for André Couvreur, author of *Les Mancenilles*, he addressed a long letter to the editor of the *Chronique Médicale* in which he expresses his unreserved approval of Brieux's play:

Dear Monsieur Cabanès, It would be very rash to treat this serious matter of the banning of *Les Avariés* in only a few lines and as hastily as you ask me to. Remember that your question embraces the whole issue of the social value of the theatre, and that it warrants a well-documented and well-thought-out book. Having already exposed the dangers of syphilis in one of my novels, I can only rejoice at seeing it translated onto the stage. I believe that the play which warns and informs is an excellent means of raising moral consciousness. Those who find the theme uninteresting or repugnant are at liberty to sasifsy their aesthetic inclinations at the café-concert where they can inhale the stench of the dirty stories . . . . As for me, I have already heard some such from official sources. 'Enough doctors, enough pathology in the theatre!' some shouted at me. No, there is never enough! The doctor is a social priest, who will in the future be responsible for the foresights, health measures and prophylaxis which will influence our lives; and pathology is a cult which is beginning to be respected, whereas its predecessor, which is based purely on faith and credulity, is waning from one day to the next. That is why necessarily, inevitably, science is destined to become intimately involved with dramatic art.

Whatever happens, concludes Couvreur after this fine diatribe, Brieux's play will be staged, and many more will be staged besides.[45]

Meanwhile, the play was read on 11 November 1901[46] by the author in person before a selected audience which gave him the best possible reception. Above all, it was a tremendous publishing success,[47] thanks in no small part to the fuss caused by its being censored. In March 1902 it was performed in Liège and Brussels. The ban was finally lifted in France, and the play was performed in Paris for the first time at the Théâtre Antoine on 22 February 1905. The success of *Les Avariés* was no mere flash in the pan, for in 1913 it was staged on Broadway after a 'Sociological Fund' created for the purpose had collected the necessary monies to put on this militant play. There was even a special performance in Washington before President Wilson and the members of Congress – a political act intended to make an official break with the conspiracy of silence deplored by the American medical profession. In 1914, admitted in a somewhat different context, the Austrian Minister of War had the play performed in all the military schools of the Austro-Hungarian empire.[48]

With such a spectacular launch, *Les Avariés* collected a following, as much because of the word itself as because of the idea of using the theatre in the prophylactic campaign against syphilis. The only note of dissent was the indignant criticism made in the journal *Le théâtre* that the theatre was becoming confused with the operating theatre. In 1906 Dr H. Mireur collected together a series of popularizing articles which had appeared in *Le Petit Provençal* under the title *L'Avarié, étude d'hygiène sociale*, a work which he dedicated, appropriately enough, to Eugène Brieux who 'has done more on his own, in the three acts of his play, than all the health-care specialists for half a century',[49] and Dr Monnet had published his *Conseils aux Avariés* in 1902. As for the theatre, it increased its anti-syphilitic repertoire from 1907 onwards with popular soirées at the Éden Saint-Denis where the programme included a play in two acts *L'Immolée* (about a case of syphilitic sterility) followed by a medical slideshow.

In the United States, a formidable campaign of anti-syphilitic screening and propagandizing which was organized in Chicago in

1938 had as its principal support a play performed at the Federal Theatre: 'Spirochete, a living newspaper'. Without plot or characters, it was a retrospective view of the struggle against syphilis, a celebration of the Bordet-Wassermann test (which everyone was invited to undergo afterwards), and a vigorous condemnation of the hypocrisy of silence. 'Spirochete' was subsequently performed in Boston, Seattle and Philadelphia. One of the organizers wrote: 'If nothing else it is the most audacious and spectacular public relations move that has ever been made in syphilis. It will enormously increase syphilis consciousness.'[50]

So now the theatre, even more than the novel, had become the spearhead of the formidable anti-syphilitic crusade which was to reach a climax between the two wars. Up until that point, no disease had mobilized people's energies and 'talents' to such an extent. At the turn of the century, Dr Burlureaux, a colleague of Alfred Fournier's, had told the young but promising Société de Prophylaxie Sanitaire et Morale that they should not be worried about encouraging the obsessions of their fellow citizens; his goal was realized only a few years later. The obsidional fever of syphilis had begun.

7

Madmen and Hérédos

General paralysis is a form of madness

General paralysis, that is to say meningoencephalitis of tertiary syphilis, received its birth certificate in 1822 in a thesis submitted by Bayle, an intern of Royer-Collard at Charenton ('Recherches sur les maladies mentales'): 'I will have achieved my goal,' he writes, 'if this part of my work can prove that chronic arachnitis exists and that it gives rise to the symptoms of mental derangement' (he underlines this double proposal).

At the end of the eighteenth century, Chiarugi in Italy and Haslam in England had described forms of madness which consisted predominantly of grandiose delusions associated with a diffuse paralysis. Haslam even anticipated future developments by giving a description of general paralysis of the insane:

The paralytic affections are a much more frequent cause of madness than is generally supposed, and they are also a very common effect of mania. The paralytics usually exhibit lesions in their locomotive system independent of their madness; speech is impaired, the mouth is twisted, the arms and legs are more or less deprived of voluntary movement, and in the majority the memory is considerably weakened. These sorts of patients are not, in general, aware of their state. Though weak to the point of being scarcely able to stand upright they proclaim themselves to be extremely robust and capable of the greatest efforts . . . . None of these patients has shown any improvement in hospital, and, according to my research in the special establishments where they have later been put away, they always die suddenly of apoplexy, or else they lapse into imbecility or profound apathy as a result of repeated attacks.[1]

But for Haslam, as for Esquirol, who twenty years later described 'paralytic dementia', paralysis and dementia were two distinct, though associated, conditions. It was this dualist conception which Bayle denied in 1822.

In new studies devoted exclusively to this question which he published in the following years,[2] in effect Bayle reduced the problem of chronic arachnitis (chronic phrenesis) to a general and incomplete paralysis and a derangement of the intellectual faculties which is mainly characterized by delusions of grandeur. Its terminal stage is marked by 'a state of dementia and an increase in the general and incomplete paralysis'.

Whilst Esquirol's dualist theory continued to inspire research at the Salpêtrière (particularly under Baillarger in the middle of the century), the unicist conception was developed and refined at Charenton by Calmeil, who gave a complete description of the new morbid entity which he calls 'diffuse chronic periencephalitis',[3] asking in particular whether the principal anatomical lesions might not be much more serious than those described by Bayle. Likewise, Parchappe, at the Saint-Yon asylum near Rouen, describes what he calls 'paralytic madness' as a specific mental alienation 'in which there is a simultaneous disruption of the intelligence and motility; which generally has an acute onset, though it can enter a chronic state; which always has an unfortunate outcome, and which coexists with several pathological alterations in the encephalon, amongst which the softening of the cortical layer is a constant pathognomic factor'.[4]

The general paralysis thus defined might have done no more than figure in psychiatric nosography (though difficult to situate in the nosography of Pinel and Esquirol) had it not fitted in so well with the arguments of those who believed that the etiology of madness was necessarily organic . . . For the first time, then, 'something' had been discovered in the brains of the insane! Moreover, these anatomo-pathological lesions were not only to make general paralysis the model of organic mental diseases, they were also to swing the psychogenetic conception of madness, as defined by Pinel and Esquirol, towards an organogenetic conception (a shift led by Moreau of Tours, who considered madness to be 'a nervous affliction pure and simple').

Consequently, by the second half of the nineteenth century, general paralysis occupied as important a place in theoretical psychiatry as in the preoccupations of the statisticians who were beginning to establish their long reign of power. The 1874 General Report on the insane[5] shows 2,619 general paralytics in the asylums, which was 6.22 per cent of the institutionalized population. In fact, certain establishments like Charenton specialised in the treatment, or at least in the admission, of such patients, and had, at that date, 34.7 per cent of them.[6]

In 1884, the official dictionary of medical science[7] definitively established the specific character of progressive general paralysis. The onset[8] is of variable length, with intellectual enfeeblement and disturbances of the personality and the moral sense, and it is marked by an apoplectiform ictus or a particularly violent fit of mania. Then follow the classic symptoms of impaired speech, pupillary inequality, disruption of movement (particularly in locomotion) and delusions of wealth and grandeur. There are fairly long periods of remission, but the symptoms reappear and worsen until they produce a state of dementia interspersed with epileptiform or apoplectiform attacks which end up killing the general paralytic, unless he ends his life in a state of profound cachexia.

This same dictionary endeavours to distinguish this general paralysis of the insane from a 'general paralysis of syphilitics' whose symptoms are approximately the same, but whose lesions may be different. In fact the official doctrine was always that the only profound lesions of the tertiary stage of syphilis are those of the periosteum, the bones and the viscera (liver, kidneys).

A syphilitic madness

Because of the predominance of male cases of general paralysis, Bayle and his successors listed amongst its causes, obscure though they were, the influence of 'sex', but without for one moment suspecting syphilis (even though it had been diagnosed in certain cases). Approaching the problem from the opposite angle, it had been commonplace since the beginning of the sixteenth century to mention madness amongst the many avatars of syphilis. But these references can hardly be counted as inspired intuitions, and the prevailing opinion at the end of the eighteenth century was, in fact, that the brain was one of 'those vital parts which may well not be susceptible to the action of syphilis' (Hunter).

Although in the nineteenth century madness continued from time to time to be ranked as a possible consequence of syphilis[9] and the syphilitic antecedents of numerous general paralyses were increasingly often demonstrated,[10] the etiology of general paralysis remained uncertain, suggesting multiple causes (for Magnan at Sainte-Anne it was alcoholism). In 1857, however, Esmarch and Jessen affirmed that syphilis was the cause of 'GPI', and in 1868 Jespersen and Kjelberg put forward the idea that, conversely, an organism free of syphilis cannot develop GPI. But despite these enlightened thinkers, doctors continued to distinguish GPI from a 'pseudo-general paralysis' of syphilitics.[11]

From 1879 onwards, Alfred Fournier endeavoured to destroy

this fallacious distinction invoked by psychiatrists.[12] He had already, a few years earlier (in 1876), given syphilis a role in the genesis of the locomotor ataxia (tabes) described by Duchenne de Boulogne. Avoiding a direct confrontation with psychiatrists unwilling to examine the theories of a syphilologist, Fournier began by prudently retaining the term pseudo-general paralysis. But his masterstroke was to show that this pseudo-GPI was a frequent complication of late syphilis. He then stated his theory more and more clearly, demonstrating, for example, the etiological connections between GPI and tabes in a communication to the Académie de Médecine in 1894.

For several decades, Fournier and his successors, Morel-Lavallée and Belières, had to contend with general incredulity. 'Several times,' confesses Fournier, 'I had the experience of having to diagnose syphilitic madness[13] in the presence of very competent and justly famous psychiatrists; and almost invariably my opinion was received as a hypothesis which was possible, rational, perhaps tolerable, but singularly adventurous and tainted with heresy.' This led to a battle of statistics in which the two camps busied themselves enumerating the syphilitic antecedents of patients with GPI. In support of Fournier's thesis, work such as that of Régis at Bordeaux, together with a large number of medical theses, claimed percentages ranging from 65 to 80. In the opposite camp, Magnan of Sainte-Anne was, in 1888, willing to accept only four certain cases of syphilis and five possible ones in a hundred general paralytics of the male sex.

The quarrel continued beyond 1900, and Fournier accumulated arguments: cases of general paralysis in juveniles (here he was attempting to discredit the causes invoked by his adversaries, such as alcoholism, overwork, and the influence of the passions), and new statistics on 4,700 cases of tertiary syphilis, by far the largest sub-group of which was 2,009 cases in which the cerebro-spinal system was affected[14] – whence Fournier's aphorism: 'the nervous system is the victim *par excellence* of tertiary syphilis.' (Michel Corday in *Vénus* puts it more colourfully by making Léon Daudet's doctor friend say that the brain is syphilis' choice morsel, its treat.)

The question was once more brought before the Académie de Médecine in 1905, when Fournier and Raymond were opposed by Lancereaux, Duchenne de Boulogne and, most importantly, Joffroy, a former pupil of Fournier's to whom we owe the haughty remark: 'I acknowledge the existence of general paralysis *in* syphilitics, but I do not acknowledge syphilitic general paralysis.'[15]

Fournier, then, was still far from carrying conviction, either in

France or elsewhere. In England, for example, in Hack Tuke's *Dictionary of Psychological Medicine* in 1892, it is cautiously suggested that general paralysis does not necessarily have a syphilitic origin, but that syphilis is one of its most frequent causes. However, in 1907 Plaut used the recently perfected Bordet-Wassermann test to obtain positive results in the blood and the cephalo-rachidean fluid of general paralytics. But it was not until Noguchi and Moore's discovery of the treponema in the cerebral cortex of general paralytics in 1913 that Fournier's doctrine was to triumph definitively.[16] The psychiatrists who had previously not been prepared to acknowledge syphilis anywhere were from then on to see it everywhere; simultaneously, the interesting problem of the authentic cases of pseudo-general paralysis disappeared.

Maupassant's 'GPI'

Although Maupassant's doctor was right to say that the writer's disease was 'neither more nor less interesting than that of any other subject',[17] it nonetheless interests us here in that it showed itself right in the middle of the debate on the syphilitic origin of general paralysis. As we have seen, Maupassant was infected with syphilis, perhaps from the early 1870s. Around 1879–80, as he was approaching thirty, he experienced the first attacks of a precocious neurosyphilis, with a paralysis of the accommodation of his right eye. Ten years later, after reading *Horla*, Frank Harris[18] began to wonder about his friend's mental health:

– Your *Horla* is astounding, I told Maupassant when I saw him again. The terror you must have experienced and which inspired your account proves, however, that your nerves are in disarray . . .
Making fun of me, he interrupted gaily:
– My health has never been better.
Some years previously, in Vienna, I had studied venereal diseases, and I was just finishing reading a recent German work on syphilis in which it was demonstrated for the first time that this ailment causes paralysis in certain subjects between the ages of forty and fifty, at the precise moment when their vital forces are beginning to decline. An idea crossed my mind.
– Have you ever had the pox? I asked him.
– Oh yes, all the infantile diseases, he exclaimed, laughing. Everyone catches it when they are young! But for ten years I haven't had a trace of it. I have been free of it a long time now. It was in vain that I related the German specialist's discovery to him, he gave it no credence. He hated everything German, and considered the reputation of their science to be vastly exaggerated.

No-one else suspected the onset of general paralysis at a time when psychiatrists, and even many syphilologists, were united against Fournier's theory. Thus, for example, at the very moment that *Horla* appeared, Charles Mauriac, head of department at the Hôpital du Midi upbraided 'over-eager pathologists . . . who have dreamed up and taken to the extreme the conquest of the brain by syphilis'.[19] Meanwhile, Maupassant's strength was declining and Harris, increasingly anxious about his state of health, urged him to have done with 'all these orgies'.

However, he still craved the fatal caresses. Had syphilis weakened his moral fibre? Many of us have succumbed to nervous depression between the ages of forty and fifty; but uncompromising abstinence, moderate exercise and a change of environment have restored health and reason. In Maupassant's case, the fact that when young he had idled his time away on the boats at Bougival, and his frolics with Mimi and Musette, had loaded the dice against him.

According to Harris, Maupassant had had 'a sort of presentiment of an impending and unexpected end' ('He knew, three years in advance, that the indulgence of his sensual desires was dragging him inescapably to madness and death'). We know the outcome: the bout of suicidal madness in January 1892 which caused him to be interned in Dr Blanche's sanatorium[20] where he died eighteen months later. It was Albert Lumbroso who first mentioned Maupassant's syphilitic madness: 'Maupassant's mistake was to have made his condition worse; he accelerated his madness by his way of life.'[21]

Hereditary syphilis

Hereditary syphilis, which had been recognized since the sixteenth century, had been the subject of a good number of writings at the end of the eighteenth century, both on the question of the process of transmission and on that of the threat which syphilis of newborn children posed to the human race.[22] After a long eclipse due to the theoretical and therapeutic stagnation of anti-syphilitic medicine during the first two-thirds of the nineteenth century the subject gathered momentum as the campaign against the venereal peril developed.

Since Swediaur, the three means of transmission of syphilis to newborn children which were envisaged were the infection of the infant at birth, the infection of the fetus by the mother whilst in the uterus, and infection by the father at the moment of conception. This latter, which today appears preposterous, was the explanation which was the most favoured at the time. A corollary of this view was that the mother of a newborn syphilitic infected by the father could remain unharmed ('Colles' law', 1837).[23] Although hereditary syphilis of paternal origin had a few opponents[24] it occupied a key position in Alfred Fournier's work. The latter, in spite of (or because of) his countless works on syphilis, was particularly interested in the question of hereditary syphilis, which fitted in perfectly with his prophylactic and moral crusade.

Once again, Fournier thoroughly reexamines the question, beginning by endeavouring to give a complete clinical picture of hereditary syphilis. Amongst the signs he describes, the three most frequent make up what is generally called 'Hutchinson's triad': nerve deafness, interstitial keratitis and dental deformations (in particular, 'Hutchinson's teeth') – all of which are characteristic manifestations of hereditary syphilis in later childhood. But there is an infinite variety of other signs and syndromes: respiratory, circulatory, osteo-articulatory. As for the neurological symptoms, they naturally occupy a key position in Fournier's descriptions and those of his school: infantile hemiplegia in particular, but also infantile epilepsy, chorea, convulsions, etc.

A distinction was made between manifest hereditary syphilis, which differs from acquired syphilis in having the symptoms sketched above, and cryptic hereditary syphilis, which is detectable solely by the dystrophic stigmata which Fournier said would require a whole volume to describe.[25] The archetypal sickly syphilitic baby is described as follows:

Born at seven months of an equally syphilitic father and mother, it was a sickly creature of miniscule dimensions, a dirty yellow in colour, and so lifeless and emaciated that it hardly seemed worth taking care of it. This miserable creature was wrapped in warm wadding and placed in the best possible conditions, to prevent it from getting chilled. It could hardly swallow a few drops of sugared milk or water.[26]

It is interesting to note that in the work in which this description figures, which dates from 1918, the treatment prescribed is still Van Swieten's liquor, whose 'miraculous influence', states the author, gave this sinister and sickly creature the strength to suckle and subsequently to put on weight.

From the end of the nineteenth century onwards, 'hérédo-syphilis' (hereditary syphilis) assumed a growing importance, not only as a disease, but as a cause of degenerescence. The term was not used at first, although in 1841 one could read in the Annales d'hygiène publique that

Syphilis is slowly and surreptitiously sapping the strength of succeeding generations. It does not kill outright, but it prevents people from living. It attacks the very essence of life, poisoning it at the source and grinding down the spirits.

The more it infects individuals, the more it poisons families, the more it insinuates itself into the masses, the more it brings about the degradation and degeneration of the human race.[27]

In 1886 Fournier introduced the notion of 'late hereditary syphilis' as follows: 'Finally, a possible but definitely much rarer consequence of hereditary infection consists of more or less serious arrests in intellectual development. Nowadays it is a well-authenticated fact, albeit little-known and not generally accepted, that the progeny of syphilitic subjects are sometimes intellectually deficient.'[28] In 1901, Bourneville, a psychiatric doctor at Bicêtre, where he had set up a department for idiot and epileptic children, supported this idea by taking syphilis to be influential (though not as crucial as alcoholism and 'a number of insalubrious professions') in the production of idiocy, epilepsy and psychiatric disturbances in children.[29]

In 1905, Freud himself acknowledged hereditary syphilis in the Dora case: 'Her father had fallen ill because of the licentious life which he had led, and she thought she had inherited his disease from him. I took great pains not to tell her that I too, as I have already mentioned (p. 12, no. 1) considered the descendants of syphilitics to be especially susceptible to grave neuropsychoses.'[30]

Freud also wrote in his *'Three essays on the theory of sexuality'*:

In more than half of the severe cases of hysteria, obsessional neurosis, etc., which I have treated, I have observed that the patient's father suffered from syphilis which had been recognized and treated before marriage, whether there was evidence of tabes or general paralysis, or whether the anamnesis indicated in some other way the presence of syphilitic disease. I should like to make it perfectly plain that the children who later became neurotic bore no physical signs of hereditary syphilis, so that it was their abnormal sexual constitution that was to be regarded as a last echo of their syphilitic heritage. Though I am far from wishing to assert that descent from syphilitic parents is an invariable or necessary etiological condition of a neuropathic constitution, I believe that the coincidences which I have observed are neither accidental nor unimportant.[31]

As he had done in his case for the syphilitic origin of general paralysis, Fournier weakened the opposition before going in for the kill (1904):

It emerges from recent research that syphilis can, because of its hereditary consequences, debase and corrupt the species by producing inferior, decadent, dystrophic and deficient beings. Yes, deficient; they can be physically deficient . . ., or they can be mentally deficient, being, according to the degree of their intellectual debasement, retarded, simple-minded, unbalanced, insane, imbecilic or idiotic.[32]

Soon all the doctrines of hereditary degenerescence expressed by Buchez and, above all, Morel,[33] senior doctor at the Saint-Yon asylum, came together in the notion of hereditary syphilis, which itself widened to cover dementia and psychoses. Here too Fournier (and also his son Edmond)[34] played a decisive role, introducing the notion of juvenile general paralysis (a notion on which unanimity was still far from being achieved), adding to the list of 'those who are deficient in intelligence' as a result of hereditary syphilis those with nervous problems (neuropaths, hysterics, neurasthenics, epileptics, etc.), and even allowing a further extension of hereditary syphilis to the etiology of infantile schizophrenia.

Although the concept of degenerescence began to be criticized in the aftermath of the Great War (even though since Morel it had been the stock explanation for mental diseases), that of hereditary syphilis persisted, and in fact replaced it. 'Through the notion of hereditary dystrophy, syphilis allows us to "medicalize" degenerescene rather than suppress it' (Nicole Valleur). The myth was born, and was to gain ground between the wars:

Any child whose 'physical or intellectual' development is abnormal, any child who manifests a pathological state, no matter how long it persists, or the least abnormality (a straightforward strabismus or some sort of adenosis) or which cries at night, or which is not cheerful, or which is highly-strung, or coughs, or has gastric or intestinal problems without an obvious alimentary cause, is suspected of having syphilis.[35]

And even when hereditary syphilis was not the most important factor, it could always be claimed that it was a contributory one.

From then on, all sorts of fantastic ideas were mooted: a biologist, for example, wanted to see syphilitics obliged to testify to their condition, so that even if syphilis jumped a generation (the idea of 'second-generation heredity') the inevitable effects of hereditary syphilis could be linked to their true cause;[36] a doctor identified, in addition to the banal and pitiful category of pupils who owed their scholastic failures to hereditary syphilis, the special, and antipathetic, category of 'the rowdy dunce excited by his treponema'.[37] But there were moral judgements as well as these medical frivolities:

Fournier's oeuvre is peppered with references to the syphilitic weakling, the valetudinarian child, debasement, degeneration, inferiority and decadence, echoed by authors who talk of degenerescence . . . In this respect, hereditary syphilitics were to become the living symbols of a past transgression (a curse on two generations), or rather, their perverse behaviour is both a sign of the punishment and a reminder of the crime. (Nicole Valleur)

As Alain Corbin concludes in an article devoted to 'hereditary syphilis, or the impossible redemption',[38]

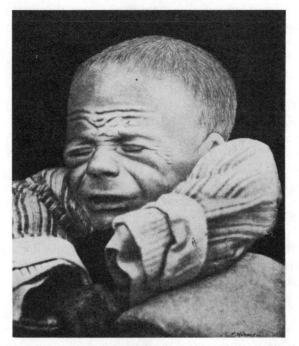

PLATE 13 The myth of hereditary syphilis racked a whole generation between the wars, feeding on the very real phenomenon of congenital syphilis. Here we see the archetypal 'syphilitic runt' with a head like an old man's, destined for either premature death or degeneration. (*Traité de pathologie médicale et de thérapeutique appliquée*, vol. XX, 'Syphilis II'; Private collection)

it was as if doctors were translating the bourgeois fantasies of their time into scientific language . . . . Even more serious in nature than syphilis, hereditary syphilis struck most often in the upper classes since, according to Alfred Fournier, the fatal diasthesis is essentially of paternal origin. This was because in the bourgeoisie, male infidelities were much more common than female ones. The lower classes thus transmitted to the bourgeois male, via their womenfolk, a virulent syphilis which metamorphosed into a germ fatal to the whole line. Despite the purity of the wife-mother, the race – for which one should read 'the bourgeois family' – finds itself threatened by a rot which has its origins in the street or on the sixth floor.'

The obsessive terror with which the bourgeoisie of the nineteenth century greeted the idea of this corrupting irruption (in every sense of the term) from the suburbs[39] forms, we may recall, one of the climactic moments of *Les Avariés*: in the third act, Henriette's father says in effect that the Avarié has inflicted on his daughter 'the supreme insult by, in a manner of speaking, forcing her into contact with the streetwalker', which has 'created I know not what mysterious link between her and this woman'. However, we go

well beyond mere physical contamination with this final reflection:
'He sullies the imagination and thoughts of my little one.'

'The hérédos'

As the great fear of syphilis, so successfully instilled during the
Belle Époque, developed between the two World Wars, there
appeared an archetype which was to be baptized with the striking
name of 'hérédo'. It is under this description – 'Marc Vanel,
hérédo' – that a bore who is visiting a famous painter is presented
in a novel by Jean Moyë published in 1939:[40] He is carrying under
his arm an autobiographical manuscript (*La vie d'un hérédo*) when
Olga, a pretty girl and chief clinician at Sainte-Anne to boot,
enters. The subject interests her, and she immediately puts the
hérédo at his ease: he is not to worry, he is talking to a doctor ('If,
like me, you were to look after the mentally ill, you would be
astonished at the number of secret tragedies which are concealed
by respectable families'). The reading can now begin.

Marc Vanel belongs to an old bourgeois family. As a child he
had been hypersensitive and sickly until a visit to the doctor finally
raised the fateful question: Are there any syphilitics in the family?
No names are mentioned, but everything is clear when we learn
that the father tumbled the maids in spite of (or because of) his
own nervous weakness. Marc then went to the Beaux-Arts,
moving in various circles where there were many people who, like
he, combined elegance of spirit with physical decrepitude – in a
word, hérédos. Next we see him in the army, and we are presented
with a new series of medical tableaux. Here, instead of being pale
and interesting, people are 'edgy' and shut up in huts. Marc's state
is not improved by this environment. In a fit of delirium he throws
himself out of the barracks window – which leads to his being put
with the madmen, and then with the serious neurotics, before
being invalided out at last. After operations and relapses, Marc
wonders if he is mad, and in fact a Bordet-Wassermann test reveals
that he is afflicted with GPI. His mother then confesses:

My darling child, you have syphilis. Your father didn't want me to tell you, he
wanted to have you treated without saying anything so that you wouldn't think
badly of us. I told him that I would tell you the truth, and I didn't think I had the
right to conceal from you a disease which, if not properly treated, would lead you
to paralysis and death. My darling, for too long no-one realized how serious your
disease was, people said that you were mollycoddling yourself, but now it is clear
that you were right. I am just an old woman who adores you, but I promise to
cure you!

After years of struggle and new sufferings the hérédo does in fact recover (or at least, the Bordet-Wassermann test becomes negative), though his mother dies amidst edifying sufferings. His father dies too, an alcoholic corrupted by his maidservant. But this is all to Marc's benefit. From now on his life has meaning, for he is going to be able to testify and thereby prevent others from suffering what he has suffered: 'O heredity, thought Marc Vanel, you have done me a great deal of harm, and now you are doing me some good.'

This dreadful novel sets out the principal characteristic of the hérédo: he is a sufferer who testifies through his own suffering. But this testimony is also an accusation, like that produced by Louise Hervieu in *Le crime*,[41] a feverish and disjointed novel which contains a series of tableaux written in an incantatory style which are worthy of our attention: 'Born of man and woman, not of goose and gander, we have behind us ranks of ancestors, their testimony and their mystery. How can we escape the heredity of our Species? We are hérédos . . . . In the white races the disease concentrates on the most vulnerable parts, the overworked and enfeebled nerve centres. It produces people who are mad, half-mad, quarter-mad, unbalanced, obsessed.'

After a denunciation of 'the hypocrisy' which leads everyone to deny being a hérédo ('and we all are'), a 'dance of fools' and a 'plea for peace' (in which we are asked to pity 'our faults, the little sallow and sticky-eyed children, the retarded and degenerate ones, the pale ones, those who are undesirable and undesired, the children who are wretched!'), we are treated to a grand finale, the 'plea to women', those fountains of life who alone have the power to break the terrible chain of heredity by refusing to make their marriage a lottery: 'You are no longer ignorant, you know that everything can be cured, and that a loyal man, even when he is sick, remains worthy of your love. You must wait for him, and remain for him his dearest hope. By treating himself he is already working for you and the home, as if he had gone to fetch you a fortune from some fabulous mine. Let this not be the end of a world, but the beginning of a new race!'

Whilst waiting for this message of hope to be heard and for the *avariés* to return cured from their 'fabulous mines', hérédos continued to parade like 'thin and fleshless poultry', as Sanchez had put it so well in the eighteenth century.[42] The hérédo is the rachitic and pitiful cupid with drooping wings depicted on the cover of *L'Assiette au Beurre* of March 1905, in an issue specially devoted to *Les Avariés*, a worthy echo of Brieux's play which was taking Paris by storm at that time. But whereas a single hérédo excites pity, hérédos as a group tend to be somewhat awkward for the collective state.

On the eve of the First World War, Léon Daudet, who is also, as we shall see, one of those who spread the notion, denounced the misdeeds of the hérédos: 'In sum, the vast majority of neurasthenics, melancholics, misanthropists, lypémaniaques and, in a word, misfits, are hérédos, a product of that terrible miniature destroyer which is also called the pale spirochaete.'[43] Following on from this broad definition, it is the literary type which, as we might have expected, most exercises the verve of the author of *Les morticoles*:

> In literature, the hérédo is characterized by a manifest predominance of verbal facility over quality of thought. Too many words for too few ideas, that is the recipe. It results in a somewhat wild superabundance which leaves the critic in no doubt once he is aware of it. To take a concrete example, the romantic school of 1830, with its turgidity, its giddy whirl of images and its nonsensical philosophical wanderings, is a prize collection of hérédos. They were drawn together by that natural propensity which abnormal people have for joining forces. I beg you not to see any blasphemy or tasteless raillery in what I have said. We are in the domain of objective observation, nothing more.

With such a fine pedigree, the breed proliferated in the inter-war period. There they are, swollen with pride and ideas of grandeur, invading not only literature but also painting, the theatre and the cinema. In painting it is the hérédos who have 'ended up imposing on the dumbfounded masses the undeservedly celebrated new style of painting which is so outrageous, so grotesque and, above all, so devoid of all decorative sense, artistic character and pictorial technique'.[44] All the other arts are affected too. The hérédos are synonymous with decadence. Humanity is under threat, and the Treponema is triumphant.

Syphilis and genius

The myth of the hérédo was so powerful that it could produce entirely contradictory theories. Alongside the hérédos who were impostors in the arts and responsible for their decadence we also find the syphilitic genius. As we have seen, Spanish authors had, at the end of the sixteenth century, touched on the notion that the pox was the enemy of the flesh and therefore the friend of the soul, and that the chancre produces a pale and melancholic subject more useful to the Republic than the ruddy, gluttonous, unimaginative drinker, in short, than the high-liver – an Aristotelian idea (pox excluded) which Lombroso revived at the end of the nineteenth century: 'The great thinkers pay for their huge intellectual powers in degenerescence and psychoses' (*L'homme de génie*).

As regards syphilis, the theory once more took form with reference to general paralysis. GPI, explained Régis in 1879 (the same year that Fournier had asserted its syphilitic etiology), classically regarded as weakening the intelligence from its onset, could in certain cases assume an expansive form resulting in 'overfunctioning of the intellectual and affective processes'. Although GPI is a tertiary, and therefore late, symptom of syphilis, argues a medical thesis in 1932,[45] the meninges are affected at the primary stage, and the character can change from this point onwards. The expansive period, when present, may last two years or more. 'The expansive form of the first period of general paralysis has been attributed to meningoencephalitis; toxaemia seems to play a crucial role in it. It acts by stimulating the neurons.'

Here we have the 'syphilitic toxin' promoted to the rank of a stimulant: 'The increased appetite becomes bulimic . . . . The psycho-intellectual functions are generally or partially enhanced. It produces the archetypal cripple endowed with superior intelligence – Velasquez' dwarf, with the most penetrating gaze that painting has ever reproduced.'[46]

Once more it is Léon Daudet, Daudet the sceptic, whom we find taking this thesis with the utmost seriousness. *Les Morticoles* and *Devant la Douleur* might give the impression that Léon Daudet the doctor believed in neither doctors, medicine nor Science – all of which he lumped together as what he so appropriately called 'the Stupid nineteenth century'. Daudet's scepticism, however, was not total. He concludes *Devant la Douleur*, not by proclaiming the bankruptcy of science, but by calling for it to be applied anew. In contradiction to the school of inaction, he looked forward to human intervention in heredity, an idea which he developed in the course of *L'hérédo*, an often confused work in which heredity appears as 'a constant and permanent attribute of life, like the principal force which moves animate beings'.

We can now understand why Léon Daudet, the friend of Edmond Fournier, unhesitatingly embraced all the theories of hérédo-syphilis. Daudet, who made such fun of Pasteur's 'little animals', believed fervently in the treponema and in its power to produce genius – and with what verve!

The microbe of the terrible disease, the treponema, since we must call it by its name, is as much the power behind genius and talent, heroism and wit as that behind general paralysis, tabes and almost all forms of degenerescence. Sometimes exciting and stimulating, sometimes deadening and paralyzing, the hereditary treponema pierces and worries the cells of the marrow and the brain; it brings with it congestions, manias, haemorrhages, great discoveries and scleroses; strengthened by the interbreeding of syphilitic families, it has played, plays now, and will continue to play a role comparable to that of a Fate of antiquity. It is the spirit, invisible but present, which moves the romantic and the madcap, the sublime-looking misfit, the pedantic or the violent revolutionary. It is the yeast which raises the somewhat heavy dough of the peasantry and refines it in two generations. It makes a great poet of a maid's son, a satyr of a peaceful bourgeois, an astronomer or a conqueror of a sailor. An age such as the sixteenth century, with its splendours and its depravities, its gallantry, its amorous frenzy, its formidable expansion, appears to the initiated observer as an incursion of the treponema into the elite and the masses, as a sarabande of hérédos. From the very first line of his famous dedication Rabelais has seen the truth of the matter, and he himself was undoubtedly part of it, with his dazzling language and his continual whirl of frenzied and brilliant images. The majority of the degenerescence, the majority of the misdeeds attributed to alcoholism can be imputed to this spiral whose agility, ductility, penetration and congenitality, if one can say such a thing, remain a mystery . . . . As thrusting and as acrobatic as the propagator of life which is associated with it in many a conception by hereditary transmission, the treponema fosters at once the dramatic intensity of life, the sterility which is its opposite, and the hardest of scourges.[47]

Another theory went even further: since, despite our hopes of controlling it, we must give up the idea of completely eradicating the terrible spirochaete, could we not at least exploit it? The idea was particularly prominent in a novel of the inter-war period (*Tréponème*), by a doctor who wrote under the pseudonym of Marc La Marche. His theory is simple: since in 99,999 cases out of 100,000 the treponema causes madness, senility and death, and only in one case does it produce a genius, what we have to do is to revive the psychic centres which it has atrophied or made latent. The same author repeats his idea in a poem entitled *Syphilis*, in which, after a long list of the thousand-and-one infirmities caused by the terrible malady, we come to the question of genius:

> Are you not, Syphilis, the great go-between
>   Working to put man in touch with his genius,
> The source of powerful thoughts, the transmitter
> Of the seeds of art and science, the inspirer
>   Of delightful follies?
> . . . .
> Crush with sobs the lyrical breast
>   Of the sublime musician'
> Inspire the weary metaphysician,
> Shape the harrowed eye of the wretched painter
>   And the voice of the tragedian.
> The world still awaits torches and kings,
>   The ambassadors of the Chimera.

You can give them to us . . . If we must put up crosses
To get them, we accept your laws
O Syphilis, salt of the Earth![48]

Undoubtedly we must make allowances for irony, but to what extent? Such theories have been made possible by famous examples: Maupassant's GPI, and that of Nietzsche (currently disputed), as well as those who are too ready to promote the idea that their general paralysis coincided with their most creative period – which is false, like the more general proposition that GPI can produce genius, however ephemeral.[49]

However, a biography such as that of Karen Blixen[50] does reopen the debate about syphilis and literary creativity. Karen Blixen was infected by her husband at the end of 1914, when she lived in Kenya. Although she was treated with salvarsan in a hospital in Europe, syphilis assumed a growing importance in her outlook as a writer. 'Now that I have endured this too,' she said later, 'I am even closer to great things.' Karen Blixen did not develop general paralysis, but she did develop tabes, which soon reduced her to a living skeleton. It was then that she began to become a literary success with *Seven Gothic Tales*, *Out of Africa* and *Winter Tales*.

Syphilis seems to have been the price she had to pay for mastering her art. Likewise, one of her heroines rediscovers her lost humanity by contracting syphilis, chastely, after kissing the foot of the statue of St Peter in the Vatican.

8

Syphilis Everywhere
(Between the Wars)

The age of the dispensary

By intermixing populations on a huge scale, the First World War produced (amongst other misfortunes) such an increase in the incidence of syphilis – not to mention gonorrhea – that the disease once more assumed epidemic proportions. But even so, can we really believe the statistics of the time[1] which claim that there were between 700,000 and 800,000 new cases of syphilis in France during this period? We will be returning to the delicate question of medical statistics later, but one thing we can say with certainty is that this sudden upsurge hampered to some extent the intense prophylactic campaign begun in Fournier's time and provoked a new wave of anxiety.

Contemporaries were struck by the comparison between the dreadful war which had killed millions of men, the 'Spanish' 'flu of 1918 which had killed as many or even more, and syphilis (and hereditary syphilis in particular) which would finish off those who remained: 'Yes, the treponema threatens to wipe out humankind.'[2] It is in this context that we must consider the extraordinary development of the myth of hereditary syphilis in the inter-war period analysed in the previous chapter. There were, so to speak, two horribly complementary catastrophes, both fatal: on the one hand the catastrophe of healthy men mown down by the war, and on the other that of the hérédos who were to populate, or rather depopulate, the France of the future. There was therefore no question of relaxing the campaign begun before the war.

In 1913 the Paris health authorities had created a number of dispensaries for outpatient treatment, but because of the increase in cases of syphilis both at the front and at home the Undersecretary of State for Military Health and the Council for Welfare and Public

Hygiene had jointly set up a new category of dispensaries called '*services annexes*'. The first of these came into operation in Bourges in 1916; so as not to embarrass its clients it was a place which, like its name, was very discreet. It offered free daily consultations (and occasionally an additional evening surgery to fit in with 'the hours of rest of the working class'),[3] check-ups in a small laboratory with an ultramicroscope and equipment for the Bordet-Wassermann test, and outpatient treatment or hospitalization in a small department containing a few beds for patients whose condition posed a threat to those who came into contact with them (until their lesions had cleared up).

With the coming of peace, all that remained to be done was to increase the number of these flexible dispensaries and, most importantly, to bring them within a national state-financed programme for the first time. It was also necessary to substantially reorganize anti-venereal prophylaxis, basing it on centralized institutions financed and controlled by public authorities.

In 1919, the Inter-Allied Congress on Social Hygiene took place in Paris, and doctors like Henri Gougerot set out a complete programme for the struggle against the venereal diseases. Shortly afterwards, the Ministry of Hygiene and Social Prevention was set up and the Commission for Anti-venereal Prophylaxis, which was reorganized under its aegis, voted a resolution (4 May 1922) inviting the Minister to ask central government for the funds necessary to create and run the anti-syphilitic dispensaries. In 1923 almost two hundred '*services annexes*' modelled on the one which had been set up in Bourges in 1916 were in operation in France.

Thus the worker finds, during his hours of rest, free consultations given in discrete surroundings, where he can be sure of receiving care of as high a standard as that which the most affluent bourgeois can afford. Except during such time as the symptoms are too contagious, syphilis does not in fact necessitate hospitalization, and outpatient treatment which allows the worker to continue with his job without losing time seems in the light of experience to be more and more the ideal weapon for the struggle against the spread of this scourge.[4]

At the same time, the prophylactic institute set up in 1916 had a central dispensary, laboratories and numerous dispensaries in Paris and the suburbs (there were 800,000 consultations between 1916 and 1925).

The elaboration of the network of dispensaries was completed by the setting up of the Central Service for Prophylaxis Against Venereal Diseases and the National Office of Social Hygiene, which were answerable to the Ministry of Hygiene and responsible for the masterminding of the anti-venereal struggle in France. At the same time there was a proliferation of Leagues: the 'Anti-Venereal League of Alsace and Lorraine' (1919), the 'League for the Abolition of Syphilis' and, most importantly, the 'French National League Against the Venereal Peril', which was founded in 1923, and which opened numerous dispensaries in the suburbs of Paris, founded the School of Sociology Applied to the Study of Syphilis and organized the Conference Against Hereditary Syphilis (Paris, 1925) and the Conference for Social Defence Against Syphilis (Nancy, 1928). As for the French Society for Sanitary and Moral Prophylaxis founded by Fournier in 1901, it continued its activities and set up a subsidiary in 1925, the Committee for Female Education, which pursued the impossible dream of educating young women.

In accordance with the wish expressed at the Second International Conference for Prophylaxis Against Syphilis in 1902, societies on the model of the French Society for Prophylaxis were set up in Belgium (which seemed to be very much in the forefront of this mobilization of prophylactic forces), in Italy, Germany, Denmark, Canada and, a little later, in Japan. The Red Cross was also active, and founded, also in 1919, the League of Red Cross Societies, which brought together the numerous national societies which had been set up since 1864. It gave rise to the Pan-American Conference on Venereal Diseases in Washington in December 1920 and the Conference of Western European Countries on Venereal Diseases held in Paris a year later.

Shortly afterwards, Belgium, which remained in the forefront of the prophylactic struggle,[5] took the initiative in the setting up of the 'International Union Against the Venereal Peril', which was intended to establish links between the various nations with a view to taking common and concerted measures against venereal diseases. This body, based in Paris, had thirty-four member nations in 1928. In June 1922, a first 'Congress of French-speaking Dermatologists and Syphilologists' took place in Paris at the Hôpital Saint-Louis. The second congress took place the following year in Strasbourg, and led to the foundation of the 'Association of French-speaking Dermatologists and Syphilologists'.

In addition to these great international congresses there were regional efforts, such as the Conference on Social Defence Against Syphilis held in Nancy from 29 to 31 May 1928 on the initiative of the French League Against the Venereal Peril. Nancy also had an 'Anti-Venereal Branch of the Office for Social Hygiene of Meurthe-et-Moselle', and thanks to the personality of Dr Spillmann[6] this city was set to become one of the capitals of militant anti-syphilitic activity. The regional press, symptomatic of the times, gave its active support to this effort initiated by the Prefect, aided by several Superiors of the Order of the Sisters of Saint-Charles, presidents of societies for the aid of wounded soldiers, and pupils of the regional school of nurses, not to mention prominent ladies who, commented the press, 'were eager to be present at this first meeting so as to show that they had not hesitated to lend their precious help to the struggle being waged against the venereal peril'.

It was, moreover, in the long-neglected provincial towns that we can best see the effects of the anti-venereal struggles. The anti-venereal dispensaries whose importance Alfred Fournier had been the first to appreciate[7] appeared in all towns with over 10,000 inhabitants in a variety of forms: autonomous dispensaries, mixed dispensaries (often in conjunction with anti-tubercular dispensaries), or dispensaries annexed to a general hospital.[8] At the same period, the special hospitals, henceforth considered ignominious, disappeared. It should be noted that although these new dispensaries were in principle free, the patient was required to have a letter from his doctor, who took good care only to send those who were unable to pay.

Paris was not to be outdone, however, and in order to strengthen the anti-syphilitic campaign which culminated at the beginning of the thirties set up, in 1932, the Alfred Fournier Institute (Alfred Fournier was born in 1832) at the instigation of the indefatigable French National League Against the Venereal Peril. In a vast building which then dominated the Boulevard Saint-Jacques the Fournier Institute housed several dispensaries, laboratories for teaching and research, administrative departments and departments for the production of anti-venereal propaganda. We shall have more to say about this body, which is still in operation today.

At that point there emerged a worthy successor to Alfred Fournier, who died in 1914: Professor Jeanselme, who succeeded to the chair in the treatment of syphilis at the Hôpital Saint-Louis in 1918. Amongst other works which we owe to Jeanselme is a voluminous treatise on syphilis published in 1931, a work which is indispensable to the modern historian.[9] Here is how, a few months before his death in 1935, he tells the story of the reform of the dispensary of the clinic over which he presided.[10] In 1918 there was nothing but a makeshift dispensary (and this is at Saint-Louis!), relegated to a corner of the radiotherapy ward, and inadequately separated off from it by a scanty curtain stretching from one wall to the other. Not only did this dispensary fail to operate satisfactorily as far as the patients were concerned, but it was also impossible to provide the teaching which students and trainee doctors were entitled to expect. Once the department had moved into the hospital, things began to go differently. There were 10,178 consultations in 1920, and 33,480 injections of novarsphenamine were given (and only 49 mercurial injections, which speaks volumes about mercury's fall from favour). In 1933, after a further reorganization, the dispensary comprised a head of department, two assistant doctors, six externs, two social workers (to 'follow up' the 30 per cent of patients who did not return), three nurses and a 'dresser', not forgetting a secretary whose duty it was to keep the sacrosanct index, which was the real keystone of health surveillance. There were 57,521 consultations there that year, and 555 cases of syphilis were treated.[11]

Should one rest content with waiting until syphilitics decide of their own accord to come to the dispensaries? Of course not. They must be systematically tracked down, in the first instance amongst the patients of medical practitioners (and the public health authorities had high hopes of the collaboration of general practitioners, pharmacists and social workers), and also in maternity hospitals, for which, because of hereditary syphilis, special provision was made, including the creation of their own dispensaries.[12] Special measures, centring on systematic examinations, were also agreed upon for what we would now call high-risk groups: railway company workers, merchant seamen, guest workers, servicemen and, most importantly, prostitutes, always regarded as the major source of venereal infections.

But despite all these measures, most doctors lamented the lack of specific laws to combat syphilis, and the fact that prophylaxis continued to depend on the goodwill of patients. Some went so far as to propose to make contagion a criminal offence.[13]

Propaganda

In the absence of sufficiently restrictive laws, the anti-venereal institutions created just after the First World War developed syphilitic propaganda which is truly astonishing to the late-twentieth-century observer, and which went far beyond that introduced in the Belle Époque – though the motivations in both cases were the same. It is impossible to give a complete account of anti-syphilitic propaganda in the twenties and thirties, with its thousands of posters, tracts, press articles and pamphlets, not to mention lectures, radio programmes, the theatre and the cinema. But what exactly was this propaganda? According to one writer it 'stands to disease as advertising stands to commerce and industry.'[14] There is another image, inherited from the First World War: in the general offensive which had just been launched against syphilis, doctors could thenceforth advance, strongly supported by the artillery of propaganda.

There was certainly no shortage of 'lectures', which were sometimes published subsequently, and which were from this time onwards aimed at more specific readerships than young men and women, often on the initiative of local or regional organizations. (We should note in this connection the pilot role given to the recently reconquered eastern regions). Servicemen were the favourite target, but they were also aimed at railway workers, or at future farm-wives at colleges of domestic science, as in this 'eighteenth and final lecture' given to the Eure mobile college of agricultural domestic science on 20 May 1928 under the evocative title *Le baiser malsain*.[15] This lecture is interesting because it seems that the 'close to nature' side of the future farm-wives gave its author the revolutionary freedom to address young women, to whom doctors had always refused to direct their anti-venereal discourses:

'Young housewives and future farm-wives, teach yourself to detect syphilis in your cooks and servants. Choose your cowherds and cowgirls carefully. Learn the signs.' Be suspicious of headaches which do not respond to treatment; hard frontal lumps (extosis); partial loss of hair; red eyes; roseola ('your servants will wrongly attribute it to having eaten fish or crustaceans'): copper-coloured spots along the hair-line ('this is Venus' diadem'); a dirty-looking neck covered in white blotches ('this is Venus' necklace'); white spots on the lips; hoarseness ('husky voice in your servants: the sore throat of secondary syphilis'); a nasal voice ('perforation of the palate by a syphilitic gumma'); a white line in the middle of the eyebrow, or particularly at its tail and ('this is Professor Fournier's "signe d'omnibus"'); a thinning beard; a nose like the foot of a cooking-pot (congenital flattening of the base of the nose because of hereditary syphilis); badly-formed teeth, and particularly half-moon-shaped clefts in the two upper incisors (these are Hutchinson's teeth, a sure sign of hereditary syphilis); jaundice, especially in drinkers ('perhaps it is the combination of a liver complaint and syphilis'), etc.

And that is not all. Future farm-wives must also beware of butchers' hands, and in particular their spittle, of the hairdresser, of the servants' linen (which must be disinfected with copper sulphate before being given to the women in charge of the laundry), etc. Does this mean that syphilis is more of a threat to country-dwellers than to town-folk? No, the threat of contagion is far greater in the town (hotel sheets, 'water-closets', office implements, etc.), but in the country syphilis often passes unnoticed because the peasant seldom calls the doctor (this at least is undeniable) – which gives rise to a form of syphilis which the author of this particularly 'muscular' lecture calls 'malignant syphilis', whose primary, secondary and tertiary symptoms all occur simultaneously, and which is capable of killing a man in less than a month. (Cases of malignant syphilis, which is rapidly fatal, were indeed possible.)

In some scarcely less dramatic instances, 'undetected cases of syphilis in the country' can lead to extra-genital syphilitic contamination in children of the same family, or even progressive general paralysis. This latter leads the author, who is in decidedly brilliant form, to formulate comparisons which are, to say the least, somewhat curious: 'It is particularly prevalent in intellectuals, the state of whose blood plasma serum, and even of the nervous tissue itself, differs from (1) that of the peasant who lives in the open air and uses his muscles much more than his brain; (2) that of the Arab who drinks nothing but water, eats nothing but couscous, fruit, dates and bananas, and who has nothing to do but to bask in the sun.'

Other 'practical advice' is addressed to young men, whether or not they are serving with the colours. That which Dr Bernay[16] dispenses requires both science and audacity. Those who have remained unwounded should carefully inspect the terrain as they march into battle. (Memories of the First World War are still fresh.) They should put on their most fetching smile and caress the lady's neck, feeling at the same time for swollen glands under the skin. They should express enthusiastic admiration of her mouth and teeth, but take particular care to glance at the lips, gums and tongue. They should praise the bosom, but examine the skin for possible suspicious blotches. And that isn't all. Having completed these preliminary inspections (and, we might be tempted to add, provided the woman, if she is a prostitute, hasn't sent the investigator packing) it remains necessary to assure oneself with one's own eyes that at the gateway there lurk neither tigers nor snakes (ulcerations, mucous plaques, purulent secretions) which might bite one as one passes. And the act should not be prolonged overmuch ('to linger is dangerous'). No kisses on the mouth, either; all one has to do is claim to have a horror of makeup.

Doctors sometimes preferred to appeal to the healthy and sporting side of French youth. 'Young sportsmen, read this', appeals a tract from the early twenties which reminds the reader in an epigraph that syphilis and gonorrhea kill 150,000 Frenchmen a year, 'the toll of the Marne, or of Charleroi'. The best way to avoid venereal contamination is continence, followed by marriage, followed by conjugal fidelity. But instinct speaks louder than reason. Thus

we doctors, putting aside the moral issues, must speak to you of the physical dangers. And as a sportsman I am speaking in particular to you, my fellow sportsmen, you who represent the élite of the race, you for whom a single moment of imprudence can destroy the benefit of many years of training. We begin from the principle that all sexual relations carry a risk, leaving aside, if you wish, questions of feeling. You meet a woman, perhaps even one of good breeding, who one day gives proof of delicious abandon. Beware. This beautiful flower may be poisonous!

There follows the usual hygienic advice, and in addition to the classic battery of protective measures the author recommends the carrying of a pocket-size container of 'Préventyl' or 'Salvatyl' to allow a discreet post-coital toilette. And if, despite everything, syphilitic contamination does take place, 'I hasten to tell you: nothing is lost . . . . But above all, if you have had a misfortune you should make a highly moral resolution, and promise not to have any sexual relations, even with a prostitute, until you are sure that you are completely cured. He who, knowing himself to be contagious, has no scruples about contaminating a woman, is more than just a dishonest man, he is virtually a murderer.'

The press played a decisive role in this propaganda campaign, maintaining the public in a state of alert by keeping syphilis continually in the news. In 1926 alone, 15,000 articles in the popular press were recorded, not to mention the numerous scientific journals; these latter added to the number of medical articles relating individual cases, thereby informing practitioners and ending the isolation of the provinces. There were also journals which specialized in the study of, and the struggle against, venereal diseases – *La prophylaxie antivénérienne* (the official organ of the French Society for Sanitary and Moral Prophylaxis and the French National League Against the Venereal Peril), *les Annales des maladies vénériennes*, etc.

At a time when there was an unprecedented increase in publicity, the poster, far more than the pamphlet or tract[17] distributed in the dispensaries, was a favoured medium for anti-syphilitic propaganda. A case in point is a particularly evocative poster issued by the Ministry of Hygiene, 'Defend yourself against syphilis', in which the disease, represented as a death's head is being fended off by a shield held by a powerful arm. There is also a poster issued by the National Committee Against Respiratory

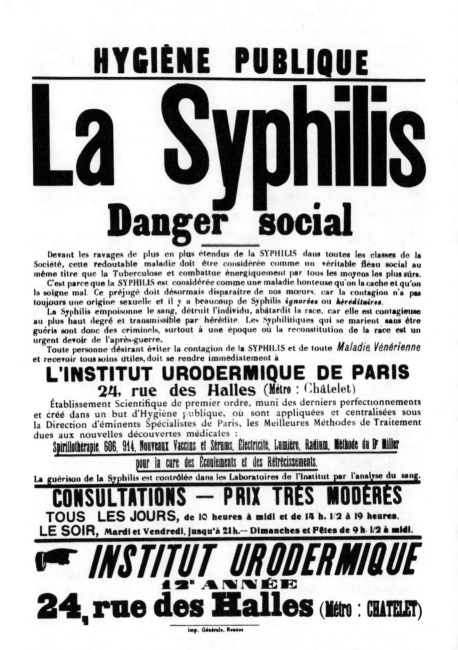

PLATE 14 During the first half of the twentieth century there was a huge poster campaign (posters were even hung on the walls of men's urinals), warning of the dangers of syphilis. (Private collection)

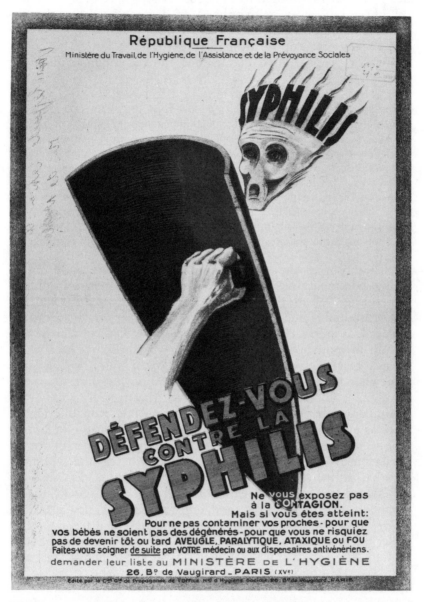

PLATE 15 A particularly effective and long famous poster produced by the Ministry of Health and Social Prevention. It appeared just before the First World War. The slogan alone is a whole programme in itself. (Bibliothèque Nationale, Paris)

Diseases and Tuberculosis[18] entitled 'The race to death'. Under the eye of Death, who stands in place of the winning-post, we see the racehorse 'Tuberculosis' beating 'Syphilis' by a head ('150,000 deaths a year as opposed to 140,000'). A long way behind, almost out of sight, 'Cancer', with only 40,000 deaths a year is barely even galloping. (A notable absentee is alcoholism, whose ravages people had already given up recording.)

Certain propagandists condemned the technique of inducing fear.

The majority of posters on syphilis published in all the countries of the world leave a nightmarish impression in the mind of anyone who has seen them. Here are some examples: a couple kiss each other on the mouth in front of a death's head; a man and woman, ardent nudists, dance in the midst of a flock of crows before Death, who is playing the violin . . . . And that is not all, there are yet worse ones. I consider that these posters foster panic and turn public opinion away from the right path. The poster which seems to me to be the most successful is that which is published by the 'Save Mothers and Babies' Association. It depicts a happy couple holding a beautiful child, with the expressive text: 'We were ill, we went for treatment, and now we have a beautiful baby in spite of everything.'[19]

In addition to the 'tub-thumping' posters there were others giving administrative information about the operation of the dispensaries.[20] Both the former and the latter covered the walls of public buildings and urinals. If they were torn down they were replaced, as in Paris in 1929, by metal plaques, 5,000 of which were put up in municipal urinals and factory washrooms. As always, after a brief delay, the provinces followed suit (though in a somewhat lower key). As for anti-syphilitic prophylaxis in the colonies, colonial doctors considered that pictures of death accompanied by menacing phrases had no effect on the natives who, as everyone knew, were fatalists. Scenarios of the following type were suggested as alternatives: A man in good health arrives quickly in front of a fine plateful of food, whereas the syphilitic, who has difficulty in walking, is always late for his victuals.[21]

Between the wars, Brieux's *Les Avariés* continued to be imitated. There was a novel[22] and, more particularly, new plays. *Le mortel baiser* was performed for the first time in Paris in 1923[23] under the patronage of the Minister for Work, Hygiene and Social Welfare, the International League Against the Venereal Peril and the 'Save Mothers and Babies' Association. The story is an interesting variant on *Les Avariés*. The situation is identical in origin, but just as the marriage is about to take place in spite of the doctor's entreaties the outraged nurse rushes to the window under which the procession is passing and calls out 'Stop! That young man is a syphilitic!'[24] The play was immediately criticized by the medical profession, who could not accept seeing confidentiality betrayed in this fashion, even by a nurse. The spectacle which concluded the show, and included a great many screens with projections of the face of the patient, hideous although he had been treated for two years, upset them even more: 'It is a crude medical error which falsifies the entire play. It may be perfect Grand-Guignol, but it is most certainly bad anti-syphilitic propaganda.'[25]

We must also mention *Presque tous*, performed in 1933, whose theme is hereditary syphilis, and whose explicit objective is to denounce 'the universal conspiracy of silence which everyone voluntarily maintains on this question'. There was also *La Statue en délire*,[26] whose audacity and excesses make *Les Avariés* seem somewhat anodyne. Narcisse Grandhomme, a nouveau riche who is unaware that he has syphilis, has the misfortune to have a pretty daughter who is engaged to a young war hero, Raymond Gircourt, himself a syphilitic. The latter, though he has been cured by Dr Talmen, wishes, before marrying, to be honest and warn his fiancée, but though she is a modern girl she sends him packing. During the first three acts we witness the development of general paralysis in Grandhomme. Above the action rises the noble figure of Dr Talmen; his nurse, Danièle, is not afraid of accepting Raymond's love, though she postpones his demonstrations of it until clinically more auspicious days.[27]

Anti-syphilitic propaganda did not only use traditional media, it also availed itself of the new media, radio and the cinema. Although sixty anti-venereal lectures were broadcast in 1926, the radio was eventually used only with reluctance, because of the impossibility of targetting particular listeners and the resultant danger that it would be counterproductive. The cinema, however, soon struck the propandists as a choice weapon, combining 'the impact of words and the shock of photographs'. The first of the genre (*Il était une fois trois amis*) was shown in 1927 at the Sorbonne to an audience of 3,000 in the presence of the Minister of Hygiene. The story concerns three friends who return from an amorous expedition with syphilis. Only the first, who is correctly treated, has fine children after marrying. The two others cannot have any until each has been treated in his turn. Another film in the same style, *Le baiser qui tue*, tells the story of a young sailor who gets engaged in Brittany before leaving for far-off seas. He catches syphilis in a port of call, and the ship's doctor advises him to wait two years before getting married. The sailor does not heed his advice, marries, infects his wife who gives birth to an idiot child, and finally sinks into alcoholism. He dies in an asylum. Fortunately, it was only a bad dream. In reality the sailor follows the doctor's advice, signs up for two more years and, after two years of treatment, gets married in perfect safety. 'Everything turns out for the best, and the syphilitics who see this film have no reason to despair', the medical critics concluded.

Another film, *La mille et deuxième nuit*, was filmed especially for the Maghreb. But observers complained that when Mohammed Ben Chegir staggered and fell because syphilis had taken hold of him the audience giggled, saying that it was because he was drunk. It seems that in this field, as in many others, the British obtained better results by making anti-venereal films on location (notably in India) and taking more account of the traditions of the country in question.

Independently of these films shown in public cinemas, the National Office of Social Hygiene made available to dispensaries and lecturers short films which popularized medical themes, and whose impact was undoubtedly greater than that of printed material. (Twenty or so films figure in the 1926 catalogue.) In the army, obligatory sessions immediately after enlistment often provided the first sexual and prophylactic education received by young recruits. These horrifying and badly-made little films were probably enough to put anyone off love (i.e. sex) altogether. But as far as the hygienists were concerned, perhaps, they served a useful purpose for that very reason.

There was just as much propaganda against syphilis and gonorrhea in the American army. From the First World War onwards it was a question of protecting the health of the troops, in other words the fighting potential, but also of protecting the moral standards of men who were far from their mothers, sisters, fiancées and spouses and were therefore more likely to indulge their baser instincts. On 17 April 1917, only eleven days after the declaration of war, the War Department's preoccupation resulted in the setting up of the 'Commission on Training Camp Activities', which embarked on an astounding programme of activity. It provided a wealth of readings and lectures accompanied by horrifying medical photographs, the intention being to engender the ultimate prophylactic reflex: continence (a subject to which we shall return). 'Over-exercise or excitement of the sex-glands may exhaust and weaken a man. The sex feelings are so powerful and the risk so great if they are turned loose, that it is common sense not to play with fire.'[28]

The CTCA even produced a film, '*Fit to Fight*'. The script of 'the first motion picture to tell the truth about the cause and effect of venereal diseases' is the archetype of the genre. A group of army friends of different social backgrounds and temperaments are, like so many others, drawn into frequenting prostitutes. Their destinies vary according to whether or not they follow the prophylactic advice given to them by the army. Two of them get syphilis, one gonorrhea, whilst one lucky survivor fleetingly tempted by the brothel is moved by his prophylactic muse to declare 'I wouldn't touch a whore with a ten-foot pole!'[29] After the war this film, whose title was changed to '*Fit to Win*', was declared obscene by the New York State Board of Censors – which says a good deal about the extreme relativity of values as far as the topic of sexuality was concerned.

The army's solicitude for its boys was even greater when it came to setting foot in the Old World. The 'Social Hygiene Division Army Educational Commission' produced a series of posters which were liberally displayed in army billets and hostels (there was no risk, therefore, of shocking chaste young girls). The most effective were those which broached the theme of returning home in shame. 'Go back to them physically fit and morally clean' proclaims one of these posters, in whose foreground a small-town mother is engaged in making a cake. Those who were unmoved by this sentiment were given a clear warning by another poster showing a departing steamboat trailing a billow of smoke in the shape of a question-mark: 'officers and enlisted man returning to the United States will be subjected to a physical examination previous to embarkation and all those found to be affected with venereal disease in a communicable stage will be detained and placed in segregation camp.'

As in Europe, the prophylactic campaign against venereal diseases, and against syphilis in particular, reached its peak between the wars, especially in the 1930s with the activities of Thomas Parran, appointed Surgeon General in 1936 by President Roosevelt. Allan M. Brandt, author of '*No Magic Bullet*' is right to see Parran's campaign as part and parcel of the 'New Deal'. For the sake of both the public health and the economy it was necessary to face up to these problems squarely, without worrying about conventions or propriety. Parran was wont to recall that in 1934 he had refused to take part in a CBS broadcast because he had been asked at the last moment not to refer to syphilis and gonorrhea by name. In 1936 a sensational article of his entitled 'The next great plague to go' appeared in the Reader's Digest, which at that time already had 500,000 subscribers. Some shocking pictorial statistics set alarm bells ringing: 'Out of every ten adults syphilis strikes one.' The illustrator depicts an arrow of retribution piercing one of a row of ten silhouettes.

In '*Dr Ehrlich's Magic Bullet*', a Warner film released in 1940, Edward G. Robinson exchanges his usual role as a gangster for that of Paul Ehrlich in honour of this noble cause. The film hails the discovery of Salvarsan, but it also gives Dr Ehrlich the opportunity to make some substantial diatribes against the conspiracy of silence

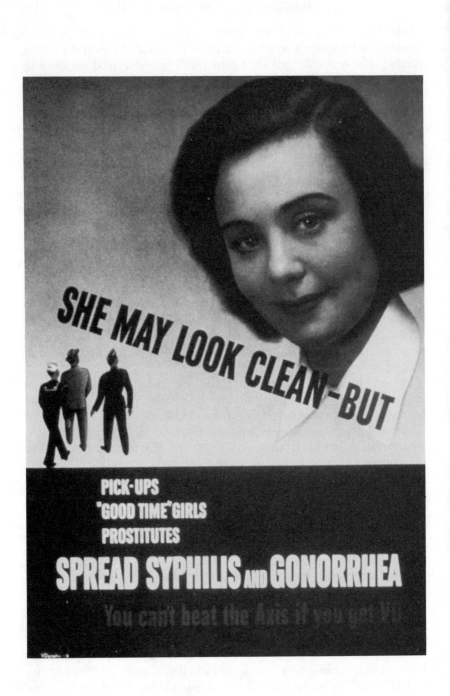

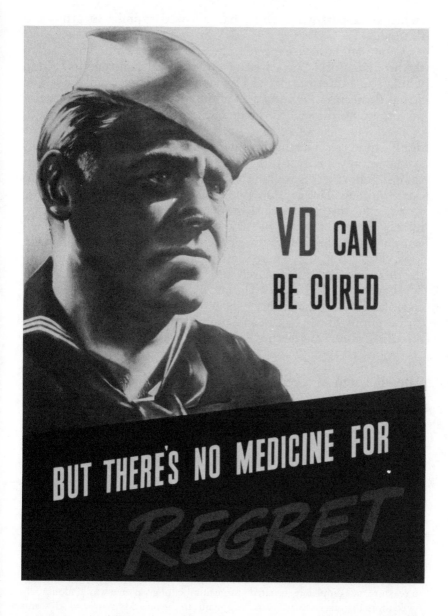

PLATES 16 and 17 During the two World Wars the American army's reputation as 'the cleanest army in the world' was threatened by the problem of clandestine prostitution and the resulting ailments 'the gin problem'. It lead to an incredible campaign of antiveneral propaganda which cullminated in the slogan: 'Sex exposure without prophylaxis is a help to the Axis'. (Allen M. Brandt, National Archives and Records, Washington)

(which still persisted) which had allowed syphilis to grow and flourish.

As one might have expected, the entry of the United States into the Second World War gave the anti-venereal campaign its second wind. The 'American Social Hygiene Association', aided by 'The Social Protection Division', set about a renewed bombardment of posters against the soldier's libido. 'Sex exposure without prophylaxis is a help to the Axis', says one. On another, a woman with a death's head (representing syphilis, or rather VD, for the Americans systematically confused the struggle against syphilis with that against gonorrhea) is walking with Hitler on one arm and Hirohito on the other. The caption is the succinct comment: 'VD is the worst of the three.' As well as these subtle allusions to contemporary history there were other posters which struck below the belt, such as that which showed a little brunette with a shy smile: 'She may look clean – but . . .'. There is also the sailor who stares sadly into the distance: 'VD can be cured, but there's no medicine for regret.' We have come full circle. The newly-arrived penicillin might be capable of curing the primary chancre, but the moral chancre of the indiscretion which has been committed remains. Anti-venereal discourse is not merely medical, but moral.

The obsession of a generation

It is not surprising, then, that the whole inter-war generation was literally obsessed with the fear of syphilis. Amongst the many authors who echo it is Gide, who recounts the fear of 'getting pickled' by an 'Andalusian star' of doubtful reputation which possessed him when a friend of his convinced him to accompany him to a brothel – a fear which his friend took pleasure in encouraging:

And when I exclaimed that he might have warned me while there was still time he protested that the disease, whose effects I would probably soon feel, was in fact nothing to be afraid of, and that one might as well accept it as a tax on pleasure, and that to seek to avoid it was to try to put oneself above the common law. Then, to reassure me completely, he cited a large number of great men who undoubtedly owed more than three-quarters of their genius to the pox. My alarm, which seems rather amusing to me now, when I think of the face I must have made – and of course I know now that I was worrying needlessly – was not at all amusing to me at the time.[30]

As for Julien Green, he relates that as he was accompanying his friend Ted, a great ladykiller, to the doctor's, Ted suddenly confided that it was a girl who had given it to him, and I didn't understand immediately, but little by little the horror dawned on me, slowly but surely. I found what Ted had just told me interesting, but I was anxious, as if I was seeing smoke rising from under a door – what lay behind that door? Suddenly my ears began to sing, because I was frightened. This was the disease about which my mother used to talk, covering her face with her sheet, when she told me the story of my Uncle Willie. My terror suddenly became something enormous, I was afraid of Ted, I was afraid to breathe the same air as him, I wondered whether having touched his hand by accident might not have given me the disease with which he was infected. All these men around me were being punished for having made love. The wages of sin is death . . . . I no longer know if I stayed or not, but when I arrived home I washed my hands and face furiously, endlessly rubbing my skin with soap. My mother had warned me, and now Providence itself had arranged things so as to teach me a lesson, to save me. It is better to die than to be defiled, Père Crété used to tell me, but being defiled leads to death. I promised to myself that I would be pure, that I would not touch anyone, or myself either. I wouldn't see Ted any more.[31]

There was also Roger Martin du Gard, on whom Régis' précis of psychiatry made a strong impression, and who let himself become obsessed by the idea of general paralysis. 'There are some days,' he wrote to Jean Schlumberger in 1933,[32] 'when I almost long for death, or some unexpected accident to deliver me! Revolution? General paralysis?' Nine years later he wrote to André Gide: 'This euphoria to which I am so little accustomed is almost terrifying! Is it the prelude to GPI?'[33]

Julien Green gives a particularly good picture of what it was like to be terrified of syphilis at that time:

Syphilis – the disease was the terror of our youth in the twenties. He saw it everywhere. Nowadays it is difficult to imagine the dread which the mere mention of this scourge struck into young men's hearts. The awful consequences of this ever-present contagion, the brain affected, one's entire life ruined in a shameful way. One of my university friends told me that his father had taken him to a hospital in which men afflicted with the unmentionable disease were treated, the object being to cure him of his sexual cravings. If we may be permitted to make light of these matters, I will recall that my sister Éléonore, who always took things to extremes, insisted on wearing gloves to read *Bubu de Montparnasse* because this novel by Charles-Louis Philippe is about syphilis. On learning that someone or other had contracted the 'great disease' she would immediately say 'That's what comes of taking one's meals in a restaurant: forks and spoons are contaminated.' These notions were idiotic, but they nevertheless give an idea of the latent panic into which we were thrown as soon as the subject of physical love came up. There was a curse on carnal pleasure outside wedlock, and yet . . . The notion of the punishment of sin inevitably entered the minds of some of us. I could have been counted as one of them. A kiss on the mouth could lead to madness and death. Sensual ecstasy was followed by the torments of fear, but we have changed all that.[34]

We should not conclude from what we have just read that the terror was the prerogative of the upper middle classes, homosexual or otherwise (though we can in fact hypothesize about how one might have led to the other). Moreover, according to certain syphilologists, 'in meticulous patients the fear of catching the disease is frequently the powerful argument which makes their sexual apragmatism complete'[35] (which brings us back to the beginning once more).

Some were so terrified that they refused to face the truth, as this anecdote from the memoirs of a country doctor illustrates.[36] A lady, 'elegant but showy, distinguished but affected', came to consult him. She was worried about a spot which had been on her upper lip for some time. On examination the excrescence proved to be accompanied by large ganglions beneath the jaw (Ricord's pleiade)! There was now very little room for doubt, and the doctor, somewhat embarrassed, got tangled up in his explanations, which were fairly clear nonetheless. Suddenly the lady understood, and cried out in outrage 'that's not possible, I am the wife of a Prefect and my husband is of the highest breeding.'

Erich Maria Remarque – whose fine novel *Der weg Zurück* (1931) describes the difficult, if not impossible, task of reintegrating themselves into society which faced young men returning from the holocaust of the Great War – accompanied Ludwig, his comrade in the trenches, to the doctor's:

'Is it . . .?'.
The doctor nods encouragingly. 'Yes, we have the results of the blood test. Positive. Now we're going to have to start doing something about the deuced thing.'
'Positive,' mumbles Ludwig, 'that means . . .'.
'Yes,' replies the doctor, 'a little course of treatment is required.'
'So that means I've got syphilis?' – 'Yes!'
A large fly buzzes about the room and crashes into the window. Time seems to stand still. The air in the room seems viscous. The world has been changed. A frightful anguish has been transformed into a frightful certainty.
'Couldn't it be a mistake?', asks Ludwig, 'Couldn't they do a second test?'
The doctor shakes his head. 'It is best to start the treatment as soon as possible. You are in the secondary stage.'
Ludwig swallows. 'Can it be cured?.'
The doctor brightens. His face is almost jovial with reassurance.
'Completely. You see these little ampoules? Injections for six months at first. After that, we shall see. Maybe there won't be much to do then. Syphilis can be cured nowadays.'
Syphilis, that hideous word which hisses like a thin black serpent.
'Did you catch it at the front?', asks the doctor.
Ludwig indicates that he did.

'Why didn't you go for treatment straight away?'
'I didn't know what it was. That sort of thing was never mentioned in those days!'

Hygiene for the syphilitic

It is but a short step from being unable to acknowledge to oneself that one has syphilis to being unable to acknowledge it to others.[37]

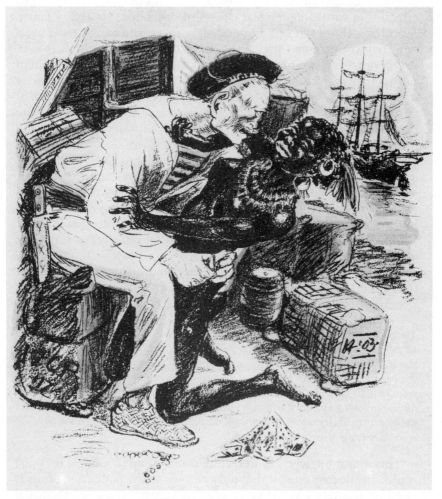

PLATE 18 Like alcoholism and 'fevers', syphilis raged in the colonies. The libertarian press quickly made the connection between 'civilization' and 'syphilization' though it was by no means certain that the contamination was all in one direction. (Drawing by Grand-Jouan, *L'Assiette au beurre*, 9 May 1903; Bibliothèque Municipale de Caen)

Syphilis was more shameful than ever, and could be endured to the death without the sufferer ever saying anything to his spouse or mistress. The doctor was therefore often obliged to treat these latter in a conspiracy of silence, a situation of which he was frequently critical.[38] Unless, which was even worse, the person who was infected knowingly allowed the disease to develop in another (or others) without saying anything. It was no longer a question of disease but of prohibition, a sexual taboo reinforced by its very failure – Eros and Thanatos fiendishly reunited.

The medical profession which since Fournier had been so effective in spreading the fear of syphilis therefore set about gently reassuring those who had nonetheless fallen and might have been tempted to think that they were no more than living dead. It is in this context that we must understand the advice addressed to them by doctors in various works of which the archetype is *L'hygiène du syphilitique*, which appeared in 1897.[39] It is primarily concerned with a 'moral hygiene'. It is necessary to 'act as a confessor to the patient' in order to reduce what another author calls 'the moral pains of syphilis'.[40] Against the wishes of many doctors their role was therefore extended, even exalted: 'There are hardly any other instances in which the doctor fulfils to such a high degree this dangerous and admirable role of arbiter of our destinies. He is, in fact, the only one who can know, understand, forgive and cure on both the moral and the physical levels. More than anyone else the syphilologist must be a psychologist and an observer, a diplomat and an upstanding man.'[41]

And the doctor, as an 'actor in the venereal drama', must not overlook the role of the woman, that victim of ignorance in matters sexual:

> The moral affliction of the man is actually in large part due to the woman, and vice versa . . . . In the man . . . fear of the pox is the beginning of wisdom . . . he thinks about it constantly. The woman never thinks about it. What in the man often leads to an obsession or a phobia is reduced to something altogether vague in the woman . . . . Though she often sees love in many affairs she seldom perceives the disease in love. Capable of complex understanding in the first instance, she proves to be of a simplicity which borders on indifference in the second. This is why she is so dangerous when she is infected.[42]

This moral hygiene can in fact be summed up in a single message which the doctor must unfailingly convey to the patient: syphilis is curable. But this was a dogma which was actually more of a moral one than a medical one, for although the arsenicals and bismuth had a treponemicidal power that was infinitely superior to that of mercury they were not always a fail-safe remedy for syphilis.

There were few doctors who dared to put things so bluntly at the time, or even to acknowledge the facts of the matter to themselves, so great were the hopes raised by the discovery of '606'. But close inspection reveals that the same medical treatises which emphasize the necessity of reassuring the patient of the curability of syphilis pose elsewhere the question of whether or not there were infallible signs of recovery. Those doctors who believed that there were chose their terms so prudently that it leads us to suspect a rather forced optimism: 'a case of syphilis treated at the chancre stage, with a Wassermann test result which is negative or even slightly positive, can, after a prolonged monitoring of the patient and the disease, be considered cured.' Likewise: 'any syphilitic, even if he is considered to be cured, should, once a year at the minimum, follow a course of treatment comprising arsenicals or bismuth in the first instance, and later on mercury.'[43]

Even a negative blood-test should not be too readily taken as a proof of recovery. To do so would be to overlook the dormant period, whose length varies from one individual to another, which follows the 'first overt signs of destruction'. (Certain doctors with poetic leanings wondered what became of the treponema during this period when it kept a low profile. 'It is claimed,' says one of them, 'that the treponema settles in by taking shelter in inaccessible regions such as the spleen and the bone-marrow').[44] By general consent, the sole proof of freedom from syphilis was the capacity to be reinfected – which boils down to saying that one must catch syphilis for a second time to have sure proof that one has been cured of the first dose![45]

Some medical journalists – of whom, fortunately, the general public was unaware – drew the inevitable conclusion from this:

It seems, therefore, that at the present time we are being told that syphilis is definitely incurable and that neither a negative serological reaction nor the absence of lesions or other obvious symptoms means anything. The syphilitic must be treated for the duration of his life, and he is lucky not to be forbidden to marry. All the precautions, time limits, treatments and tests are nothing but a thinly-disguised prohibition. Here's a fine thing – medicine, and humanity at large, checkmated by the pale treponema.[46]

A certain Zeissl added, half serious and half joking: 'Anyone who has contracted syphilis will die a syphilitic and will be resurrected a syphilitic in the valley of Josaphat.'

Health care for syphilitics moved in the direction of general health care: no overeating and, of course, no venereal excesses (though what sexual athlete would dream of such a thing in such painful circumstances?), and above all no alcohol, whose role in exacerbating syphilis had already been emphasized by Fournier and Barthélemy.[47] Syphilitics discharged from the Hôpital Cochin were even schooled in what the head of department wittily called their 'catechism':[48] a treatment to be followed for four years (the idea being to continually 'wash' the syphilitic blood with a series of injections of novarsphenamine and bismuth); no alcohol as we have already seen, but also no tobacco ('A syphilitic who neither smokes nor drinks alcohol is halfway to being cured'); sexual contacts to be confined exclusively to women who already had syphilis (were women treated to this catechism in which men were thus apostrophized?): separate eating utensils and washing kit; and no marriage during the four years of obligatory treatment.

This treatment was based on the arsenicals, which reigned supreme in the treatment of syphilis between the Wars. The first-generation trivalent arsenicals, novarsphenamine in particular,[49] were gradually replaced by the pentavalent arsenicals (Stovarsol, Tréparsol, Acétylarsan and typarsamide), which were considered to be less toxic. They were administered in a number of different ways (by intravenous, subcutaneous or intramuscular injections, orally or as frictions) and in combination with various other substances (bismuth, iodine, mercury).[50] There were a few who objected to the arsenicals on the grounds that they were significantly toxic, and who vainly proposed substitute medications such as 'vamianine, the treatment of the future',[51] a 'vegeto-metallic' compound which brought together past remedies in a single dragée: depurative vegetable substances, mercury, gaiac, sarsaparilla (now known as 'salsepyl'), not to mention traces of gold and silver.

Since traditional therapy had proved to be inefficacious in the treatment of general paralysis, the malariatherapy recommended in 1917 by the Viennese psychiatrist Wagner von Jauregg appeared to be truly revolutionary. This treatment, which won its inventor the Nobel prize in 1927, consisted of injecting the patient with malaria (impaludation); it produced undeniable results, although there is still no explanation of how it works.

As for the Bordet-Wassermann test, it was increasingly accused – and with good reason – of being unreliable. One of its opponents, Dr Vernes, also known for his contributions to anti-syphilitic prophylaxis, proposed replacing it with, or at any rate supplementing it with, his own method: syphilometry. This rather complicated method of detection, which consisted in measuring differential reactions with the aid of a 'photometer', did not meet with the huge success which its promoter and a few supporters envisaged for it.[52] However, this method reveals the desire to bring to light, by frequent checks, a supposedly omnipresent syphilis thought to be associated with alcoholism, tuberculosis and even cancer because of its hereditary consequences.[53]

Inflationary statistics

The inter-war period (and especially the twenties) was marked by an intense thirst for statistics to chart the progress of syphilis in the aftermath of the First World War. In 1925 the Ministry of Health's Commission for Prophylaxis against Venereal Diseases issued figures which are astounding today: four million Frenchmen infected (one-tenth of the population), 20,000 children killed each year (and twice the number of abortions), 80,000 deaths, not to mention the indirect consequences of syphilis.[54] In 1929 the number of syphilitics in France was put at eight million, and it was calculated that syphilis had killed 1,500,000 Frenchmen in ten years, 'as many as the war in four years'.[55] The situation was judged to be even worse amongst the troops and the indigenous population in the colonies (in Senegal a doctor estimated that eight out of ten of the native population were syphilitics).[56]

Common sense suggests that these statistics are inflated, though undoubtedly the number of cases of syphilis which were detected and treated increased everywhere in the decade 1920–30, correlating with the increase in the activities of the dispensaries (see figure 1). But it is difficult to distinguish between new cases of syphilis and old cases brought to light by a better system of detection. Nonetheless, the increase in the number of cases was by no means uniformly distributed across the regions of France (see figure 2): more departments showed a decrease than showed an increase, although the latter were more densely populated. But if we add to the departments which showed an increase those in which the number of cases remained stable we are obliged to admit that, whatever the actual figures involved, syphilis was certainly not in decline, despite the intense prophylactic campaign which had been under way since the beginning of the century. This fact was all the more worrying given that other European countries were being rewarded for their efforts with a marked reduction in the number of cases.[57] Moreover, the short-term picture was somewhat different; in the Hôpital Saint-Louis, for example, the increase in the number of cases during the 1914–18 war was followed by a sharp decrease from 1921 onwards, then an upturn from 1924 to 1927 (similar fluctuations, interesting from the epidemiological standpoint, were observed in many provincial cities – Lyons, Marseilles, Bordeaux, Le Havre, Lille, Nancy, Strasbourg).

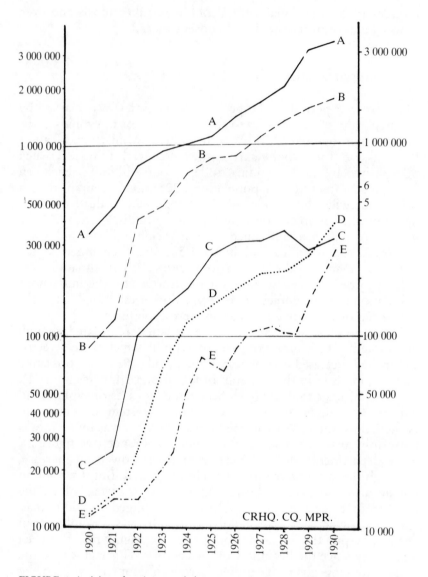

FIGURE 1 Activity of anti-venereal departments in France, 1920–1930. A: number of consultations at the anti-venereal departments; B: number of injections of arsenicals, bismuth or mercury administered; C: number of serological and bacteriological examinations performed by the laboratories; D: total number of consultations (including consultees free of disease; E: number of first-time consultees (including those free of disease).

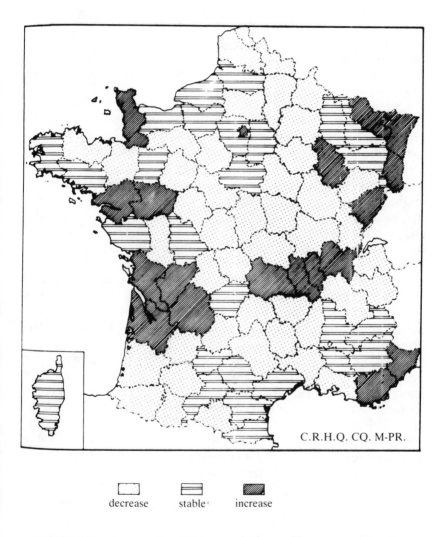

C.R.H.Q. CQ. M-PR.

decrease   stable'   increase

FIGURE 2 Development of syphilis in France, 1926–7 as compared with 1923–4.

In fact the question of the reliability of the statistics was already being raised. For one thing, medical practitioners were not keen to fill in the statistical returns. In 1927, for example, a medical enquiry on new cases of syphilis was sent to all doctors in every department of France (excepting Seine). Despite the enthusiasm for prophylaxis with which public authorities and doctors alike were imbued, and although the most eminent syphilologists and health-care specialists had agreed to act as departmental investigators, the number of responses obtained was very variable, and the information provided was often vague and imprecise. This was in defiance of a call to order which suggests that this lack of enthusiasm was nothing new: 'In conformity with the resolution adopted by the Health Congress of 1925, the attention of doctors has been drawn to the care with which they must fill in these statistics; exact figures are required, not approximations.'[58]

Similarly, people were beginning to call into question what one might call 'the great era of GPI'. There had been a tendency to see the insane (in mental asylums in particular) as general paralytics and to take abnormal children to be hereditary syphilitics, but there was a growing realization in the thirties that statistics should be seen in relative terms, if only because of the numerous cases of 'diluted GPI' and, more especially, because the majority of cases of general paralysis were of unknown origin. Moreover, Dr Ravaut's department at the Hôpital Saint-Louis identified only 318 cases of neurosyphilis in 6,113 records of syphilitics.[59] (GPI, furthermore, was much less frequent than tabes).[60]

These specific questions were overshadowed by the anguishing problem of how to eradicate syphilis from France, or at the very least, of how to maintain it at an acceptable level. However, the financial investment involved was considerable. It rose from 200,000 F in 1916 to 9,650,000 F in 1926 (and 15,370,000 F in 1942), which, despite inflation and an even more rapid increase in expenditure on the disabled and the insane, gives a good indication of the efforts which were being made.[61]

However, syphilologists continued to deplore the persistence of the epidemic of syphilis, putting the main blame on the ignorance and prudishness of sufferers, made easier by the absence of painful symptoms, which led them not to call on the doctor, and often to prefer the quack medicines offered in the newspapers. There were also those who believed themselves to be cured because their pox was no longer evident, and who visited their doctor only once, when the chancre appeared. These 'defectors from treatment' accounted for 60 to 70 per cent of those who came for consultation. The medical profession was also to blame to some extent, and specialists did not hesitate to point to the relative ignorance of certain doctors – or in some cases to the ill-will they bore towards the dispensaries, which they believed to be damaging their interests. Many doctors were also criticized for abandoning the arsphenamines (because they were difficult to inject and there was a risk of accidents), for which they substituted the less efficacious bismuth.

The statistics also began to register the influx of immigrants more and more frequently, the percentages in question ranging from 20 to 70, according to the dispensaries. (Noted, in descending order are the 'indigenes of North Africa' – who are the principal group – then Poles, Italians, and 'indigenes' of the colonies of black Africa and Indochina etc.) But the causal factor which was considered as being by far the most important element in the spread of syphilis remained prostitution, which genuinely upset doctors and the public authorities.

As far as England and the United States were concerned, William Pusey, professor of dermatology at the University of Illinois and former president of the American Dermatological Association, developed some very interesting theories in which statistics and moral judgements are closely combined:

The prevalence of syphilis among peoples and among classes is a matter of sexual habits. Sexual promiscuity is the source of syphilis, and the relative incidence of syphilis in any class is an index of its sexual habits. The occurrence of syphilis in an individual is not necessarily a stigma, for much of it, particularly in women, is contracted innocently, but a high incidence of syphilis in any class is a mark of low sexual morality. Because of factors which are obvious, the prevalence of syphilis varies widely in different statistics; from less than 1 per cent to 20 per cent or more of the population examined for syphilis. A large number of the more conservative statistics of Great Britain and the United States indicate that the incidence of syphilis is from 6 to 10 per cent . . . . When you analyse syphilis according to classes, most of them social, you get striking evidence of the relation between syphilis and sexual morality. In our civilization it is commonest, class for class, among those who lead the 'loosest' lives. One certain indictment that can be made to hold against the use of alcohol is that, by temporarily breaking down the moral resistance of those under its influence, it is a factor for the spread of all venereal diseases.[62]

But for Pusey this figure is only an average – a huge figure, admittedly, but one which should not lead us to overlook the fact that whereas the rate was only 0.5 per cent in the rural communities of the Middle West, for example, 15 per cent of criminals were syphilitics, as were 14 per cent to 20 per cent of blacks (negroes) examined by the Rosenwald Foundation, not forgetting, noblesse oblige, between 38 per cent and 100 per cent of confirmed prostitutes. A little further on, Pusey, carried away by his enthusiasm, puts the number of new cases in the United States at 871,000 per year!

'Continence and high moral character'

The medical – or, rather hygienic – attitudes prevalent in the thirties were not so very different from the imprecations hurled by the ultra-catholics of Louis XIV's time who refused to teach the general public to protect itself against the pox on the grounds that to do so would be to promote debauchery. There was only one solution, namely continence outside marriage (and, if possible, even within marriage, except for purposes of procreation). Girls might be cutting their hair short, throwing off their corsets, showing their knees and dancing the Charleston, but the medico-hygienic stance remained as repressive as ever as far as the moral implications of the anti-venereal struggle were concerned. We have seen this in practice in the fact that anti-syphilitic propaganda could only flower freely in the army (and not always there). It was felt to be imperative that girls of good breeding, be they English, American, French or German, should be kept outside all that. There was absolutely no question of transforming discussion into education.

As for working-class girls, destined by virtue of their origins to be of 'low sexual morality' (Pusey), they were to content themselves with avoiding contaminating the bourgeoisie. In *'Partir avant le jour'* Julien Green relates how his Uncle William died from syphilis as a consequence of his amorous adventures with the servants. More shocking than the disease itself was the fact that Uncle Willie, who was so good-looking, caught the pox by sleeping with his maidservant. Green's mother went so far as to make her son promise never to speak to any servant on his own. And, as we saw, the main cause of the father-in-law's indignation against his son-in-law in *'Les Avariés'* was that by transmitting to Henriette the pox contracted from a whore he had clandestinely introduced the plague of the lower classes into a bourgeois family ('this abject creature lives in us, it is in our family, he has brought it to sit at our hearth'). As for the family doctor, his moralizing role is made clear by the single question which he puts to the disgusted father-in-law, a question which is also the decisive argument of the play: 'Have you yourself never sinned?'

A great many doctors, unafraid to tread on what would now be considered very dangerous ground, responded to this highly evangelical notion that only he who is without sin is entitled to throw the first stone by saying that the solution is simply not to sin. Thus William Allen Pusey, the inventor of 'low sexual morality' and the defender (and not the only one) of the idea that there is an obvious correlation between 'syphilis and sexual morality', wrote that without seeking to minimize the effects of information and anti-syphilitic (and, more generally, anti-venereal) prophylaxis,

it surely makes for the reduction of venereal diseases to inculcate the importance of high standards of morality and the hygienic value, to say nothing of other things, of clean living. It is the duty of society to protect its youth and its young manhood and womanhood, as far as possible, from the temptations that arise from improper suggestions and surroundings and associates. It must be said that society as a whole makes no apparent effort in this direction. Rather its literature, drama, fashion of dress and social forms stimulate sex in every way that prurient ingenuity can devise. Society is derelict in that, but nevertheless the traditions of high living that prevail in the sober intelligent part of society and that result in high moral standards are now the only factors that have great effect upon the prevalence of syphilis. Continence is the only insurance against syphilis. Intelligence and high moral character are the best prophylactic measures that we have.[63]

Since sexual activity and venereal disease had become synonymous, the solution was continence, in spite of the thousand-and-one invitations to debauchery offered by modern life. Until only recently we could make fun of the attitude which prevailed from the appearance of syphilis at the very end of the fifteenth century to the end of the Second World War, and even beyond it. (From what point can we date the much-vaunted permissive society? The sixties? The seventies?) But what can we say now that AIDS has appeared? Admittedly no-one would ever again preach continence in the name of high moral character, but there remains continence inspired by fear. As for those who are without fear, it is because they lack imagination.

Vichy, or the dictatorship of prophylaxis

Despite the misfortunes which deluged France in 1940 – and perhaps even thanks to them – the hope welled up in certain quarters that there would be a new world, a world regenerated not only politically but morally and physically. It would be superfluous to dwell on the characteristics of the new French state which, trying to forget (and make others forget) the collaboration with the occupier, substituted for the motto 'Liberté, Égalité, Fraternité' the undeniably more constraining, even expiatory, one of 'Travail, Famille, Patrie'. These three watchwords signal a concern with the idea of *mens sana in corpore sano* which is very far removed from the former attachment to 'liberties' which had had such disastrous consequences. In such a context as this it was not surprising that syphilis was once more the focus of blame, especially considering the ultimately disappointing results of forty years of unrelenting prophylaxis.

In 1943, the darkest hour of the Occupation, optimism had vanished:

Syphilis alone kills 200,000 Frenchmen each year (in particular, a high proportion of infant mortality was attributed to it), peoples the asylums with madmen and the terminally ill, empties cradles and robs town and country of more than 300,000 births per year because it condemns to celibacy or childless marriage a huge number of procreators who have been badly informed because they have not received proper treatment. Even so, this has not prevented us from being inundated with degenerates.[64]

The key word here is 'degenerates': France has become a country of degenerates because, amongst other things, of syphilis (though also because of Jews and aliens). Of course, the Germans had managed to preserve themselves from syphilis, as Louise Hervieu, who was severely afflicted by hereditary syphilis and who became a passionate exponent of uncompromising prophylaxis,[65] clearly explains in the preface to *Que sais-je* (1942), dedicated to *Le Péril Vénérien*: 'However, those peoples who have reconquered their youth, and who include those who have punished us, had first purified themselves of the venereal scourge.'

A new age was dawning:

From afar, held back as I am by my infirmity, I imagine myself going up onto the terrace of the Rouen dermato-venereological centre [it was there that the author of the work thus prefaced worked before the war], there to see the coming of the age which the incurably ill, the suffering and the bedridden, those most wretched of all wretches, had paid for with their sufferings, which had been misunderstood and mocked . . . . At that time, in the bosom of a France which has been restored and healed, children will grow up beautiful and free, for syphilis, the old hereditary enemy, will have been vanquished for ever . . . . Master, you and those like you are preparing for the coming of a new world.[66]

Dr Payenneville, who was a little less exalted but rather more politic, wrote as follows:

Under the aegis of the Marshal who has so courageously undertaken to regenerate our Country we shall, we hope, also succeed in eliminating most of the factors in the propagation of the venereal diseases which have just been enumerated . . . . We are conscious of the fact that, having supported to the utmost the organization of the anti-venereal struggle in this country, we have made a substantial contribution to the work of rebuilding and regeneration of France, to which Marshal Pétain has dedicated himself with so much courage and self-denial.

With the arrival of a strong régime, numerous syphilologists (supporters of Pétain or otherwise) hoped to see the introduction of the set of strict regulations for which they had been pressing for a long time, all the more so since the war had necessarily brought about a recrudescence in the number of cases of syphilis.[67] Even before the installation of the Vichy régime, however, a statutory order dated 29 November 1939 was made in accordance with the special powers conferred on the Government (by the law of 19 March 1939, which in fact only granted these special powers for measures necessary for the defence of the realm). This order reorganized anti-venereal prophylaxis along very much stricter lines. Every doctor was to inform the victims of venereal disease they treated of the provisions of the decree in question, and alert the health authorities if it was judged that the patient was exposing others to contamination; any person against whom there were 'serious, definite and concurring presumptions' could be required by the health authorities to produce a medical certificate stating that they were not suffering from a contagious venereal disease; any woman who, knowing herself to be syphilitic, breastfed a child, and anyone who allowed a syphilitic child to be breastfed, would be punished by law; any person (prostitute or otherwise) who refused to go for treatment could be punished and forced by the tribunal to undergo treatment; in the fifth year of their studies, student doctors were required to take a practical course in an anti-venereal department, and so on.

The Vichy régime reinforced these new measures which, it must be observed, were taken at a time when the executive was more powerful. First there was article 4 of the law of 16 December 1942,[68] which required those who wished to be married to obtain, not more than one month before the marriage, a medical certificate attesting that each of the future spouses 'had been examined with a view to being married, and that no counterindications had been discovered' (the two tests performed from this date onwards were an X-ray of the lungs and a Bordet-Wassermann test). A law of 29 July 1943 extended these provisions to pregnant women undergoing prenatal tests.

In the United States, the prenuptial examination (once again, the Bordet-Wassermann test) was introduced in Connecticut in 1935 in order to track down the sinister treponema. Other states quickly followed this example, encouraging future spouses with posters

('Get full medical examination for VD before marriage'). As regards prenatal detection of syphilis, the state of New York introduced it in 1938 ('Baby health bill'). At the same period, mass detection was attempted in Chicago, and large-scale publicity campaigns were used. The American Social Hygiene Association and the various health associations, of course, regarded these measures as a guarantee of future victory over syphilis.

To return to Vichy France, it was the law of 31 December 1942 'relating to prophylaxis and the struggle against the venereal diseases'[69] which was most important in reinforcing the provisions of the order of 29 November 1939, though it did not in fact refer to it. The treatment of any person afflicted with the symptoms of contagious venereal diseases was made obligatory; it was also made obligatory for the health authorities to declare, either preserving anonymity or not, if the venereal patient refused to start or pursue treatment, if he or she caused others to run a serious risk of contamination, or if he or she was involved in prostitution. Moreover, any doctor who did not seek out the agent of the contamination was to be fined.[70]

These diverse measures naturally raised the question of medical confidentiality. A stringent anti-syphilitic prophylaxis and an effective set of health regulations had been constantly limited, as we have seen, by the absolute necessity of professional confidentiality, even so far as relations were concerned – article 378 of the penal code punishing doctors, surgeons, pharmacists, midwives, etc. who did not respect this confidentiality. Too bad if the patient's interests conflicted with those of society at large. Doctors therefore strictly respected medical confidentiality, even though, from its introduction, the Penal Code made provisions for exceptions (article 378: enumeration of sanctions 'except in cases where the law requires them to declare the facts').

However, a new law (that of 29 November 1939) authorized every doctor to alert the health authorities if he had evidence that a venereal patient was putting one or more individuals at risk of contamination. Hence the modification of article 378 ('except in cases where the law requires them to declare the facts'). However, it was the Vichy régime which most eroded the guarantee of medical confidentiality, and, interestingly enough, it did it in the name of the Order of Doctors, which it had itself founded, and one of whose principal functions was precisely that of encouraging respect for medical codes of conduct. In fact the law of 31 December 1941 modified and completed the law of 7 October 1940 instituting the Order of Doctors: article 2 'Doctors formally entered on a departmental roll of the Order of Doctors are released from the professional confidentiality introduced by article 378 of the Penal Code vis-à-vis the Supreme Council and the Departmental Councils of the Order of Doctors as regards all declarations or depositions made to these bodies.'

There were other proposals for strict prophylactic measures against venereal diseases. With the exception of the struggle, which had begun before the war and was as yet unsuccessful, to make medical records compulsory ('we should have a man's pedigree, just as we have that of a racehorse'),[71] and to exclude syphilitics from medical cover (or, at least, those who had voluntarily exposed themselves to the disease), it was the idea of making contamination a crime which was taken up again with most vigour under the Vichy régime.

As early as 1870 Dr Armand Desprès wrote:

In the act of the transmission of syphilis, whatever the place and the time in which it occurs, whatever the moral circumstances of the individuals who contract this virulent disease, there remains the moral fact that an individual is communicating to his fellow man a series of ills and misfortunes without the letter's consent, and that these are for him an unanticipated catastrophe. An individual is sick, he knows himself to be sick, he is well aware how he has contracted his illness and how it can be transmitted, his doctor has given him all the appropriate warnings but he neglects them and, quite remorselessly, there being no danger of punishment, he knowingly exposes those from whom he conceals his state to infection. He is thus committing a crime, a crime against health, in other words, other people's lives.[72]

Whence the idea of a law (which some people nowadays would like to see introduced in respect of AIDS) making the offence of knowingly transmitting a contagious disease punishable by between six months and two years in prison.

The following was one of the resolutions of the 1887 sub-commission on the 'regulation of prostitution in Paris':

We must, for example, punish, or seek to punish those truly loathsome people who, scorning all morality and even railing at the wise counsels of science, have no compunction about knowingly infecting their fellows, be they husbands or lovers, wives or mistresses. And the husband who infects his wife is doubly vile, since his first victims are often their children . . . . Therefore we would like this crime to be punished in all cases, and most severely [introducing the idea that 'the knowing transmission of syphilis constitutes a crime].[73]

We find the same preoccupations thirty years later, in 1933:

Protection from syphilis would therefore be easy, and syphilis would disappear in a very short space of time if it were not that we are dealing with men and women, that is to say careless, undisciplined, wicked and perverse beings who would not conform to rules for the preservation of public health were it not for the constraints of the law. And we would undoubtedly have made infinitely greater progress towards stamping out syphilis in France if the medical profession had had the support of the law – if treatment had had a penal sanction as a corollary in cases of refusal to conform![74]

A parliamentary bill had already been proposed in 1924 and, in 1903, the civil tribunals of the Seine had decided in favour of a request to make a contaminator liable for damages. But on the eve of the Second World War there was still no defence against the 'dispensary deserters', and health workers had to winkle them out of their homes by their persuasive powers alone.

In the end, contamination was never made a crime in France, even under the Vichy régime. This may seem astonishing considering the general desire to improve anti-venereal prophylaxis, and considering that it had been made a crime in many European states – Denmark, Sweden, Czechoslovakia, 'Soviet Russia'.[75] Belgium, in the lead as ever, extended the crime of contamination to procurers (with a seven-year prison sentence) – which led a Belgian minister to remark: 'We have no more pimps, they have all left for Paris!'[76] But this brings us back once again to the question of prostitution.

9

The Pox and the Prostitute

Regulationism

As we have seen, the role played by prostitutes in the transmission
of syphilis was emphasized from the moment the disease appeared
in Europe. Up until the time of the Revolution, however,
prostitutes got away rather lightly, apart from those who were sent
to the general hospitals or the beggars' prisons. Under the
Consulate, though, the measured and pragmatic repression of the
Ancien Régime was to give way to the *police sanitaire* which Restif
de la Bretonne had suggested in 1769.

In fact it was a decree of the government of 5 Brumaire of the
year IX (27 October 1800) which first made it compulsory for
police officers to 'supervise brothels and those who reside there or
who are found there, and to furnish the means of preventing and
containing contagious diseases'.[1] The obligatory registration of
prostitutes in 1802 and the quasi-official organization of brothels
two years later completed what from this time onwards can be
described as 'the vice squad'. From now on it was a matter of
regulating prostitution, that practice recognized as a necessary evil
in Augustinian thought ('Eliminate prostitution and the world will
be overturned by passions; treat prostitutes as honest women and
the universe will be blighted by infamy and dishonour').[2] In
consequence, regulated brothels ('the keystone of any special
policing') became numerous during the Empire and the Restoration.[3]
'Regulated brothels,' wrote Cullerier in 1821, 'are tolerated and
organized by the authorities to prevent the seduction of honest
women.'[4]

Those who supported regulatory controls lacked a theoretician
who could link moral considerations with sanitary and administrative
ones. They found one in Parent-Duchatelet, who in 1836 brought

out his work: *De la prostitution dans la ville de Paris, considérée sous le rapport de l'hygiène publique, de la morale et de l'administration*,[5] which was to have an enormous influence in the nineteenth century. The most serious, most dangerous and most fearsome of contagious diseases is syphilis, maintains Parent-Duchatelet.[6] Our forefathers did nothing to arrest its progress, whereas we struggle at great expense against epidemics which may be more spectacular but which are no more dangerous. The main propagators of syphilis are prostitutes. It is therefore right that they should be subjected to medical examinations, whether they like it or not. 'Are prostitutes entitled to do whatever they want? In other words, can we, must we, deprive prostitutes of (their) individual freedom? . . . They make themselves unworthy of that freedom by abandoning themselves to their unbridled passions and all the excesses of a dissolute life. Freedom in this case amounts to licentiousness, and licentiousness destroys society.' Prostitutes therefore have no claim to individual freedom ('they have abdicated their rights'). They must be governed by a special law. But this law does not exist. Unlike the Lieutenant General of Police under the Ancien Régime, the Prefect of Police has no power to punish people on the spot, laments Parent-Duchatelet.

In short, prostitutes are a race apart, and only regulation of their professional activities can ensure that they remain in the marginal position appropriate to them.[7] Numerous studies during the period attempted to define the characteristics of this marginal state. Prostitutes had different moral standards, of course (Parent-Duchatelet sketched out a whole anthropological study of the prostitute based on her *modus operandi*: street whore, soldiers' whore, 'fille en numéro', etc.),[8] but they also differ psychologically, being debauched to a degree bordering on mental derangement.[9] Whilst other writers went so far as to wonder whether there was some physical peculiarity in the sexual organs of prostitutes,[10] syphilologists noted that in prostitutes and those who frequent them

the depravity of the senses has become so universal . . . that vaginal coitus is almost an exception for them; hence the pressing need for the visiting doctor to examine the mouth, anus, armpits, etc. as well as the vulvo-uterine passage. The areas between the fingers and the toes, and the hair, can also provide important evidence. In short, no external regions can be overlooked, for the venereal virus, like certain dogmatic beliefs, rules everywhere and nowhere.[11]

It was around 1798 (?), Parent-Duchatelet informs us, that the idea of subjecting the prostitutes of Paris to a medical examination was first thought of. A first 'dispensaire de salubrité' was set up in

December 1802, but produced no results. It was reorganized in 1810, under the aegis of the Prefecture of Police. Inspections could be made at the dispensary (twice monthly), at a police station, or even in a regulated brothel. The systematic inspection of prostitutes or of girls suspected of being prostitutes who spent the night at the station for one reason or another had the advantage of enabling the monitoring of a large number of unregistered prostitutes. But we should have no illusions about this form of monitoring, since the average distribution of examinations performed in the early 1830s was as follows: 43 per cent in the dispensaries, 53 per cent in regulated brothels, and only 4 per cent at the police stations. As for the total number of examinations, it rose during the same period to nearly 100,000 per year, reaching 155,897 in 1854, a number which even Parent-Duchatelet himself considered prodigious. It was certainly a huge number considering that, on the admission of the administration itself, many unregistered prostitutes, and even registered prostitutes, escaped inspection.

Leaving these figures aside, there was unanimous agreement in the middle of the century that the keystone of regulation should be the registration of as many prostitutes as possible, whether they operated from a regulated brothel or not, based on an obligatory periodic medical examination.[12] However, even if in certain places these proposals had been anticipated,[13] the medical examination which was at the heart of regulationism often left a good deal to be desired. We will be returning to the key issue of the prostitutes who avoided this examination. However, its effectiveness was cast into doubt by Ricord himself in 1838. The speculum, which the prostitutes of the Maghreb poetically called 'the government's penis',[14] and which Ricord considered to be an indispensable 'instrument of medical control' was not used systematically. Ricord also criticized the frequency of the examinations:

If examinations of prostitutes, using the speculum or not, are to furnish any sort of guarantee they must be repeated at least every three days, for I have found by experience that on the third day, and sometimes even the second day, following infection the pus of the chancre is contagious. Given this one can appreciate how dangerous and inadequate the examinations are; in Paris, prostitutes 'en carte' who live alone are examined once a month, and those who operate from brothels once a week![15]

On the same subject and at the same period, Parent-Duchatelet points out an unexpected obstacle to the medical examination. The examination was performed on a sort of table, rather similar to the modern gynaecological table.

According to all the doctors I have consulted on this matter, the advantages of this table are undeniable, particularly so when the speculum needs to be used to complete the examination; it allows doctors to make a close examination of the state of the anus, and in particular of the groin, whose sensitivity can often indicate to experts the presence of various irritations of the neck of the uterus or of deep-seated local vaginitis. Despite the advantages of this apparatus it has been impossible to use it in the dispensary for a very singular reason. Many harlots wear hats, and the fear of crumpling them by lying flat on their backs would have obliged them to assume a posture that was uncomfortable for them and which prevented a thorough examination. Had this drawback been ignored they would inevitably have been put off the dispensary, and the number of recalcitrants and unregistered prostitutes would have increased. It has therefore been necessary to make do with a raised chair with a back which is greatly reclined, but not sufficiently high to restrict the movements of the head and neck.

This one anecdote gives an insight into the gulf which separated the strongly-voiced principles of regulationism from their application in practice.

The hospital

At the beginning of the nineteenth century, when the debate about regulationism was unfolding, prostitutes with venereal diseases could only be hospitalized with the greatest difficulty, for the hospitals refused to admit this category of patients just as they had refused to hospitalize the first pox-victims at the very end of the fifteenth century. A special department for prostitutes was set up at the Hôpital des Vénériens in 1811 and at Saint-Louis in the following year.[16] With the increase in venereal diseases due to the occupation of Paris in 1814, the Prison de la Petite Force was hastily converted back into a hospital which evoked the gloomiest days of Bicêtre. This anticipated what Parent-Duchatelet was to explicitly formulate: a symbiosis of the prison and the hospital.

During the July monarchy, the hospitalization-imprisonment of prostitutes was clearly evident in Paris with the specialization of the venereal hospitals – men at the Hôpital du Midi (the former hospital for venereal victims),[17] so-called 'civilian' women at the Hôpital de Lourcine,[18] and prostitutes at Saint-Lazare. Much has been written about Saint-Lazare which was dreaded by prostitutes until its demolition in 1940. Saint-Lazare was a leper-colony in the Middle Ages, a convent and work-house belonging to the priests of the Mission from 1632 onwards (we are reminded of des Grieux's escape), and an ante-chamber for the guillotine during the Terror (André Chénier awaited death there); from the time of the

Consulate onwards it became a women's prison with an entrance at the top of the Rue du Faubourg-Saint-Denis. In 1836 an infirmary was added to it, and this gradually became the prison-hospital of Saint-Lazare of sinister repute. At the end of the nineteenth century it consisted of two main sections, the judicial section in which the condemned and the accused could be treated in an infirmary which included a maternity wing and a venereological department, and the administrative section consisting of the Special Infirmary with its 300 beds.[19] It was here that registered and, more especially, unregistered prostitutes were forcibly sent when they had been arrested by the vice squad and found to be sick. Chancres and secondary symptoms of syphilis rubbed shoulders with other venereal afflictions: soft chancres, vulval and anal growths, metritis and, of course, gonorrhoea.

Apart from the administration of mercury and potassium iodide, the régime at Saint-Lazare was that of the toughest prison: appalling food, no heating whatsoever, forced labour, lamentable hygiene and a mixture of strict confinement and promiscuity (particularly in the upper floors of the old convent) which increasingly gave Saint-Lazare the reputation of a school of vice. Inadequately 'blanched' of their pox (a practice which Alfred Fournier vehemently criticized), prostitutes were released, but barely had they crossed the threshold before they were rounded up by recruiters for the regulated brothels, who put them beyond the reach of the vice squad.

In the provinces the situation was more confused, for every town was different. In Lyons, prostitutes with venereal diseases were locked away in the beggars' prison at the end of the eighteenth century. In 1803 the Superintendent of Police of the town 'was the first to perceive and proclaim the pressing necessity of suppressing prostitution, that hotbed of syphilis. He contributed to the creation of the Hospice de l'Antiquaille, of which he continued to be one of the most generous benefactors; he outlined the first regulations for the inspection of prostitutes.'[20] From 1806 to 1809 there were no less than 2,000 admissions of patients with venereal diseases, 50 per cent of whom were prostitutes. Although it is no longer possible to regard the term 'venereal' as synonymous with 'syphilitic' it nonetheless appears that syphilis accounted for a large number of these cases. In 1810, in fact, the doctor of this establishment stated that 'syphilis had spread to such an extent that the hospice could no longer meet all requests for admission; often when a prostitute was declared ill she was left to languish in prison until there was a vacant place for her.'[21] Patients were pinpointed by 'health visits' to the regulated brothels of the town, whose numbers fluctuated between fifty and seventy-five during the first decades of the nineteenth century.

In Bordeaux a dispensary service was set up next door to the hospital for venereal victims, and the general inspection of all prostitutes was entered in police records. From this time onwards there was a collaboration between the authorities, who ensured that the establishment worked properly, and the medical profession, which supplied assistant surgeons from the nearby hospital. The examinations were monthly, free, and compulsory. They were performed regularly from 1830 onwards, and from 1855 they were made bi-monthly. The dispensary doctors also visited prostitutes who had been arrested (by the ordinary police) in the town hall prison. 'One can understand,' wrote the dispensary doctor,

the necessity of such a measure, which has long been considered essential to public health. It must be acknowledged, in fact, that by this means alone can we hope to reduce the ever-growing number of cases of syphilis in women whose vice and poverty has set them outside society. This fact justifies the arbitrariness of the means, and makes them an inescapable necessity for the administration, given the toleration of well-regulated prostitution.[22]

In Strasbourg venereal diseases were treated in the public hospital in a department which

occupies a special isolated building; the ground floor is for men afflicted with the pox and cutaneous diseases, and the first floor is for women. Registered prostitutes with the pox are kept separately under lock and key. A second department houses prostitutes with cutaneous diseases and syphilis. For ten or more years two Sisters of Charity have run this department, and they have been of great use. Cleanliness, order and decency reign throughout, and the prostitutes rarely behave dishonestly towards the Sisters. The department dedicated to the former consists of three spacious and airy rooms, and can take forty or so beds. Unfortunately this number is too low; mostly it is necessary to have ten or so beds on the floor.[23]

Setting aside the forced optimism of these reports, sanitary conditions seem to have been very mediocre, particularly in small towns. In Nancy, Spillmann denounced the deplorable conditions in which prostitutes with venereal diseases were treated at the Maison du Bon Secours.[24] In an enquiry held in 1887, Bourneville, a psychiatrist at Bicêtre, criticized the lamentable organization of the department for victims of venereal disease at the Hôtel-Dieu de Saint-Étienne, d'Épernay, de Chateau-Thierry, de Belfort, etc.[25] Of course, the anti-clericalism of the author of these reports gives us grounds to suspect that he may have painted a particularly black picture.

In England, the Lock Hospital in London, opened in 1747,

admitted 44,973 victims of venereal disease between this date and 1836; the author who gives these statistics[26] expresses regret that the number of them who were syphilitics is not stated. At any rate, the large number of prostitutes is emphasized, as is the number of soldiers. The other London hospitals (notably Guy's and St Bartholomew's) are infested with these prostitutes with venereal diseases, whose numbers no regulations or police measures restrain. The number of beds occupied in the English capital remains a constant 500. As for the prostitutes who roam the streets or haunt the brothels while waiting to run aground in hospital, they are calculated to number no less than 13,000 (*The Lancet*).[27]

In any case, the prostitute was condemned to the hospital. It was this fate which Charles-Louis Philippe evoked in *Bubu de Montparnasse*, that masterpiece, if not archetype, of populist literature.[28] In 1898 he met Maria Texier, and began a liaison which he recounts in his novel.

Tired of her existence as an unemployed worker she wants to become a prostitute. To some extent she already is one, but she wants to go into it in a big way . . . . How I remonstrated with her! I told her about the vice squad, about syphilis, and above all of how wretched her old age would be. Her arguments were always stronger than mine: the vice squad leaves women in silk dresses alone, for they may have powerful protectors. People don't die of syphilis. As for old age, my little Maria had no desire to live beyond forty.[29]

The inevitable happened: 'You will not be surprised to hear,' wrote Philippe to the same friend a month later, 'that the poor girl I told you about caught syphilis in the course of the wild life she has been leading lately. This poor child of twenty-one leaves hospital, falls ill again, and is soon back there. It will go on like this until she dies'.

In preparation for his novel, Philippe gathered documentary evidence, entered brothels and visited Saint-Lazare and Lourcine: 'I went recently to the Hôpital de Lourcine, and I saw many, many of them, young and old. Syphilis everywhere.' These studies are reflected in *Bubu* when Louis Buisson tries to open the eyes of his friend Pierre Hardy, who still harbours illusions as to the nature of the disease which has struck Berthe, the young prostitute with whom he has fallen in love:

I used to go to the Hôpital Broca where one of my old schoolfriends was an extern. I have seen all the whores being examined with the speculum, and what diseases they have. I have seen the local ladies laughing because they have been told 'The pox is nothing; you take pills for three years.' I have seen women who have had the pox for eighteen months tearfully burying their heads in their hands and saying 'I shall never be cured.' The doctors console them by bursting out laughing. I have seen old women spreading their legs like animals. They are so accustomed to being ill-used that they make not a murmur of complaint.

Jean Lorrain, who enjoyed frequenting the seediest parts of Paris and describing 'the magnificent decay of Paris in 1900' (Hubert Juin),[30] conjures up in *Monsieur de Phocas* the atmosphere of the hospital: 'She was at the Ospedale, in the venereal department, in the oppressive atmosphere of a large ward with whitewashed walls, its windows burnished by the sunlight of a most beautiful afternoon. She was lying amidst the off-white hospital sheets, and her auburn hair, spread out on her pillows, made her yellowish syphilitic face seem even more sallow'.

Fifty years later, with the arrival of the medical novel, these scenes of the dispensary or the hospital were still enormously popular, though it was the surgeon rather than the syphilologist (who was now beginning to be called a venereologist) who was in the spotlight. In Maxence van der Meersch's *Corps et âmes*,[31] a novel revolving around life in a hospital, the great medical issues of the forties are dramatized. There is tuberculosis and the 'san', of course, (the author was to die of tuberculosis), the introduction of X-rays, the routine removal of the tonsils and, rather discreetly, syphilis. There is a bit of GPI here, some babies with hereditary syphilis there, and, of course, the classic tableau of the ward of syphilitic prostitutes:

The prostitutes, naked to the waist, their breasts heavy and flaccid, lowered their heads fearfully and shiftily and continued to wash, to tuck up their skirts, to pass scraps of soapy towels under their nightdresses, without replying. This was the eyesore of the hospital, the most difficult ward to handle. They often arrived drunk. Sister Angélique often had to force them into bed with a few slaps across the face. Moreover, certain of these syphilitics were covered with purulent eczema. It was Sister Amélie, a tiny girl not much more than twenty years of age, who undertook to wash their sores.

The genre of the medical novel, crude in style but of irreproachable morality, reached its height at the end of the forties with *Les hommes en blanc* by André Sourbiran. This stream-of-consciousness novel, which was an enormous publishing success, mentions syphilis, particularly insofar as it destroys Love with a capital 'L'. The junior doctor describes how he was bombarded with anti-syphilitic propaganda during his adolescence (the film *Le baiser qui tue* had particularly terrified him), then his initial training seeing women in the dispensary, the examination table ('the deep and disquieting trap of which the speculum gave a glimpse . . . the visceral side of beauty'), the sessions of anti-syphilitic injections: 'There there were none but syphilitics, two hundred perhaps, waiting their turn to go into a cubicle and receive, behind the white curtain, their dose of arsenic, mercury or bismuth; my previous terror returned, for although there were old prostitutes with raucous voices in this crowd there were also many young faces which seemed so pure and innocent, and which concealed their corruption so well.'[32]

'Treponema machine-guns

No-one at the time would have questioned the extent of the links between the pox and prostitution. Since before the Revolution, but especially during the nineteenth century and the first half of the twentieth century, prostitution was considered to be the most important factor in the transmission of syphilis, particularly when people began to become obsessed with the venereal peril on the eve of the Belle Époque. A revealing story is related in the Goncourts' *Journal*. Two senior officials are debating whether or not to wear their decorations to the brothel. One says no. The other says yes, because that way you get women who don't have the pox.

Neisser, who twenty years earlier had discovered the causative agent of gonorrhoea, was one of the many who asserted that prostitution is the source of all instances of venereal contamination. Few whores escape the pox.[33] The estimated percentage of prostitutes who were syphilitic varied between 30 and 70 according to the time, the place, and the generosity of the statisticians; but from this point onwards there was a tendency to argue that every prostitute would inevitably be infected with syphilis after a certain number of years.[34] It was this which led a syphilologist just after the 1914–1918 war to describe prostitutes as 'treponema machine-guns'.

But can this conviction (the image of a triangle formed by prostitution, sex and the disease) be supported by the figures? In this domain more than in any other, statistics must be treated with caution, for they range from obvious underestimates to gross overestimates. Nonetheless, an administrative enquiry in 1869 demonstrated the extent of the problem: nearly 9,000 syphilitic prostitutes left French hospitals in 1864.[35]

Let us confine our attention to those few statistical enquiries which do not seek to demonstrate at any price that every prostitute is a syphilitic. A survey of 1,000 venereal victims entering Saint-Lazare for the first time between 1890 and 1900[36] reveals, in addition to the youth of the great majority of them (between seventeen and twenty years of age), an interesting distribution of venereal diseases: 651 cases of gonorrhoea, 36 of soft chancre and 421 of syphilis (some prostitutes having at least two of these afflictions). Although as regards syphilis this was less than the extreme advocates of regulationism maintained, it is nonetheless a considerable number.[37] If we reflect on these figures, as did two doctors in Lyons in 1936, we can see that there is a very high risk of contamination for a prostitute, who in a period of ten years may have intercourse 20,000 or 30,000 times ('a tidy sum, which certainly makes one think', they remarked).[38]

Not surprisingly, numerous practitioners comment on the fatalism of prostitutes on being told that they have contracted syphilis; and, indeed, the fact that they were 'pickled' represented a certain sort of liberation for a number of them, like 'being tattooed, having been in prison, knowing how to play belote or waltz back to front.'[39] The same author notes that whores were much more upset to be told that they had crabs.

Clients, however, were less philosophical, and it was important that a brothel should not be thought to be tainted with the pox. In *La maison Philibert*, for example, the brothel-keeper relates that after his house had been put out of bounds by the local clergy he received the *coup de grace*: 'One of my lady-boarders caught smallpox, and died of it in hospital, which dealt me the final blow. It was put about that my girls were infected. It was *small*pox . . . but in our business, names associated with unpleasant diseases put clients off.'[40]

This brings us back to that vein of literature in which the pox and prostitution are associated on every page, though not constituting the principal theme. A few decades earlier, naturalism would have been more discreet, and one would have searched in vain for traces of syphilis in Nana. But although the word itself is not used, the idea of the contaminating courtesan (in the widest sense) is nonetheless the main theme of Zola's novel.[41] In the drawings of his contemporary, Félicien Rops, on the other hand, the prostitute is much more clearly an allegory of syphilis. Behind the heavy makeup and the already toothless smile stand the she-demon, the death's head . . . Between the thighs of this woman who offers herself outstretched slips death with the long wings of a vampire, avidly licking her sex with its red tongue.[42]

There is no allegory in *Bubu de Montparnasse*, however, since, as we have seen, Charles-Louis Philippe wrote it as an authentic documentary on prostitution and syphilis. Berthe, a young prostitute, once thought that she would escape syphilis, just as one of her clients, the unfortunate hero of this desolate novel, once nurtured the equally vain delusion that he would make her love him and save her from her miserable plight. But ineluctable syphilis arrives on the scene to, as it were, put things in order. Berthe is forced to entrust herself to her pimp, nicknamed Bubu. Stunned, the latter wanders the streets aimlessly:

The terrible word struck him like a thunderbolt as he was striding along, and resounded, beating time to his step like a black drum. The pox, Berthe and the pox! He felt it at his side, like a red and blood-spattered companion, like an unbelievably savage master . . . . He remembered its learned name: syphilis. Implacable science, which names and dissects our ills – it filled him with fear because it throws us into hospital, because it sees us for what we are, because it cuts up our lives with its words and instruments as if we were nothing but flesh, disease and death.

But Bubu pulls himself together. You don't drop a woman because she has the pox, he is told by Grand Jules, a more experienced pimp who is surprised that Bubu hasn't already had it. They drink absinthe. Then Bubu goes off to make love to Berthe, who is highly contagious, in an infernal communion. Jules has convinced him, it is high time to catch the pox. Later, Berthe has to go to hospital and Bubu, short of money, attempts a burglary which lands him in prison. After her discharge, Berthe has to manage on her own.

She had syphilis. At that time she had a bad pain in her mouth, and I expect that all her kisses carried syphilis. Many had succumbed in this way. In hospital she said to herself, 'I don't know what I'm going to do, for I can't give my disease to other people.' She left. During her first days she thought 'I will tell him: wash yourself thoroughly.' But she had to make a living, and you can't keep feeling pity day after day. When she had been walking for a long time the paving stones became hard and she was weighed down as if with a heap of cobbles or of hearts of stone. She thought: Someone gave it to me.

In a letter to a friend (15 February 1899), Charles-Louis Philippe revealed his conclusion whilst he was still in the process of drafting his novel:

I am continuing my studies of prostitution. Have I told you that I am going to write a novel on the subject when I have finished my book on Mother? What I have discovered is appalling. Syphilis, alcoholism and villainy are daily phenomena in the lives of more than 50,000 Parisian women . . . . A prostitute, my friend, is often a poor chaste creature chosen by Destiny to do evil. She is no longer herself, but an instrument of Destiny. Every prostitute has syphilis, and generally catches it soon after entering the profession. Then she walks the street at night, laughing to attract men and give them her disease.

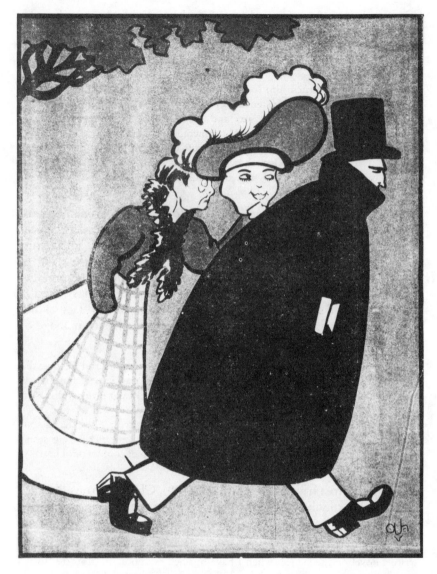

PLATE 19   Drawing by André Hellé which appeared in 'L'Assiette au beure' on 21 March, 1908, entitled 'the mask of sensual delight'. Behind the mask of the streetwalker is the true face of poverty and venereal disease. (Bibliothèque Municipale de Caen)

Countermeasures

Regulationists focused their attention almost exclusively on the institution of the brothel, the ideal being to confine all prostitutes, or at least the great majority, within brothels. But it gradually became clear that this worked only on paper. For one thing, the brothels were far from being as 'clean' as was claimed. Sanitary inspections were cursory,[43] insufficiently frequent (as Ricord had already observed), and, above all, they were of dubious value because the inmates came and went so frequently and did not follow a sustained course of treatment.[44]

But there is worse to come. Just before a sanitary inspection the madam would spirit away whores who were sick, and in particular those with syphilis. Or sometimes a healthy prostitute brought in from outside would be substituted for one who was sick – the doctor, for whom the brothel would often be the fifth or sixth he had visited that day, would be incapable of recognizing who was who. Moreover, venereal diseases could be disguised. The madam, who by this time had become quite wily, would often anticipate the official visit by making her own inspection or bringing in a midwife, or even a medical student prepared to break the rules. It was, of course, the madam who had to pay for hospitalization. But with a slightly astringent injection of red an inflamed vagina could be restored to its normal pale pink. A few chocolate pastilles could mask buccal ulcerations, and in the case of vaginal ulceration the doctor could be made to believe that the prostitute was having her period by the application of bull's blood. There were even better tricks: a few scraps of sheep's intestine cleverly stuck on and coloured with carmine would hide a chancre.[45] (Of course, it was important that the doctors performing the examination did not look too closely; but, as numerous syphilologists complained, they did not). 'Finally,' adds a practitioner from Lille,[46] 'if any persistent and over-sticky mucus remains at the neck of the womb they adroitly clean up the affected areas; this is called "the handkerchief trick", and all the experts know it. It should also be pointed out that Madame is a dab hand with the speculum, and very dexterous with the nitrate crayon. (Sometimes she actually causes damage, which serves her right!)'

These same 'filles à numéro'[47] who were so adept at concealing their venereal diseases to fool the doctor and, alas, the client knew the complementary trick of feigning scabies or a chancre (by applying a piece of caustic potassium to the genital organs) when they had been put in prison and wanted to be sent to the infirmary so as not to be separated from a girl-friend.[48] Lesbianism – something which Parent-Duchatelet dreaded even more than syphilis – was rife in brothels.

Thus it was the prostitutes working in brothels, who by definition should have been subject to the most rigorous prophylactic regulations, who were particularly adept at avoiding them – even

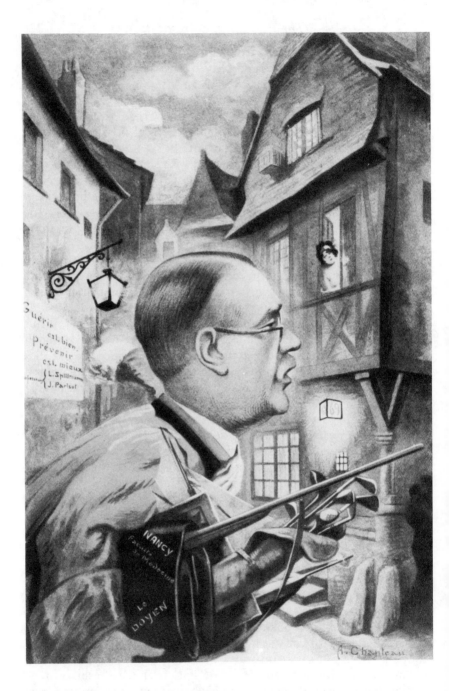

PLATE 20 Dr Spillmann, founder of the model dispensary at Nancy in the early twenties and apostle of anti-syphilitic prophylaxis, declared war on prostitutes. Here we see him mounting an assault on a *'maison à gros numéro'*. (Caricature in *Chanteclair*; private collection)

though sanitary examinations took place weekly from the beginning of the twentieth century onwards. As for the prostitutes who, though registered with the 'bureau de moeurs', did not operate from a brothel (they were called 'filles en carte'), they were subjected (again at the beginning of the twentieth century) to two sanitary examinations per month, or four if they were syphilitic. Unlike their fellow 'filles à numéro', who were inspected at their place of work, 'filles en carte' had to attend a dispensary – where, it might be supposed, trickery would be less successful. Moreover, the card which they had to present whenever the authorities required it made it possible to ensure that visits were made regularly.

But the brothels had to contend with a more serious form of competition, namely 'undeclared' whores (as opposed to 'declared' ones like the 'filles à numéro' and the 'filles en carte'). The regulations had scarcely been introduced before Gisquet, a former Prefect of Police, denounced what was eventually to prove the ruin of the system:

It was principally those of the lower sort, those known as soldiers' girls, who plied their shameful trade without restraints. Far from the places where the inspectors usually operated, it was easy for them to sidestep the police regulations. However, this group, who were frequently accessories to wrongdoing, required rigorous surveillance more than any other, in the interests of safety and public health; a huge proportion of these wretched creatures – known by the police as undeclared prostitutes, in other words unregistered and thus not subject to medical examinations – were infected with syphilis. At a conservative estimate more than a one-third of them had this disease.[49]

Soon everyone was denouncing the fact that an ever-growing band of clandestine prostitutes was defying the regulations. In 1826 in Lyons (ten years before the seminal work of Parent-Duchatelet) after a particularly acute period of unemployment 180 venereal victims were hospitalized in three months, two-thirds of whom were young clandestine prostitutes.[50] In Bordeaux in 1837 the department of venereal diseases recorded that twice as many undeclared as declared prostitutes visited for treatment:

It is now easy to point to the real home of syphilis in Bordeaux. If all the prostitutes who swarm in public meeting places could be subjected to a general examination it could be proved that the cruellest symptoms of the venereal disease are to be found amongst the large and dangerous clientele of the so-called *maisons de Passe* . . . . It is there that the syphilitic venom, protean in its forms and hydrophobic in its virulence, is engendered and communicated; it is there and only there that the shameful propaganda of vice and the appalling theory of the poisoning of society run riot, hidden and unpunished.[51]

At the end of the nineteenth century the problem became so worrying that it formed one of the main topics considered at the international congress on dermatology and syphilology which was held in Paris in 1889. At this congress speakers denounced the unchecked spread of syphilis amongst clandestine prostitutes who, according to some syphilologists, constituted more than 90 per cent of Parisian prostitutes![52] They complained that prostitutes avoided visiting the dispensaries at all so as to avoid being registered (which was automatic as soon as they were caught by the vice squad), and that it was they who had the highest incidence of syphilis. A statistical enquiry undertaken by the City of Paris Health Clinic produced the figures shown in table 1.[53]

Table 1 Distribution of syphilis between declared and undeclared prostitutes, Paris

	Declared prostitutes with syphilis (%)	Undeclared prostitutes with syphilis (%)
1859 to 1868	12	22.9
1869 to 1878	6.2	16
1879 to 1888	3.22	16.4

We can see here that although the number of cases of syphilis in declared prostitutes decreased (these statistics naturally served the cause of those who favoured regulation), the number of cases amongst undeclared prostitutes remained stable. The health clinic doctor also pointed out that since undeclared prostitutes visited much less frequently than declared ones (understandably so, since they were only inspected when they were caught) the figures relating to the undeclared prostitutes need to be increased considerably.

The view that clandestine prostitutes were much more contagious was largely corroborated by a set of figures which relate to a later period (1934 to 1936) but which are interesting because they deal with what was happening to men (these figures were gathered from the Saint-Louis and Tenon dispensaries).[54] Here 48.8 per cent of contaminations were from women encountered in the street, who were sometimes 'filles en carte', though most often clandestine prostitutes; the former, and sometimes the latter, operated from the *maisons de passe*. To this must be added 6.7 per cent due to hotel and restaurant prostitutes, who were also undeclared. Contaminations in brothels account for only 4.9 per cent, that is to say less than contaminations from casual affairs (as much as 12.7

per cent!), established mistresses (6.2 per cent) or legitimate spouses (5.7 per cent).[55]

What this proves, in fact, is that men went to the brothel less, not that brothels were less likely to cause contamination. In fact there were 235 brothels in Paris in 1841 and as few as 47 in 1903. During this time, however, the number of prostitutes increased much faster in proportion than the general population, giving more and more opportunities to 'streetwalkers' and clandestine prostitutes (out of 1,000 venereal victims admitted to Saint-Lazare for the first time between 1890 and 1900 there were 177 declared prostitutes and 832 clandestine ones).[56] 'Prostitution is changing its character, the brothel is dying out', complained a doctor in favour of regulation in 1923: 'the unbridled competition of the street has sounded their death-knell.'[57]

But who were these clandestine prostitutes who were changing the rules of the game? The clandestine prostitute is a 'little working girl' who touts herself on the boulevard, the girl in the brasserie or the tavern 'who goes upstairs'. This latter category wreaked havoc in small provincial towns, doling out pox after pox to young men out for a binge.[58] (Fourteen bars in Toulon were closed for this reason between 1921 and 1926.) Thus it was the prostitute in the provincial town who continued to follow her profession in total freedom, operating solely by word of mouth and spreading misery at markets and fairs. Luckily enough, commented a doctor from the Vosges in 1882, the peasant's instinct for self-preservation is stronger than his tendency towards dissimulation, and he loses no time in consulting his doctor.[59]

It was the mounting tide of under-age clandestine prostitution which particularly worried the authorities. Indeed, if the worst aspect of prostitution was clandestine prostitution then the worst aspect of clandestine prostitution was the issue of minors, a problem which was both medical and moral. Here we have the very dregs of prostitution, the source of the worst of syphilis. Fournier warns that 'it is syphilis in the depths of society which produces syphilis higher up . . . from the most abject hovel to the most honest hearth.' (Here we are again!) From 1835, when working as a prostitute before the age of twenty-one was prohibited, minors had gone underground, and this had resulted in their contracting the disease at an early age. Since they could not even be registered when they were caught they quickly broke all records for venereal disease. In his study of prostitution in Europe at the beginning of the twentieth century, Flexner[60] reports that 44.9 per cent of syphilitic prostitutes in Vienna were between fifteen and twenty years of age; the figures were much the same for

Berlin, Munich (where 50 per cent of prostitutes were underage), Zurich and Paris.

The paradoxical result of this was that when these prostitutes were old enough to be registered, and thus medically supervised, many of them had already been syphilitic for several years. They were all the more likely to spread the disease because they were more attractive on account of their youth; sometimes they would enter the profession before the age of fifteen, sometimes even before the age of twelve. They were so much in demand that they were admitted to brothels, from which they had to be excluded anew in 1901. But this was a waste of time, just like the law of 11 April 1908 on the prostitution of minors which prescribed the reformatory up until the age of majority (or until marriage), but which could not be applied because existing establishments were insufficient and inappropriate; there was, of course, no question of building new ones.

There was another category of clandestine prostitutes who were even more difficult to catch – 'ladies of fashion' (Flexner) who escaped all controls, and from whom their bourgeois clients nonetheless often suffered rather more than just financial damage. But where was the line to be drawn? Is prostitution a question of the number of clients? Yes and no, reply the theoreticians of anti-syphilitic prophylaxis, consoling themselves with the thought that these ladies could only infect a restricted number of victims, on account of their relative inaccessibility.

'In the wake of the regiments . . .'

From the sixteenth century onwards, public authorities had been aware that prostitutes and their favourite clients, the military, constituted two complementary factors in the propagation of the pox; indeed, it was they who introduced it into Europe during the Italian campaign. We have already seen how in the eighteenth century prostitutes captured 'in the wake of the regiments' were locked up in the beggars' prisons at the request and expense of the Extraordinary Council of War.[61]

During this period there was much royal concern for the health of the armies. 'The soldier has little option but to frequent prostitutes, which means that he will almost inevitably catch the venereal disease', wrote an official at the Toulon military hospital in 1764; following this sensible remark he sketches a project for establishments 'to treat the venereal maladies of debauched women'[62] in the towns most frequented by the troops. These establishments would be annexes to military hospitals in which care would be lavished by the army surgeon. The idea, emphasized several times, is to avoid repeated contaminations by what was in fact a limited number of prostitutes (an enquiry conducted on thirty-five soldiers with venereal disease traced the infection to just three prostitutes) – 'from which one concludes that the treatment required to treat these three women would have been less costly than that required to cure the thirty-five soldiers.' Going beyond this is the long-term idea of 'gradually purifying the polluted blood at the heart of the Kingdom'.

This was another good idea the Crown had neither the time nor the financial resources to put into practice. But undoubtedly the militarization of the country following the wars of the Revolution and Empire would make the problem more acute. Everyone deplored the fact that the pox and scabies were soon sending more people to hospital than the enemies of the Republic, numerous though they were; a decree of 24 Thermidor of the year VIII therefore proposed that hospitals intended exclusively for the treatment of scabies and venereal disease should be set up near the armies. But the Empire, which had killed a good many more, was not particularly preoccupied with the health of its armies, with the result that at the beginning of the Restoration the state of health of the military was far from ideal, despite the fact that peace had at last been restored. 'Monsieur le Colonel de la Légion,' wrote the Prefect of Morbihan to the mayor of Vannes on 7 February 1826, 'there are in the town of Vannes a good number of whores who are spreading the venereal disease to its soldiers, rendering them unfit for service.'[63]

Following on from various rulings (1818, 1831) which did no more than make the discharge of soldiers dependent on their satisfying the army surgeon that they were free of venereal disease, a decree of 10 May 1842 relaunched the struggle against syphilis in the armies: 'An affliction which deeply affects man's constitution and which damages whole generations at their source has become an object of the liveliest public concern, and the officers of the Army Health Corps are called upon to play an active role in realizing the projects which it has set in motion. It is a matter of stamping out syphilis.'[64] Soldiers were obliged to declare their disease as soon as possible, and were to be punished for concealing it. Also under threat of punishment, syphilitics were to give the name and address of the woman who had contaminated them.[65] It was thought that whilst control of prostitutes posed well-known problems, control of the military was easier, sanitary discipline being no more than one form of discipline in general. And to act on the military would be an indirect way of acting on the prostitute, since it was the combination of the two which was such an important factor in the propagation of syphilis.

However, very few garrison towns made concrete efforts to organize the struggle. An exception was Brest, where, in 1829, a dispensary was set up at the expense of the ministries of War and of the Navy. In the middle of the nineteenth century there were sixty beds almost always in use, which works out at about 350 cases per year. Sometimes sick prostitutes themselves attended a kind of infirmary called the 'violon' [violin] of the dispensary. In 1856 police records mention 344 declared prostitutes (131 attached to a brothel, 213 'en carte'), but it was estimated that there were at least twice as many clandestine prostitutes. The maritime hospital looked after venereal victims independently of this dispensary reserved for prostitutes with venereal disease. From 1850 to 1855 an average of 200 patients were treated there, one-fifth of the total of that establishment. This was a great number, especially if we accept the estimates of the chief surgeon of the Navy at Brest who concludes that, including seamen treated aboard ship, 2,144 out of 6,294 men contracted syphilis during that period.[66]

There was, however, cause to deplore a considerable increase in the number of cases of venereal disease in most garrison towns, and throughout the second half of the nineteenth century prefects were repeatedly instructed to repress clandestine prostitution (which sometimes even took place in barracks), which had long been considered to be the main cause of contagion.[67]

Things were no better in England in the mid-nineteenth century, if we can believe contemporary statistics. In a little under seven years no less than 8,032 victims of venereal disease were discovered amongst 44,611 soldiers, 1,415 of these cases being of 'primitive' syphilis (chancre).[68] The results were a little less grim in the Navy, but they were frankly catastrophic in the merchant navy, no less than one-third of whom had some sort of venereal disease. As for the examination of recruits by the militia, it showed that 25 per cent of them were victims of venereal disease (*The Lancet*, 1853). Military doctors were the first to call for urgent measures:

The perusal, in the *British Medical Journal* of 25th February last, of a report of an interesting paper by Mr William Acton, on the 'Rarity and Mildness of Syphilis amongst the Belgian Troops quartered at Brussels, as compared with its Prevalence and Severity amongst the Foot Guards in London', induces me to offer a few observations on the prevalence of syphilis in the British Army, and its possible prevention or mitigation.

From the opportunities afforded me by a service of upwards of thirty years as a medical officer in the army, I am enabled to endorse the statements of Mr Acton as to the frightful extent to which not only the Foot Guards, but the whole military force of the empire, is paralysed by this foul disease; and to express a decided belief that it is, to a certain extent, preventible, or at least capable of considerable mitigation.

I am not in a position now to refer to documentary or statistical evidence to prove the truth of this assertion, or to show the actual extent to which syphilis prevails in the army generally, or its comparative prevalence in the several commands at home and abroad, and in the different arms of the services; nor is this necessary to my present purpose, for the fact is well known. It is sufficient to state that a very large proportion of our best and most efficient soldiers are constantly confined to hospital, at heavy pecuniary loss to the state, and loss of efficiency to the army; whole considerable numbers are annually lost to the service altogether, by deaths and invaliding, from this loathsome disease. In the large garrisons of the United Kingdom, this is especially the case; and the great depôts for recruits, such as Chatham, are the fertile hotbeds where syphilitic disease is sown broadcast amongst the young soldiers.[69]

This preoccupation increased at the end of the nineteenth century, particularly as regards the troops in Indochina and North Africa.[70] Statistical evidence revealed the role of the seaman as a long-distance vector of syphilis, and merchant seamen were quickly included in many prophylactic projects. But once again these were only projects. By contrast, the great shift in prophylaxis which began around 1900 found fertile ground in the Army; the young recruit was 'bombarded' with lectures, health manuals, pamphlets, posters, films, etc. (in a few months, when the 'rookie' became a veteran it would be too late). Flexner points out that moral and prophylactic education was general in all the armies of Europe, and that it was an element in the preparation for war (he published his work in New York in 1913): 'The first nation to succeed in reducing it (venereal disease) will acquire a considerable advantage over its adversaries.'[71]

In fact it was not until the First World War that proper measures were taken. We have already seen that, thanks to the war, syphilis, which might have been thought to have been halted by the campaign begun twenty years earlier, flared up once more: it attacked the civilian population, but it made far more of an impact on the soldier, wrenched from his family and his hearth.[72] The 1914–18 war was thus considered to be 'a cause for exultation for the venereal diseases' because of the intermingling of populations, the 'feeling of the brevity and fragility of the chastest existence', and also 'the greatest degree of freedom women had yet known'.[73]

In the USA in the course of the 1914–18 War, registered brothels and bars of prostitution were banned within a five-mile radius around military camps. Subsequently the War Department extended this distance to ten miles, but it was difficult, there and elsewhere, to combat clandestine prostitution, and even more difficult to combat a particularly pernicious species, namely soldiers' girls, who weren't even venal: 'The peculiar charm and glamour which surrounds the man in uniform causes an unusual type of prostitute to spring up in time of war. Girls idealize the soldier, and many really feel that nothing is wrong when done for him. One such girl said that she had never sold herself to a civilian but felt that she was doing her bit when she had been with eight soldiers in a night.'[74]

Such was the 'girl problem' which, from the First World War onwards (though it was even more of a problem for the liberating armies during the Second World War), threatened the reputation of 'the cleanest army in the world'. 383,706 cases of syphilis and gonorrhoea were recorded in the American army between April 1917 and December 1919, causing the loss of seven million days of active service, just a little less than the 'flu.[75]

Acknowledging this massive contamination 'poisoning the most fertile springs of the nation', the Ministry for the Armed Forces took up the struggle against syphilis from the beginning of the First World War onwards,[76] endeavouring to put into effect the measures taken before the war: as many medical inspections as possible, monthly or bi-monthly; great discretion, and the end of punishment for failure to take immediate medical advice; diagnoses to be coded on hospital records; a list of names to be sent secretly to the chief doctor of the corps. In September 1916 a ministerial circular ordered that there should also be systematic medical examination of soldiers going on leave and coming off leave, and that those who were contagious should be arrested. Furthermore, numerous administrative measures designed to track down the sources of infection were taken. The great innovation, however, was the setting up in 1916 of a dermato-venereological clinic in every major military centre; meanwhile the ministries of the Armed Forces and of Public Health began to collaborate more closely than ever before. But it was not until the end of the war that this full-scale anti-syphilitic crusade (a term which, incidentally, was often used) could develop a propaganda machine of the same type – though much more muscular – as that directed at the civilian population at the time. Only a few details differed, notably the provision of sanitary posts in every garrison town and near stations and red-light districts.

Unfortunately the French soldier, unlike his American counterpart, refused to have anything to do with this type of facility. It was necessary to return to the good old individual health-care kit, with its calomel ointment, supposedly a preventative against infection. The pack also included the equally venerable 'French letter', and the majority of military doctors limited their prophylactic lectures to the following advice: 'With a condom you can be almost 100 per cent certain of not catching gonorrhoea, and 80 per cent certain of not catching the pox.'[77] Instructions, with which the Army was not niggardly, followed – but the condom remained. Was it not, after all, the best way of avoiding the impossible task of distinguishing the declared from the undeclared prostitutes, not to mention the girl 'picked up' in a bar who, at the outset at least, could equally well be a girl of easy virtue or a wily prostitute (and, of course, the former could just as well have the pox)?[78]

From the end of the Second World War onwards the military were subjected to the same régime as civilians – in other words, they were left to their own devices. This explans why no-one was particularly surprised at the reappearance of the good old condom in a Ministry of Defence circular of 1953: 'I am pleased to be able to inform you that preservatives are no longer supplied by the Health Service. Their use may well constitute an effective means of individual protection from venereal diseases, and it may well be that they will continue to be recommended on these grounds, but for many reasons it is not vital to supply them free to users, at least in peacetime.'[79] If war broke out again, then, the resumption of free supplies of preservatives would therefore provide some consolation!

Abolitionism

In the UK, as in the other countries of Europe, the increasingly worrying problem of prostitution, the principal source of venereal infection, gradually led many doctors to advocate regulatory control.[80] But prudence was necessary in the country of *habeas corpus*; the result was the first of the contagious diseases prevention Acts in 1864, which confined itself to the surveillance of some naval ports and garrison towns and the introduction of obligatory medical inspections of prostitutes. In 1866, and then in 1868, the geographical application of the Act was cautiously extended (though its application to London was never contemplated) and measures were introduced to deal with prostitutes who refused the bi-monthly examination (up to three months in prison). However, what appeared to be quite normal to the French after the Revolution and the Empire seemed almost intolerable to many Britons. The surveillance of prostitutes meant the existence of a record system, an appalling idea across the Channel.

While opposition to regulationism was growing, its supporters were expecting spectacular results; but, following the classic pattern, the health monitoring of prostitutes simply increased the number of clandestine prostitutes, thereby maintaining, if not increasing, the level of venereal diseases. In the colonies, where the Acts were introduced almost everywhere, the results were even worse, mainly because of serious abuses by the vice squad (in Hong Kong, for example). The paltry results of the Acts caused Dr Drysdale of London to tell the international medical congress held on the occasion of the Universal Exhibition in Paris in 1867 'I am convinced that the system which allows unrestricted prostitution in London results in fewer cases of syphilis than the present system in Paris'. But at the same congress a London hospital surgeon reported that in a regulated brothel in London between 1862 and 1867 twenty-five out of 109 prostitutes were syphilitics, and he called insistently for surveillance measures:

Let us therefore recommend these measures, especially in England, where they exist only in part, for the protection of the army and the navy. Let us recommend them, gentlemen, wherever they are not yet being called for, and not solely for the benefit of the masculine sex, but also to spare these wretched women, who well deserve the pity of enlightened philanthropists, from the awful consequences of the disease by which they are devoured. In London, where there are no restrictions, the people who concern us come to the hospitals in the most pitiful state, asking for treatment.[81]

In the 1860s the UK was torn between regulationism and the 'laisser-faire, laisser-passer' attitude so in keeping with its traditions. Supporters of regulatory controls were few and far between, but very active. One such was William Acton,[82] to whom *The Lancet* frequently opened its columns. A Royal Commission (The Commission on Venereal Disease) had been set up:

Although the Commission sitting at the Admiralty has now closed the inquiry upon which it has been occupied for several months, and concluded the examination of witnesses, the report cannot be completed for some few weeks. The amount of evidence taken has been considerable. Amongst the principal points established will be the usefulness of the system of examinations instituted under the Contagious Diseases Act, and a wide basis of facts will be afforded for supporting an extension of that measure. There is much evidence to show that the moral usefulness of this restrictive system is not greatly inferior to its physical utility. The women detained and prohibited from diffusing the disease are brought under religious influences while in hospital, and a proportion of them absolutely reclaimed and restored to their friends. Some doubts have been expressed as to the propriety of enforcing the provisions of that Act, as implying a recognition of the vice which is the parent of disease. But the permanent and frightfully extensive injuries inflicted on the population, and especially on the costly trained men of our naval and military forces, involve facts so serious that they cannot be overlooked, and require restrictive and sanitary measures more urgently than most other diseases of which we seek to limit the spread by legislative measures. Morally and religiously there is reason to believe that the unhappy women are likely to be materially benefited by the influences brought to bear upon them during periods of detention. The necessity for further Lock hospitals, and the advisability of an extension of the Contagious Diseases Act, will probably be amongst the most important conclusions deducible from the evidence taken. These are matters of national importance, and it was probably chiefly with a view to the solution of these questions that the authorities appointed this Commission. (*The Lancet*, 2 December 1865)

However, opposition was rekindled once the surprise had worn off. W. Acton himself revealed that he was aware of this when he wrote that: 'It is fair to say that more than one of the most eminent lawyers who have illuminated the seat of justice in this country have expressed themselves against domiciliary visitation as 'contrary to the spirit of English law'. Apart from this fundamental objection, there was an outcry against the encouragement that was being given to prostitution, and against the false sense of security flaunted by the clients of 'official' prostitutes. 'The new legislation,' said the vicar of Windsor, 'treats fornication as a necessity, since its aim is to render the practice less dangerous. The result of this is that men can sin in greater physical security and abandon themselves unrestrainedly to their whims.' A certain Dr Taylor also produced the following interesting supplementary objection: 'On the unsupported evidence of a policeman a woman may be arrested and condemned to three months imprisonment if she refuses the unseemly violation of her person with a surgical instrument.'

The struggle polarized around the 'National Association for the Repeal of Contagious Diseases Act', and there appeared a figure who was to be the guiding spirit of abolitionism: Josephine Butler, the founder of the 'National Association of English Women for the Repeal of the Laws on Contagious Diseases'. She envisaged no less than that Christians in the whole world should form sections to fight 'against the threats of the disease and to deliver the world from the wound of legalized prostitution'. Besides this puritanical opposition there were other solid arguments, such as those of the Reverend C. S. Collingwood against a proposal by a French regulationist[83] to extend the medical examination to soldiers and factory workers:

It is instructive to observe that the examination of men which is now in question applies only to men of the working classes. Officers of the navy or army and all civil servants of the crown are as much under the control of the government as the workers, and are as likely to spread syphilis as civilian workers, private soldiers and seamen; captains of merchant vessels can be as immoral as their crew, and the government has an equal right to examine either group; but there is no question of that. Why is this distinction being made if not because it is considered to be an indignity to which gentlemen would not wish to submit, and because it is a fact that no examination can be imposed unless the surgeons have the right to command those who are being examined? It is the same principle which lies behind the idea of inspecting women whilst men are generally left at liberty, namely that women are defenceless and that men who could avoid doing so would not submit themselves to it. Tyranny always attacks the weak.[84]

The first abolitionist congress took place in 1877 in Geneva. Meanwhile, the British Parliament was deluged with petitions. In 1873, 900,000 signatures had been gathered, and a first bill to repeal the laws had been defeated only by a very narrow majority. The repeal bills brought in 1875 and 1876 could not secure a majority in the House of Commons either, but in the general elections which followed the candidates had to reckon with electors who were in favour of repeal. As the *Pall Mall Gazette* remarked in 1883:

It is undoubtedly the case that in any electoral constituency dominated by the working class vote, a candidate would not have a shadow of a chance if he defended them. Rightly or wrongly, the working classes believe this law to be unjust because it stigmatizes the woman who, in most cases, is of their class; they believe, on the contrary, that this same law is very much to the advantage of the man who has brought about the disease and who is still supposed, rightly or wrongly, to originate from the upper classes in the great majority of cases. If anyone doubts this antipathy towards the Acts, he should ask a Minister or a Member of Parliament if he would like to propose the extension of this law, which at present affects only a few garrison towns, to Manchester, Birmingham or London.

In short, although those who supported regulation of prostitution tried to demonstrate that syphilis had decreased in the Army, or in those towns which had been subject to the Acts, and who predicted a frightful recrudescence of the disease if the repeal was carried (other statistics, of course, claimed to show the opposite),[85] this controversial law was repealed by the House of Commons on 21 April 1883. But the regulationists counterattacked the following year, and Lord Dalhousie produced a draft of the 'Criminal law amendment bill', passed on 14 August 1885, whose aim was to protect women and young girls (protection which included the suppression of brothels, and which was a *de facto* return to regulationism). The debate was therefore far from closed, either institutionally or medically, and even less so morally. For many abolitionists, in fact, syphilis was the natural punishment for sin (a classic theme since the disease's first appearance), and no-one was entitled to be preserved from it, and certainly not by putting a government health label on prostitutes, which would only serve to promote the corruption of young people. 'If the medical arts,' said one of these fervent abolitionists, 'should manage to lift the punishment inflicted by nature on wicked mankind, this discovery would be antisocial and demoralizing, for it would create a moral syphilization far worse than physical syphilization.'[86] Furthermore, any sufficiently structured attempt to regulate prostitution would simply consecrate the fall of woman, turning her into nothing more than a piece of merchandise.

This rather high-minded and Utopian Puritanism which aimed to save fallen women by providing refuges and patronage,[87] found its best arguments in the condemnation of regulations – the first article of the statutes of the Abolitionist Federation denounced the administration of prostitution as 'faulty hygiene, a social injustice, a moral monstrosity and a judicial crime'. Abolitionists defended the autonomy of the human subject, and its corollary, individual responsibility. They consequently condemned 'any discriminatory régime applied on the pretext of *mores*' – which was exactly what Parent-Duchatelet was imposing on prostitutes.

The abolitionists naturally objected particularly strongly to brothels, as for example did Louis Fiaux, one of the most ardent opponents of regulatory controls: 'What is this strange-looking institution? What is this huge number, these figures sixty centimetres high which label it as shamelessly as the phallic red lantern of the brothels of Ancient Rome? What are all these chained and padlocked shutters which evoke the grimness of prisons, but also the mysterious call of illicit pleasure?'[88] Once inside the door one sees the hideous spectacle of 'clusters of women sprawling on the seats, upturned against the walls, draped limply on statues, sitting astride men's knees and suffocating them with their bosoms, groping them, twining round them in attitudes which are either comically amorous or mock-cynical and brutal!' And it is best not to mention the act itself, the repetition of which leaves the prostitute 'intoxicated, dazed, dizzy, her flanks aching from the foul surfeit.' Elsewhere, this same author accuses army medics of recommending brothels to the troops, and even of requiring town councils to set them up and maintain them. Fiaux concludes that it would be better to instil 'a sexual conscience' in the soldier.[89]

This moral argument supports the Abolitionist Federation's disapproval of measures 'which, by treating the patient like a tool, have no other object but to clean it for base ends'. Besides, the State has no more justification for maintaining prostitution and the male licentiousness which causes it than for tolerating theft, for example. No, both should be universally suppressed, and continence rehabilitated: 'In several countries, an élite group of young men has undertaken to demonstrate by their own example the joy and beauty of a chaste life, that necessary prelude to the spotless conjugal union which they have set as an ideal.'[90] This confidence in the new generation surfaces once more in the following more specific appeal to female solidarity: 'All these women's efforts are directed against prostitution, of which, they rightly believe, they carry the stigmata. They abhor the regulation of prostitution as much as they would if their sex were branded on their forehead with a red-hot iron to designate them as slaves.'[91]

These considerations were just as compelling for Parisian radicals (who formed the extreme left at the time) in their campaign against the vice squad[92] and in a marxist, or even anarchist,[93] analysis which explicitly links prostitution and the economic subordination of women or even the subjugation of the proletariat, from which, as it happens, almost all prostitutes originate. But, in the end, it was medical and sanitary considerations, rather than moral, social and judicial ones which best served the abolitionist cause. Those in favour of regulation held it to be axiomatic that the brothels guaranteed public health; the abolitionists, by contrast, bolstered by the failures of the system in force, argued that the brothel was 'the conservatory and the laboratory of syphilis'. They claimed that one should look at the problem from the point of view of the prostitute who could be contaminated, and thus herself become a contaminator, by her first client after the sanitary inspection, or from the too often neglected point of view of the infectious client who ought to be abstinent, but who soon recovers his 'state of physiological turgescence' and makes for the brothel where folk are less scrupulous: 'this creates a certain sort of mentality which we can call the venereal mentality, . . . he has been syphilized and he syphilizes: he gives the opposite sex "their just deserts".'[94]

In fact it was easy for the abolitionists to prove that it was absurd and scandalous that prostitutes' clients had hitherto been ignored: 'What good is it incarcerating a few wretched women for a short while when new centres of infection are all the time appearing unchecked? For as long as regulatory measures leave men touched, new sources of infection will arise.'[95]

The abolitionists concluded that the authorities were not entitled to give prostitutes certificates of immunity and that the regulations should therefore be abolished; their grounds were that medical supervision of brothels was ineffective (indeed numerous minor epidemics of syphilis had brothels as their source) and that clandestine prostitutes were even more likely to spread infection. Of course, this would not mean the disappearance of prostitution, but at least prostitution would no longer have the state's blessing: 'Prostitution will continue after the brothels have closed, but in a less cynical, less ignominious form, one more in keeping with contemporary moral standards (Louis Fiaux).

In sum, the abolitionists wanted 'women to walk the streets freely'. In the UK, everything was taken care of by *habeas corpus*. There were some there who went so far as to minimize the disease itself, which in the context of the time was the greatest proof of love of liberty one could imagine:

Today, under the influence of an unreflective terror which has seized people's minds regarding a disease which is very much less dangerous than formerly, people have needed no encouragement to neglect the regard shown hitherto by law for the liberty of the humblest citizen. Given human nature, it can be concluded *a priori* that the power irresponsibly given to the police will be greatly abused. The history of all peoples at all times abounds with examples which confirm this hypothesis. The development of representative government is simply the development of a device intended to prevent outrageous abuses of unchecked power. Every one of our political struggles which has ended in some new progress towards free institutions has had as its object the ending of one of the most flagrant abuses of unchecked power. And now all of this is being forgotten in a total panic, artificially created, over a disease which is disappearing, and which claims only one victim for every fifteen carried away by scarlatina.[96]

In Norway from 1860 onwards, health regulations for prostitutes were replaced by regulations applying to all citizens without exception: doctors were obliged to notify the disease, and every newly-diagnosed syphilitic had to sign a document stating that anyone who knew or had reason to suppose that he was afflicted with a contagious sexual disease and who infected another person or exposed them to infection by means of sexual intercourse or immoral practices would be punished with imprisonment of up to three years.

In the United States the question of prostitution was just as worrying. In the 1870s Dr Guichet studied health and medical care in the United States and, more especially, in New York and Philadelphia, and he denounced unregulated prostitution as the principal cause of the spread of syphilis:

prostitution mirrors the town in its incredible rate of development, its rapid and remarkable growth; it wallows in the mud of the filthy, poorer quarters and conceals itself behind the flowers of the new, prosperous quarters. No police regulation forces these women to be inspected by a doctor; there are no examinations, regular or irregular, and no dispensaries; it is only when the infected prostitute is so seriously ill that she can no longer continue her ignoble trade without pain that she comes to be medically examined. Those with money are treated at home; the poor ones the doctor sends from the first hospital to the *Charity Hospital* on Blackwell Island where, after they are cured, they are made to work for a while in the *Workhouse* so that there is the best possible guarantee that they can no longer transmit syphilis. Given these conditions, one should not be surprised at the enormous figure of 61,705 victims of venereal disease, of whom 50,450 are syphilitics, out of a population of 942,294 inhabitants.[97]

For her part, Dr Katherine Bement Davis, Commissioner of Corrections for New York City, estimated that 70 per cent of the women sent to the city workhouse because of prostitution were victims of venereal disease (syphilis or gonorrhoea).

This relaunched the struggle against prostitution, with medicine coming to the aid of morality. Between 1910 and 1916 almost all American cities set up 'vice-commissions'. The 'vice-commission' of Chicago expressed itself thus in 1911:

Prostitution is pregnant with disease, a disease infecting not only the guilty but contaminating the innocent wife and child in the home with sickening certainty almost inconceivable; a disease to be feared as a leprous plague; a disease scattering misery broadcast, and leaving in its wake sterility, insanity, paralysis, and the blinded eyes of little babies, the twisted limbs of deformed children, degradation, physical rot and mental decay.[98]

Proponents of regulation formed committees in various cities: New York, Chicago, Philadelphia, Cincinnati. But often, as in Albany or Sacramento in 1884 or in Cleveland and St-Paul in 1885, attempts to regulate prostitution were vigorously rejected by the populace, and notably by women's associations who believed that it was necessary to try to eradicate prostitution but not to organize it. Thus, a New York police regulation, which in 1910 introduced, in addition to the taking of finger prints from prostitutes who had been rounded up, a medical inspection and obligatory treatment in case of venereal disease sparked off a violent campaign of feminist protest which had the regulation annulled as unconstitutional a year later. Similarly, a surreptitiously regulationist proposal which would have given discretionary powers to health committees came to nothing before the Senate.

In the end, regulation, so dear to the French (Americans at the time spoke of the 'French system'), did not take place. Like Canada and Australia, the United States turned towards a sanitarist solution, making it obligatory for syphilitics to be treated, without specifically discriminating against prostitutes, and for doctors to declare cases anonymously, except when they had to 'denounce' to the health authority a recalcitrant patient – something which of course they never did.

Uncompromisingly abolitionist countries were rare, and included only the UK, the Low Countries and Switzerland. As for Japan, it was initially opposed to all regulation, as we see from the testimony of a Belgian expressing regret about the devastating effects of unregulated prostitution in the land of the rising sun:

A strict medical control of houses of prostitution is absolutely necessary, but in Japan there exists nothing of the sort. And all my attempts to convince the government that it is its duty to extend its control meet with the reply that it is a very delicate problem, and that one cannot oblige prostitutes to live a healthy life, that everyone can do what they wish with their own bodies and no one else has rights over them, not even the government.[99]

It was not until the Meiji period that, thanks to the English doctor, Newton, the first hospital for venereal victims was created in 1868; six years later anti-syphilitic controls were officially introduced in every administrative district.

At first France (and most Latin countries) maintained the regulations despite the attacks on them. The abolitionists, in fact, were having to contend with a growing obsession with the venereal peril which was at odds with what was apparently such a liberal reform. 'The abolitionists are nihilists when it comes to hygiene', said Fournier, who emerged as the main champion of regulation in France. Also around 1900, another opponent of abolitionism described the brothel as 'a pillar of social order',[100] agreeing with Philibert, the brothel-keeper in Jean Lorrain's novel, when he says 'My establishment is a public utility ... I am maintaining order and propriety; I am even defending the health of the nation; I am the safeguard of French Morality.'

The Abolitionist Federation, which had taken the debate to the Human Rights League, was unpleasantly surprised when the latter judged in favour of regulation; prostitution, it concluded, 'must be classified with unhealthy trades and professions, and as such must, like other unhealthy trades and professions, be subjected to inspectors intended to guarantee the interests of the public at large, of which one of the foremost is public health.'

The last stronghold of those in favour of regulatory controls held firm, above all in France. An extra-parliamentary commission, which the government was obliged to appoint in 1903, and which concluded in favour of the abolitionists, ran into hostility from the all-powerful Société de Prophylaxie Sanitaire et Morale, which finally succeeded in wrecking its efforts. As for local representatives, they regularly declared themselves to be in favour of regulation, though more for political than for medical considerations. After the mayors had been consulted in 1904, and almost all had been discovered to be opponents of abolitionism, a coalition appeared in November 1936 against the abolitionist bill brought by Henri Sellier, the Minister of Health. It was a combination of the 'Amicale des maîtres d'hôtels meublés de France et des colonies' (which collected for the occasion a fighting fund of fifty million francs), numerous parliamentarians who were just as willing to disappoint their electors in this matter as on the anti-alcohol campaign whose bills they were trying to sink at this time, and, finally, the medical specialists responsible for the control of brothels who, according to Sellier, 'even if they reaped no great profits from their participation in public institutions, nonetheless received titles and decorations (?).'[101]

Setting aside the manoeuvrings of politicians, most doctors were sincere in their desire to preserve, even strengthen, the health regulations regarding prostitution. 'Believe me, young people,' wrote one of them,[102] 'it is better to frequent the brothel . . . . Nothing to fear from the old hand, her wounds have had time to heal and the virus no longer has a hold on her.' (J. Lacassagne was later to use the term 'honorary syphilitics' for prostitutes who had been thus immunised'.) 'Moreover, all these professionals are examined officially every week, and officiously each day by the deputy-madam or doctor of the establishment.' 'Far from opposing the brothels,' said the chief doctor of the health dispensary of the prefecture of Police, 'we must on the contrary recognize their utility, for they represent what is ultimately the most discrete, least scandalous and, above all, least dangerous form of prostitution.'[103]

Whilst the most optimistic continued to preach in favour of 'the healthy woman and the healthy client in the medically-supervised and hygienically transformed brothel',[104] it was easy for some of the more realistic doctors to be ironic, as was, for example, Dr Lutaud at the Congress in Lyons in 1906: 'The security you are seeking,' he told his colleagues, 'will not come about until you have turned the 85,000 prostitutes of Paris into well-drilled civil servants . . . until any candidate for an erection has been examined by a doctor.'[105] This abolitionist irony was demolished by some astonishing neo-regulatory prescriptions: in Belgium, article 14 of the health regulations on brothels stipulated that in every room there should be two bottles which were constantly replenished, one containing a solution of caustic soda for the prostitute, the other with fresh oil for the client. 'Both of the champions present must anoint themselves, in the name of public health.'[106] But this was nothing compared to Colombia, where prostitutes who had been arrested and treated had their genital areas shaved before they were freed. A circular distributed in the city streets alerted the people as follows: '*Prevencion! Mujer masurada o afeitada en sus partes genitales externas, es mujer enferma. Tenga cuidado*' ('A woman whose external genital areas have been shaved is a sick woman. Beware!')[107] It was simple, but effective![108]

In France, certain particularly active dispensaries were also bastions of neo-regulationism. Such was the public health dispensary at Nancy, set up in 1925 along the most modern lines, which specialized in the medical surveillance and treatment of prostitutes:

Each new woman brought in by the police is questioned by the medical social worker, who is always present during examinations. The information supplied is entered on a medico-social record form. These facts, which we verify by cross-checking, are extremely useful to us from the point of view of health, but also from the moral point of view, to guide us as to how to behave towards the woman (whether she is to be immediately registered or not, whether the police should be asked to mount a strict surveillance, etc.). This form also informs us as to all the detectable clinical symptoms, both of syphilis and of other afflictions. The woman is provided with a record of treatment (produced by the Health Ministry) on which are recorded the Wassermann reactions and what treatment there has been . . . . Every woman brought in (registered or not) is photographed by the police; this photograph is affixed to a form bearing the particulars of the woman and the registration number of her records . . . . Given this, any of the information can be requested from us by dispensaries in other towns, reducing the chance of error to almost nil (voluntary or involuntary exchange of records, false information, etc.). We simply send the photograph and the details.[109]

In 1932, no less than 2,200 health files on prostitutes had been created.

In Nancy, as elsewhere, doctors engaged in the struggle against syphilis could not fail to reflect the general tendency towards abolitionism: 'The general tendency nowadays is to suppress all forms of regulation. They begin by suppressing regulated brothels because, for emotional reasons, it is the easiest target to attain. Having got through this first stage, the abolitionist will try to suppress the regulations. The unfortunate epidemic at Nancy[110] proves beyond doubt what we should think of the abolition of regulation.'[111]

There were some experiments, which were abolitionist only in name, but they were hardly convincing. In Lyons in 1910 the number of single prostitutes given treatment for syphilis increased considerably (which was rather worrying as regards their previous state of health) after voluntary consultation had been temporarily substituted for the usual police measures, but the number of unregistered prostitutes treated increased only slightly. The fifteen brothels in Strasbourg were closed in 1926 (though, oddly enough, individual prostitutes continued to be registered), but, ten years

later, fatal cases of venereal disease, far from having decreased, had
grown following the reappearance of unregistered brothels and the
proliferation of clandestine prostitutes.[112]

Health care 'à la française'

During the unceasing combat between regulationists and abolitionists
from the end of the nineteenth century onwards it became
increasingly obvious that France would be incapable of making an
absolute choice between the two systems. In the first place, there
was a contradiction in French society: it wished to preserve its
health, but also, unconsciously, preserve prostitution as a sexual
outlet, despite its being the main cause of venereal contamination.
No one dreamed of eradicating prostitution, neither those in
favour of regulation, who wished to continue to reinforce the
administrative regulation of prostitutes (and all the more severely,
since it had failed entirely), nor, in the final analysis, the
abolitionists, who wished to suppress those regulations and, as a
substitute for them, to subject prostitutes to common law,
repressing public provocation of debauchary by judicial authority.[113]

These contradictions were to be brought to light during the
Occupation and the Vichy régime, which also stepped up the
regulation of prostitutes: a model decree for the occupied zone
supplemented the clauses of the statutory order of 29 November
1939[114] regarding prostitutes. As well as making a distinction
between 'controlled prostitutes' and 'prostitutes under surveillance'
(the second being those who broke the new law), a more thorough
health inspection was thenceforth to include a personal file kept by
a social worker, which could be communicated to the Prefect, the
police and the judiciary, as well as a health card and record. It
divided regulated brothels into categories (the first category
received only 'controlled prostitutes' – who in the minds of the
administration were the first choice as far as health was concerned).
Provision was also made for the licensing of places for soliciting.
Likewise, certain establishments could be authorized as places of
prostitution, as opposed to brothels.[115] Any prostitute recognized
as afflicted with a contagious venereal disease was to be immediately
isolated and treated; the 'prostitute under surveillance' could only
be treated in a special section of the anti-venereal department of a
hospital, so that she could be subjected to special surveillance.

These draconian measures coincided, as if by chance, with those
of the German army of occupation. Whereas Nazi Germany
forbade brothels on its own territory (just as it had forbidden

syphilitics to marry, under pain of sterilization), it allowed its troops to frequent certain French brothels on condition that they were for their exclusive use. Not only could a German doctor be present at the health inspection of the prostitutes reserved for the occupying troops, but in the 'German' brothels a male nurse posted at the bottom of the staircase took the names of the soldier and the prostitute who went up with him. In every room, a notice 'legible at six metres'[116] required the use of a disinfectant (potassium permanganate and a calomel ointment) *ante-* and *post-coitum*, and the use of a rubber preservative. Any prostitute who contaminated a soldier of the Reich by breaking these regulations was threatened with prison or labour camp. Pharmacists, for their part, were forbidden to sell without a prescription any medicament which could mask a venereal disease, and to German soldiers in particular – here we have full-blown regulationism.

But the pox continued to defy regulations. In 1942, in spite of the new clauses of the law of 31 December of that year[117] – that 'anti-venereal charter' which decreed that any prostitute recognized by the doctor to be infected with a venereal disease should be named – it appeared that infection by unregistered prostitutes continued to increase. Although they were the target of the decree of 24 December 1940, there were still 9,125 unregistered prostitutes to be had in Seine in 1942. In this 'département' in the same year there were 'only' 462 cases of syphilis amongst unregistered prostitutes as opposed to 205 cases amongst 6,185 registered prostitutes.[118] However, there were 3,394 declared cases of syphilis, 94 per cent of which were not referable to prostitutes who underwent health inspections; in other words, it was the prostitutes who were most ill who were most adept at hiding themselves.

After this new acknowledgement of failure, particularly embarrassing given the measures taken, regulationism was violently attacked by the 'Ligue française pour le relèvement de la moralité publique', a product of the Vichy régime dedicated to the improvement of the moral standards of the country and the defence of the family spirit. In an appeal to Marshal Pétain, this league denounced what it called 'super-regulationism', claiming that France would be revitalized if brothels were closed and the regulation of prostitution were abolished (beginning with the free zone). According to their plan of campaign, procuring would then be firmly suppressed, thus strictly applying article 13 of the statutory order of 29 November 1939 (the article prohibiting soliciting); 'male demand' would be reduced thanks to a 'climate of moral cleanliness'; 'the female invitation' would be reduced by moral surveillance (including, amongst other things, the monitoring of women's magazines, such as *Confidences*, which 'distort the minds of hundreds of thousands of young women').[119]

The Liberation brought a change of morality, but there continued to be calls for an end to a situation that was as absurd in judicial terms as it was ineffective in terms of anti-venereal prophylaxis, especially at a moment when movements of troops and people were producing a considerable upsurge in venereal diseases. It was for this reason that the muncipal council of Paris voted for the closure of regulated brothels on 13 December 1945, a prelude to the so-called 'Marthe Richard law' of 13 April 1946, a law which took its name from the Paris town councillor who supported the bill. This spectacular measure, which was taken up by the press and which stirred public opinion[120] was hailed as the triumph of abolitionism. But this was to overlook the fact that this law provided in its fifth article that 'the existing registers and records will be destroyed as a national health and social record system is established.' The system of records was introduced by the law of 24 April 1946, which received much less press coverage. The system which France put into operation was therefore a composite system in which regulationism and abolitionism were closely intermingled (although the closure of regulated brothels was more an admission of failure by the regulationists than a genuine triumph for abolitionist 'physiocratism').[121]

One might even say that the 'sanitarism' which set in from that time onwards was due to regulationism rather than abolitionism. In fact, the decree enforcing the law of 5 November 1947,[122] and also that of 1948, along with several memoranda and a law (8 July) all emphasize regulationist considerations by widening the scope of the health records; from this point onwards, for example, these had to record any prostitute convicted of soliciting.

The essential object of the sanitary and social records of prostitution is to track down prostitutes with venereal disease who wish to avoid being treated for their disease and to allow the prescribed treatments to be regularly and fully administered by doctors whose responsibility it is to inspect prostitutes. The name of the prostitute is entered on to the medico-social form. However, this form is neither an administrative document nor a police document.[123]

It was on this subtle linguistic difference that health care 'à la française' was based. In fact although the medico-social surveillance of prostitutes was in principle operated only by the health authority, the collaboration of the police was indispensable to the functioning of the health record system. The prostitutes were not taken in by this, and in 1952, the Seine health file contained only 3,000 records, although it was estimated that there were between

15,000 and 20,000 prostitutes in the 'département' (and, in fact, before 1946 there were 7,000 registered prostitutes). Moreover, its 'yield' was insignificant, for between 1948 and 1951 there were three cases per thousand of primo-secondary syphilis in Seine. By contrast, out of 189 hospitalized with secondary syphilis at Saint-Lazare in 1948, 185 had been detected thanks to police raids.[124] Things were much the same in most cities, Marseilles and Lyons in particular, where most prostitutes had hitherto escaped the periodic controls.

Having thus proved its inefficacy, the health record system was unable to survive the criticism of the abolitionist lobby, which had been strengthened by international support towards the end of the fifties. But what was to be done? The remarkable increase in sexual freedom at the end of the fifties went hand in hand with a decrease in prostitution and, more importantly, a dispersion throughout the social structure of those responsible for contamination; the public authorities therefore widely concluded that it was not logical to restrict the anti-venereal struggle to prostitutes, and that it had to be extended to the whole population. It was in this spirit that the law of 28 July 1960 was passed; this law ratified the international Convention of 2 December 1949 which prohibited all measures which discriminated against prostitutes. The edict of 25 November 1960 abolished the health record system. However, it introduced a zest for prohibitionism (another doctrine which proposed to make prostitution illegal, hoping, rather optimistically, that to make it a crime would put an end to it) to what was this time an undeniable victory for the abolitionists: stricter repression of soliciting, a legal ban on accommodating prostitutes, etc.

However, anyone who walks the streets of Paris or any of the large provincial cities today will perceive that prostitution has not disappeared for all that. Nor has syphilis, and the key question must now be as to the statistical relationship between the two.

10

The End of the Terror (1945 to the Present Day)

The legal plan of campaign

In the aftermath of the Second World War, the legislative measures of 29 November 1939 and 31 December 1943 were maintained in their entirety. In fact there was even less question of laying down arms given the recrudescence of venereal diseases in 1944 and 1945 which was linked to movements of populations, successive military occupations and, according to some, the closure of regulated brothels.[1] The laws of July and August 1948[2] re-set the parameters for the organization of the anti-venereal struggle: the dispensaries were maintained and reorganized,[3] and it was made obligatory for every contagious victim of venereal disease, and for pregnant women like to transmit hereditary syphilis, to have themselves examined and treated, either in a dispensary or in a state or private hospital, until they were no longer contagious.

Any doctor, wherever he practised, who discovered a case of contagious venereal disease[4] had to warn the patient of the disease with which he was afflicted and of the resulting dangers of contamination. Three sorts of measures were also proposed by the code of public health: as the law of 1942 had already ordered, the doctor had to send the director of the 'Action sanitaire et sociale' in the 'département' a declaration (which carried neither the identity nor the address of the patient) giving information on the nature of the disease (primary or secondary, as far as syphilis was concerned), sex, age and the presumed circumstances of contamination (prostitution, casual relationships, conjugal relations, etc.). This so-called 'simple' declaration had to be made 'nominal' (in other words, to include the patient's name and address) if the patient refused to begin or continue treatment, if he or she was involved in prostitution or if, in the doctor's opinion, there was a serious risk of the venereal disease being transmitted to one or more others because of the patient's profession or way of life. To this day these declarations comprise the only source of statistics on venereal morbidity.[5]

Moreover, a patient could be hospitalized either on the grounds of the nominal declaration or by the health authority. Finally, an ascendant epidemiological enquiry (a search for the contaminator) or a descendent one (search for one or more contaminees) had to be carried out by the health authority, starting from the names of partners which the consulting patient was supposed to have supplied. Moreover, serological examinations were compulsory upon marriage, pregnancy, naturalization, donation of blood, etc. – the Nelson Mayer test,[6] perfected in 1949, which was increasingly replacing the less reliable B–W test.

Similar measures were in operation in most countries, particularly as far as systematic declaration was concerned. Some, however, such as England and the Netherlands, did not require it. On the other hand, no 'advanced country' would dream of neglecting the organization of dispensaries, even though their effectiveness was low relative to the number of consultations (18,000 for the 'département' of Calvados alone in 1946).[7] Many venereologists believed that systematic monitoring should be extended to military recruits, civil service staff, railway employees, workers in the food industry, cafés and restaurants, merchant seamen and even applicants for driving licences.

Penicillin to the rescue

In 1877 Pasteur had noted the antagonism between certain fungi and certain microbes, predicting that this might one day have beneficial consequences for human medicine. But it was Alexander Fleming, a Scottish doctor, who in 1928 discovered the great bactericidal power of a mould, *Penicillium notatum*. In 1939 a team of Oxford researchers managed to purify this substance whilst preserving its properties. Penicillin was born. After conclusive experiments on humans in 1941, the United States immediately launched into industrial production of the first antibiotics. In 1943 Mahoney, Arnold and Harris successfully treated four cases of early syphilis with penicillin. It was a form of treatment that was effective, non-toxic and easy to use. Penicillin immediately became the miracle remedy for syphilis (amongst other things), completely overturning the use of the arsenicals, which had already come under criticism.[8] This time the 'magic bullet' which Erhlich had so carefully sought had been found.

Penicillin was first widely tested and used in the liberating armies, against syphilis and also gonorrhoea. In 1951 the US Public Health Service was in a position to publish statistics on six years of treatment of early syphilis with penicillin. Satisfactory results were observed in 98 per cent of cases, and no support was discovered for the idea that arsenic and bismuth made penicillin treatment more effective.[9] However, many European and French doctors defended this idea, advocating either using novarsphenamine as an initial treatment or combining bismuth with penicillin. In fact, although no one denied the usefulness of penicillin, it was doubted that it could cure syphilis on its own.[10] There was much debate on this subject at the conference of French-speaking dermato-syphilologists which took place at Brussels and at Liège in April 1949. At that time there were few who used penicillin exclusively, despite the excellent results obtained by injections of slow-release penicillin. What really upset people, for various reasons, was the speed of the new treatment; it worked in a few weeks rather than in several years.

However, penicillin began to be used against syphilis at the beginning of the fifties. An adequate penicillin treatment[11] proved to be effective for all stages of syphilis, both recent and advanced. It was above all in the domain of congenital syphilis that the new treatment gained the most support: pregnant syphilitic women treated with penicillin before the fifth month of pregnancy did not transmit the syphilis to their children. Thus penicillin immediately destroyed the dogma, which was so powerful between the two Wars, of hereditary syphilis.

Ten years after the triumphal advent of penicillin it seemed that the terrible disease of syphilis was finally being vanquished. The chief doctor of the departments of anti-venereal prophylaxis was resolutely optimistic in his assessment in 1953: 'The anti-venereal struggle which has been waged rationally in France for more than thirty years has culminated, in 1953, in spectacular results.'[12] In fact, cases of primo-secondary syphilis in France fell from 40 per 100,000 in 1946 to 5 in 1953 and 4.5 in 1952.[13] There was a similar rapid decrease in cases of congenital syphilis, which fell from 7,114 in 1946 to 1,804 in 1952. 'Which proves,' concluded the doctor, 'that syphilis really is disappearing.'

This almost miraculous drop is explained by contemporaries as much by the general adoption of antibiotics as by the strict application of the venereal legislation which had been in place for ten years. However, the considerable diminution in the number of syphilitic contaminations recorded in the fifties had the effect of slowing down the activity of the dispensaries. Should those that were not financially viable be closed? No, replied those in charge, who, although they did not believe that a recrudescence was likely in the near future, thought it prudent not to dismantle an infrastructure which had taken so long, and been so difficult, to set up. However, fifty years of terror suddenly gave way to a medical optimism which was soon reflected in the population at large. Would syphilis finally disappear?

Many people believed that it would: in 1955 a paper to the Société Médico-Psychologique was entitled 'Neurosyphilis vanquished, GPI an historical disease'. The same year, at the Congress of French and French-speaking psychiatrists and neurologists held in Nice there was a paper which was bold enough to speak of 'the end of neurosyphilis': 'It is in fact exciting to think that, because of the revolutionary development of medicine since the beginning of this century, we are, perhaps, a generation privileged to witness the disappearance of certain major diseases under the influence of our treatments.'[14] It concluded: 'Penicillin above all, and for ever.'

In the United States, thanks to penicillin, 'the result of the mass treatment of syphilitic disease was overwhelming. The determination of the United States Public Health Service to rid the world of syphilis almost succeeded, and then all those who had to do with syphilis rested upon their oars, except the United States Public Health Service. Syphilis and gonorrhoea are on the rise again, and rather rapidly so.'[15]

The eternal return

Whereas the 1950s had been characterized by the feeling, supported by a rapid diminution in the number of cases, that syphilis was finally destined to disappear, the years 1964–5 brought a sudden end to the general optimism, both in France and throughout the world. In France, after a peak in 1946 of approximately 15,000 registered cases, the arrival of antibiotics brought a rapid fall to 1,874 in 1954. At this point, with only three cases for every 100,000 inhabitants, it seemed that syphilis was going to be definitely eradicated. After a period of relative stability in the years 1955 to 1958 the number of cases began to grow from the beginning of the 1960s. This upsurge peaked in 1964 and 1965, but thereafter fell only slowly and partially, and to the present day there has only been a slight diminution to an average of around 4,000 cases per year (8 per 100,000). The low point of 1954 was never regained (see figure 3).

The national average hides fairly substantial regional differences: at the clinic for cutaneous and syphilitic diseases at the Hôpital Saint-Louis, the upsurge emerged as early as 1957.[16] The same thing happened in the army, where the number of cases of syphilis began to rise from 1959 onwards.[17] On the other hand, in the dermatological department of the Centre hospitalier in Tours[18] and in Reims[19] the 'return' did not begin until 1968–9. But although the figures for each 'département' are not necessarily directly comparable (a fact to which we shall return), it was certainly the case that no region was spared.

Most other countries in the world had the same experience, beginning with a low point in the middle of the fifties: there was scarcely one case per 100,000 inhabitants in Canada, Sweden and the United Kingdom, and the figure was as low as 0.38 in Belgium, in 1958.[20] At the Geneva clinic of dermatology cases of early syphilis had likewise practically disappeared in 1957 and 1958.[21] There followed a sudden upturn at the end of the fifties, and in several countries the figures for the sixties and the seventies matched or surpassed the maxima recorded at the end of the war.[22] In short, syphilis, after having suddenly yielded to the attack of antibiotics, returned throughout the world from the beginning of the sixties, nowhere giving any sign of a new retreat.

Although in the United States an article in the 1951 edition of the '_American Journal of Syphilis_' was entitled 'Are Venereal Diseases Disappearing?', the findings on these matters soon had the health authorities worrying again:

When these cases of congenital syphilis began to appear the health authorities knew that there had to be an increase in acquired syphilis. How did this situation arise? The doctors as well as the public thought that the venereal diseases had been eliminated. Medical educators were ignoring the subject, and still are ignoring it. Medical students were unaware of its existence. The Congress cut the appropriation to such a small proportion that the Public Health Service had to curtail certain educational efforts. Public education concerning these matters had been dropped and the teenagers, among whom the toll is greatest, were unaware of the dangers of free love, thus the venereal diseases began to increase. Small epidemics began to appear in many communities as well as in the metropolitan cities.[23]

As for France, for the last twenty-five years, it has seen an increase in cases of syphilis of proportions which had until then seemed to have been confined to eastern countries (the situation was stable in West Germany, the United Kingdom and Belgium): furthermore, France was leading the industrialized nations, together with Poland. Even though the statistics produced by the WHO

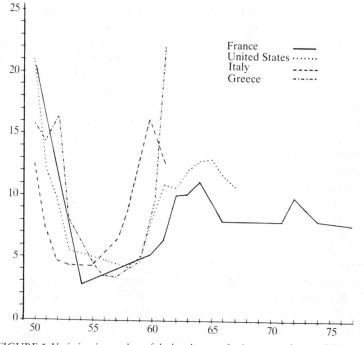

FIGURE 3 Variation in number of declared cases of primo-secondary syphilis per 100,000 inhabitants.
Sources: INSERM; Société Française de Prophylaxie Sanitaire et Morale; Ligue Française contre le Péril Vénérien; Institut National d'Hygiène; US Public Health Service; Brandt, *No Magic Bullet*.

(World Health Organization),[24] which are often based on national figures (France amongst other nations rarely responding promptly), are erratic, partial and, above all, very much lower than they should be, the facts cannot be denied; and, unlike in the fifties, no one today would dare to announce the definitive disappearance of syphilis. Quite the contrary, everyone is now resigned to the fact that syphilis is endemic and likely to flare up in propitious circumstances, and it is now assumed that in times of great population movements syphilis will exceed its present reassuring incidence of 10 cases per 100,000 inhabitants. And, of course, we can only be fully reassured by this statistic if we know it to be reliable.

Unfortunately, this is not the case, for in France as elsewhere the data relating to syphilis in private patients are incomplete because of the more or less conscious reluctance of practitioners to play the role of health police. We shall see from the epidemiological enquiry that patients were even more resistant. In the United States, for example, an experiment undertaken on the initiative of the American Social Health Association in 1961 revealed that private doctors had, in the preceding months, declared only 11.3 per cent of the total number of cases of syphilis, although they had actually treated 75 per cent.[25] This, together with the fact that there were 100,000 new cases a year led epidemiologists to estimate that there was an untreated reservoir of at least 350,000 cases. In France, an enquiry conducted by *Le Quotidien du médecin* (13 August 1985) was unequivocal: only 9.1 per cent of doctors questioned systematically declared STDs to the DDASS; 54.5 per cent declared them 'sometimes', and 18.2 per cent never.

Although this under-recording still allows us to see the general tendencies within each country, it makes it impossible to compare region with region or state with state. On a world scale, the rates given per 100,000 inhabitants (when there was a response) for the period 1969–71 varied from 1,342 for Mali to 0.1 for the Philippines. This clearly makes it impossible to produce any serious world total. In 1954, when the figures were at their lowest, the WHO estimated that there were 20 million with venereal syphilis throughout the world (not counting non-veneral treponematoses which will be mentioned later). Today the figure must be at least three times as great.

We encounter the same difficulty if we try to compare the French 'départements'.[26] If pressed we can accept that between 1980 and 1982 there were 57.86 syphilitics per 100,000 inhabitants in Paris, whilst in the peaceful agricultural area of Creuse the figure was only 0.7. But any was the figure for Essonne 13.86 as opposed to only 0.6 in Val d'Oise? Or 10.86 for Orne as opposed to 0.6 for Manche? It must be said that these figures are hardly serious – we shall see in respect of serological syphilis (which does not figure on the obligatory declaration) that the real incidence of syphilis was substantially greater.

Whatever the case, the return of syphilis was accompanied by a continued level of cases of neurosyphilis[27] whose virtual disappearance, however, had led to its being dropped from the diagnostic classification of INSERM and the WHO from 1968 onwards. However, a 1982 enquiry[28] uncovered evidence of new cases, albeit few, of GPI in various hospitals. The classic symptoms had altered somewhat,[29] with fewer cases of delusions of grandeur and with atypical forms[30] in which difficulties with memory, irritability and dysarthria predominate. These new forms of GPI, often associated with a history of alcoholism, continue to strike mainly at men of fifty or so who are unaware of the source of contagion. These GPIs are mostly discovered by chance, which leads us to suppose that their actual number is far greater. This 'unprompted appearance' of GPI (Dr Th. Gineste) is another example of the thousand and one tricks of syphilis.

Syphilis today

It is now time to sum up the facts about syphilis as it is today. It is an important disease whose pathogenic agent is, as we know, the pale treponema; it belongs to the group of spirochaetes, which are spiral, mobile, transversally divided bacteria. Without going into details of the constitution and antigenic structure of the pale treponema, it can nonetheless be said that this fragile organism, which divides every hour or so in its active phase, cannot survive outside the body for more than a few hours: this means that today as ever, despite a good deal of effort, it is impossible to make an *in vitro* culture of it for a sufficiently long time, and consequently numerous mysteries remain concerning it (the possibility of infravisible forms, for example).[31]

This extremely virulent pale treponema is almost always transmitted from one human body to another by sexual contact (in at least 95 per cent of cases), by percutaneous contagion if there is the least erosion, and even across a healthy mucous membrane. The classic incubation period is three weeks, but this can be shorter (fourteen days) or much longer (up to three months), notably in cases of local or general intercurrent antibiotic treatment. Following the incubation period, which cannot be detected either clinically or serologically, during which the treponemas diffuse throughout the body by means of the lymphatic system, the primary period is characterized by the appearance of a chancre, the first clinical manifestation, which is situated at the point of inoculation and accompanied, four to five days later, by a local adenopathy consisting of numerous, hard painless ganglions. The chancre is a round or oval ulceration which is indurated, has a red, smooth, varnished surface and secretes a clear serous fluid. It is painless and, if not treated, cicatrizes in a few weeks, often leaving no trace (though the adenopathy may persist for several months).

Since the 'Ancien Régime' whole volumes have been written on the multiple local signs and specific appearances it may assume in each case: genital chancres (often on the male balano-preputial furrow and on the female *labia majora*, *labia minora*, or on the neck of the womb – when it is perceptible) and extra-genital chancres (on the lips, tongue, tonsils, anus, to mention only the most common). But the 'fine' textbook chancres are nowadays being displaced by atypical forms[32].

The primary period, which lasts between three and eight weeks, gives way to the secondary period at least forty-five days after the appearance of the chancre (two months after contagion), though often later. It lasts for two or three years, and has numerous clinical symptoms: cutaneous lesions, with roseola (increasingly atypical and discreet) being found most often on the thorax, followed or accompanied by papulous syphilides of very diverse forms, mostly found on the palms of the hands and the soles of the feet; mucous lesions of the mouth, genitals or anus (the famous 'mucous plaques'), which are painless but extremely contagious; alopecia (often patchy); and, finally, visceral symptoms; meningitis, hepatitis, renal and osseous symptoms, etc.

The primo-secondary period is succeeded by what is known as latent syphilis; this has fewer (or more deceptive) symptoms, and is not contagious, though the potential for infection is still there. Only a positive blood test,[33] sometimes performed by chance, reveals it. Due to processes which are still poorly understood, this stage can last indefinitely or become symptomatic at a later stage in the case of a disease not treated in the first stages. Symptoms of the tertiary stage appear a minimum of five years after the first symptoms, but sometimes as much as twenty or thirty years later. In such cases lesions are far more serious: destructive cutaneo-mucous gummas (common in the first centuries of the disease, but exceptional today), lesions of the bones and joints, cardiovascular lesions (syphilitic aortitis and aneurism of the aorta in particular), gastric lesions, hepatic lesions, etc. But the most formidable complication remains neurosyphilis (principally tabes and GPI), which has become less frequent than it was before the war, but whose quiet and insidious return we have already mentioned.

However, untreated patients do not necessarily proceed through the whole cycle. This interesting issue was explored at the beginning of the century by a somewhat unethical experiment. Boek, completely convinced of the inappropriateness of the treatment given at the time, abstained from treating 2,000 patients with primary and secondary syphilis between 1891 and 1910.[34] The general public, if not the patients themselves, were safeguarded by the hospitalization of the patients until cicatrization was complete. Boek's successors followed up the experiment in 1929 and again in 1949. They found that only 25 per cent of patients had relapsed into the secondary stage, 15 per cent had benign tertiary local symptoms (of skin and bones), 14 per cent had cardiovascular symptoms, and only 10 per cent had neurosyphilis. They concluded that two-thirds of the patients had lived with their syphilis with a minimum of discomfort, even though it had not been treated. Nonetheless, they thought that syphilis should be treated, for its outcome in a given subject could not be predicted, and it could lead to serious problems in 30 to 40 per cent of cases, and could be transmitted to offspring.

Even today, penicillin or, in the case of allergy, other antibiotics (chlortetracycline or oxytetracycline) is the favoured method of treatment for syphilis in all of its stages. (And it is thanks to penicillin that congenital syphilis had become very rare in Europe until five years ago when the number of cases, which are often difficult to detect, increased rapidly.) Penicillin is a powerful bactericide, acting on the cell walls of dividing treponemas. There is no indication at present that the treponema will become less susceptible to this action (unlike the gonococci, which are gradually becoming resistant).

In principle, therefore, a seven to ten-day course of treatment during early syphilis, and fifteen to twenty day treatment during latent syphilis, is enough to effect a cure. Syphilis may also be cured using the 'instant treatment' technique, in which the necessary quantity of slow-release penicillin is administered in a single injection. This type of treatment is very advantageous from an epidemiological point of view, for it makes mass campaigns possible and also simplifies the treatment of subjects whom the practitioner, for various reasons, has little chance of seeing a second time. But this raises once more the question as to what are the criteria of being cured.

For a long time it seemed that the idea that the 'pox virus' could lie dormant and reappear after a long period was based more on fantasy than on the facts of the matter. But the intuitive view now seems not to have been so far wide of the mark (if the disease is allowed to develop and is left untreated): the treponema might, it seems, be able to penetrate all cellular elements, including the nerve cells and the nuclei, just like a virus.[35] Now it is not certain that the concentration of pencillin is as high in the tissues as in the external lesions or the blood. Consequently it is still possible to find treponemas in the tissues, the cephalo-rachidian fluid and the lymphatic ganglions after treatment of late syphilis which has resulted in a negative blood test and therefore a theoretical cure. These treponemas, which have lost a good deal of their virulence, remain inactive in the tissues, but can become pathogenic once more in circumstances which are not yet fully understood.

In short, a 'clinical cure' can be claimed when syphilis is treated at a late stage, but there is no absolute microbiological criterion for cure; thus some practitioners prefer to say that the disease has been 'correctly treated' rather than that it has been cured. They also recommend a long period of post-therapeutic monitoring, and have thus taken up once more the cautious attitude of their predecessors, who had good reason to regard syphilis as a slippery character. However, the uncertainty of cure following treatment may be more important in theory than in practice, for therapeutic failures are usually due to reinfection by untreated partners. Nowadays, moreover, the increasing number of cases of reinfection in the same subject following the disappearance of immune protection (whatever that is) is enough to justify caution. Thus penicillin has not completely eradicated syphilis, not so much because of any therapeutic inadequacy (when the treatment is late) as because it will not be possible to study the biological behaviour of the pale treponema, and thereby fight it better, until we can make a culture of it.

The existence of other treponemas which are not transmissible by venereal means but which are closely related to the pale treponema (*I. pertenue* and *I. carateum*, for example) also complicates the picture. It was in the early fifties, when the incidence of venereal syphilis had dropped so much that it was thought it would disappear, that the attention of the WHO[36] was increasingly drawn to the existence of numerous tropical and equatorial regions where endemic non-venereal treponematoses were becoming more serious.

Although these diseases were less serious than venereal syphilis, they affected large proportions of the local populations. The most important of them was yaws, which raged in the hot, humid regions of Africa, South-East Asia and Central America. Before the WHO embarked on a full-scale crusade against this endemic it was estimated that around 50 million people were affected by it, half of them in Africa. There was also pinta in South America and bejel in the Middle East, increasingly often associated with endemic syphilis, a disease long confused with yaws,[37] found in hot, dry climates (particularly in Africa).

These endemics have certain common characteristics. They are found in rural districts where hygiene is particularly poor;[38] contamination is non-sexual; there are few or no primary symptoms (what symptoms there are being confined to cutaneo-mucous disorders); a good general state of health is maintained, except in the infrequent case of late lesions of the tertiary type, especially of the bones.

Thanks to mass campaigns initiated by the WHO penicillin markedly reduced these endemic treponematoses, just as it had done with venereal syphilis. Paradoxically, however, in areas where endemic syphilis is diminishing or has disappeared, venereal syphilis is tending to replace it. This is so, for example, in the south of the Sahara, where following the disappearance of endemic syphilis a new generation of adolescents – which, unfortunately, provides the bulk of urban prostitution in the country – is now susceptible to venereal syphilis.[39] Taking advantage of the Pyrrhic victory, venereal syphilis, that 'artefact of civilization',[40] seems to have found a new place of residence.

In any case, these non-veneral treponematoses raise the possibility of a common origin in a single type of treponema which subsequently differentiated. But what was the original disease? And why shouldn't it have been an animal treponema? This brings us back to the dispute about the origins of syphilis waged around particular bones, such as the cranium found in 1939 in Iraq which seems to date from the first millenium BC and which bears gummatous osteo-periostitic lesions.[41] It is therefore certain that some sort of treponamatosis was part of the pathological history of Eurasia, but that this was yaws and not syphilis,[42] as is proved by the existence of little-known epidemics of non-venereal syphilis in Europe between the sixteenth and eighteenth centuries. Thus the problem remains unresolved.[43]

Epidemiology

Prophylaxis against syphilis today [in France] depends on the declaration made by the doctor to the Direction Départementale de l'Action Sanitaire et Sociale and the epidemiological enquiry which follows it, which must be performed by social workers responsible to the medical inspectors of each 'département'. Unfortunately, as we have seen, these declarations are always incomplete, particularly as regards private patients, and the epidemiological enquiry raises many difficulties. In fact the patient often refuses to answer questions (when, by some chance, the doctor decides to ask them) as to the precise sexual practices involved and the number and identity of partners before and after the contamination.

All epidemiologists deplore this situation. At the Lausanne University Clinic of Dermato-Venereology in 1963[44] barely more than half of enquiries went ahead; their results, moreover, were disappointing (125 cross-examinations produced only thirteen new patients). In the same 'département' during the period 1960–73, 200 patients gave 381 contacts, of which only 182 could be tracked down, 'the information about them given by our patients being incomplete or false'.[45] But doctors sensibly preferred 'half-full' to 'half-empty' bottles, judging that the 199 contacts identified brought in 80 new cases of syphilis, 'which, had they not been traced, would have gone untreated'. At the Saint-Quentin dispensary, only 12 per cent of cases of primo-secondary syphilis were detected through epidemiological enquiries (as opposed to 65 per cent of cases where the patient had discovered the chancre himself and 23 per cent of cases where he had been warned directly by his partner).[46] In Strasbourg at the beginning of the seventies only 35 per cent of epidemiological enquiries produced a result through the contaminator indicating contacts of his own accord; the enquiry produced results in 100 per cent of cases for contaminations due to conjugal relations, in 36 per cent of contaminations due to prostitutes, in 24 per cent of contaminations due to casual relationships, and in 9 per cent of contaminations due to homo-sexual relationships.[47]

However, well-conducted epidemiological enquiries[48] can produce excellent results, allowing the construction of a chain of contamination which can sometimes be spectacular. That produced by the anti-venereal department of Maine-et-Loire in 1971[49] is often quoted as an example. Beginning with the discovery of a chancre in a single patient it is possible, provided the enquirer be sufficiently penetrating and the patients sufficiently forthcoming, to establish an entire chain of contamination. In the example given here (see figure 4) it was possible to track down both earlier and later stages in the chain, revealing no less than thirty-four subjects with primary or secondary syphilis! In this particularly fruitful enquiry the fact that the subjects were of modest social position or belonged to the world of procuring and prostitution made it possible to push enquiries further than would have been feasible or desirable in more affluent circles. This instance undoubtedly represents the limit of epidemiological enquiry.

However, the results are far from negligible, especially in those departments which are more active. In Toulouse and the surrounding region 242 enquiries were possible out of 365 cases diagnosed in

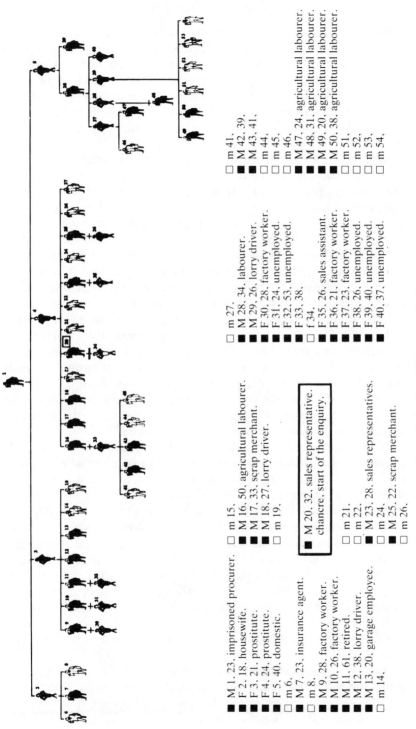

■ M 1. 23. imprisoned procurer.
■ F 2. 18. housewife.
■ F 3. 21. prostitute.
■ F 4. 24. prostitute.
■ F 5. 40. domestic.
□ m 6.
■ M 7. 23. insurance agent.
□ m 8.
■ M 9. 28. factory worker.
■ M 10. 26. factory worker.
■ M 11. 61. retired.
■ M 12. 38. lorry driver.
■ M 13. 20. garage employee.
□ m 14.

□ m 15.
■ M 16. 50. agricultural labourer.
■ M 17. 33. scrap merchant.
■ M 18. 27. lorry driver.
□ m 19.

■ M 20. 32. sales representative. chancre. start of the enquiry.

□ m 21.
□ m 22.
■ M 23. 28. sales representatives.
■ M 25. 22. scrap merchant.
□ m 26.

□ m 27.
■ M 28. 34. labourer.
■ M 29. 26. lorry driver.
■ F 30. 28. factory worker.
■ F 31. 24. unemployed.
■ F 32. 53. unemployed.
■ F 33. 38.
□ f 34.
■ F 35. 26. sales assistant.
■ F 36. 21. factory worker.
■ F 37. 23. factory worker.
■ F 38. 26. unemployed.
■ F 39. 40. unemployed.
■ F 40. 37. unemployed.

□ m 41.
■ M 42. 39.
■ M 43. 41.
□ m 44.
□ m 45.
□ m 46.
■ M 47. 24. agricultural labourer.
■ M 48. 31. agricultural labourer.
■ M 49. 20. agricultural labourer.
■ M 50. 38. agricultural labourer.
□ m 51.
□ m 52.
□ m 53.
□ m 54.

FIGURE 4 Chain of syphilitic contamination.
Source: Service antivénérien de Maine-et-Loire, 1971

1962 and 1963.[50] In the Amiens dispensary a single chain of contamination allowed the identification of sixteen cases of syphilis amongst twenty-six contacts (one woman alone, pinpointed by the ascending enquiry, having contaminated seven subjects).[51] But these cases are somewhat exceptional, and in general epidemiological enquiries were not pushed as far in France as in the United States, where one-third of new cases of syphilis were discovered in this way.[52]

Whatever the case, these enquiries, like the information furnished by the all-too-rare declarations, allow us to draw up a picture of present-day syphilis. The first thing to note is that syphilis is essentially an urban phenomenon, and one of startling proportions: 54.4 per cent of cases in Copenhagen in 1967, although this city accounted for only 15 per cent of the population of the country; 15.1 per cent of cases in New York in 1969 (4.2 per cent of the population); 59.3 per cent in London (central) in 1967 (6.8 per cent of the population).[53] In France, Seine alone declared one-half of the total cases of primo-secondary syphilis in the country.

This phenomenon goes hand in hand with an epidemiology linked to large-scale population movements like tourism (it henceforth became classic that STDs peak during the summer); thus town-dwellers were contaminated away from home,[54] when it was not as a result of a partner who was passing through. Consequently syphilitics are predominantly single (64.3 per cent in Geneva in 1969 and 1970)[55] or alone (75 per cent single, widowed or divorced in Lausanne between 1960 and 1973).[56]

Men diagnosed as syphilitic are, today as in earlier times, more numerous than women: two out of three in Belgium and three out of four in France. But this raises the problem of the time of the diagnosis as it appears on the declaration form. Since primary syphilis is mainly detected in men, it seems that diagnosis happens later in women, and is often made at the secondary stage; in other words, in women the chancre is only infrequently discovered, and women can thus remain contagious without knowing it for several weeks or even months before being diagnosed. Yet it seems that women are contaminated at an earlier age than men (in one of the dispensaries of the Hôpital Saint-Louis[57] the peak age for men is 24 and for women is 19), although this does no more than reflect the fact that women are more sexually precocious than men (see table 2).

Are the young proportionally more affected? The press supported this view when the numbers increased in the 1960s,[58] particular studies putting the percentages for the 15–19 age group between ± 10 per cent (Great Britain, Denmark) and ± 20 per cent (USA,

Table 2 Age distribution of subjects with early syphilis for the period 1971–1980, France

Age	Men (%)	Women (%)	Average (%)
15 to 20	7.8	14.7	11.2
(of whom 15 to 17)	(0.9)	(2.3)	
21 to 29	42.2	44.0	43.1
30 to 44	37.5	28.6	33.1
45 and over	12.5	12.7	12.6
	100.0	100.0	100.0

France) or even 30 per cent (Czechoslovakia, Sweden).[59] But that was 1968, and nowadays we have cause to revise these figures downwards, on condition, of course, that in the case of France we stick to the figures provided by the declarations.

Those under twenty continued to form a sizeable group, despite the maximum falling (logically enough) between the ages of twenty-one and twenty-nine, an age-band corresponding to the greatest sexual activity and the greatest frequency of change of partners. But to return to the young – who pose a problem, as we shall see, because of a scarcity of information which is astonishing in our day and age – it is interesting to note that female precocity is confirmed (twice, and nearly two-thirds the number for the fifteen to seventeen age-band). This phenomenon is equally notable in the United States where syphilis amongst the under-twenties is currently increasing faster in women than in men.

It is much more difficult to assess the socio-professional groups which are affected, since this information does not figure in the declarations. It is not surprising to see at the top of the 'hit parade' manual workers, detainees and, above all, immigrants; the latter have no choice but the dispensary, whereas the middle classes avoid becoming statistics in the secrecy of their private consultations.

The role of immigrants is often emphasized, and therefore merits our attention here. At the Saint-Quentin dispensary 40 per cent of the syphilitics are immigrants, although immigrants form only 2.5 per cent of the population of the town.[60] At the Valenciennes dispensary immigrants, the majority of whom are from the Maghreb, account for more than 50 per cent of patients.[61] But before they became a privileged category of contaminators the immigrants had become the privileged target of prostitutes. This is the sad phenomenon of itinerant prostitutes, some from the most sordid red-light districts of Paris, who come to ply their trade in the camps for immigrant workers on pay day. But this raises the old question of prostitution, and, more generally, that of contaminators (see table 3).

Table 3 Means of contamination of infected subjects, 1971–80

Means	Men (%)	Women (%)	Trend
Non-venereal	1.8	1.1	→
Conjugal contamination	2.5	18.5	↓
Prostitution	6.7	9.6	↓ ↓
Casual relationships	89.0	70.7	↑ ↑

Source: INSERM

Although official statistics are valuable, they are misleading for two reasons, both related to the difficulty of assessment: one is the omission of homosexuals, the other the existence of a considerable and fluctuating number of 'casual relationships' which are in fact new types of prostitution. But before we return to this matter it should be observed that there is no cause to question the great predominance of contaminations from casual relationships, in other words the casual fling, the one-night-stand: this is the phenomenon which some doctors have described as 'sexual vagabondage' or 'door-to-door sex',[62] and others, though fewer, have gone so far as to describe as a psychopathological behaviour.[63]

This enormous category is the bugbear of epidemiologists, for it is here that they encounter the most barriers to their enquiries: 'Both the person contaminated and the contaminator are frequently inaccessible, either because they have left town or because they have moved on (hitchhiking). This, at least, is what patients tend to say. In fact these are evasions which conceal the unspoken desire to bring the enquiry to a halt.'[64] This is particularly notable in homosexuals, amongst whom epidemiological enquiries almost always fail. However, their numbers are far from negligible (insofar as we can estimate them): 9 per cent in Strasbourg,[65] 11.9 per cent in Geneva,[66] 14.7 per cent in Lausanne.[67] In Doubs in the period 1970–80, contaminations due to homosexuality were higher than those due to female prostitution.[68] However, the proportion is probably well in excess of the 10 per cent usually given, if we include undeclared homosexuality. We have already mentioned the

42.4 per cent of cases of primo-secondary syphilis contracted in men in the United Kingdom between 1971 and 1977 through homosexual relationships, with an evident preponderance in London.[69] Equally high proportions are found in Australia and the United States, where syphilis in young homosexual males quadrupled during the seventies. As with AIDS, these figures reflect the almost exponential rate of contamination which results from the fact that homosexuals have a large number of different sexual partners. Moreover, the rates of reinfection are very much greater in homosexuals and in prostitutes.

There remains the question of prostitutes, whose contribution appears to be relatively small from the statistics (less than conjugal contamination by the husband!).[70] But figures gathered from clinical practice paint a very different picture. In Toulouse the upsurge of syphilis in the sixties can be largely attributed to contamination through prostitutes.[71] Of prostitutes, 58 per cent had syphilis and 80 per cent of servicemen with syphilis were thought to have caught it from prostitutes.[72] Also at the time of the upsurge, 88 per cent of servicemen in Toulon contracted syphilis because they were privileged victims of prostitutes and barmaids.[73] At the Valenciennes dispensary prostitution and casual relations had an equal share (36.1 per cent). At the Hôpital Saint-Louis the rate of contamination by prostitutes grew steadily, and even predominated in cases of syphilis in men over thirty.

And this is to reckon without a new category of prostitutes, namely 'occasional' prostitutes. These are often married and ply their trade only intermittently, often to make ends meet at the end of the month; they operate as offices and shops close, even in the housing estates, a common locus of contamination unknown to the health authorities. These occasional prostitutes are much less well informed about the different risks of venereal diseases than the professional prostitutes. It is this fringe which has artificially swollen the category of 'casual relationships' to the detriment of that of 'prostitutes'. At the Brocq dispensary of the Hôpital Saint-Louis, for example, there are three distinct groups of contaminators who account for far more contaminations than conjugal or homosexual ones: prostitutes (36 per cent), chance acquaintances (27 per cent) and regular partners (21 per cent).[74] It is clear that a good proportion of these 'chance encounters' are in fact prostitutes when one reflects that many patients prefer to say that they have 'had an encounter' rather than that they have 'gone with a prostitute'.[75]

This, combined with the problems of mounting an epidemiological enquiry (imagine a social worker asking questions in the little bars of the Rue Saint-Denis), has led many epidemiologists to mourn the suppression of the health record system, all the more so because the order of 25 November 1960 was premissed explicitly on the improbability of an upsurge of the disease, whereas what actually happened was precisely the opposite. Henceforth the prostitutes, though they remained agents of contamination (it is rare not to find one or two in chain of contamination), have deserted the dispensaries and escaped post-therapeutic control. But should we for all that demand the return of regulation?

A final aspect of the epidemiology of syphilis to which doctors are devoting more and more attention is the monitoring of blood tests; this permits a more reliable evaluation of the incidence of syphilis than the declarations of primo-secondary syphilis. These examinations – which are legally performed as part of pre-marital and pre- and post-natal checkups, and systematically on detainees, immigrant workers, blood donors, certain cases for hospitalization, etc. (and which, in fact, are more and more frequently performed in a random fashion on various sectors of the population) – are giving very alarming results.

In the dispensaries it is not rare to find that the proportion of syphilis detected in blood tests equals or even exceeds that of early syphilis.[76] This proves that there are a large number of unrecognized cases of syphilis, as for example at the Hôpital Pasteur in Colmar where 299 cases of syphilis revealed in blood tests led, following enquiries, to 118 completely unrecognized cases of syphilis.[77] At the national level the various samples of the population which have been examined give positive blood tests of rates which far exceed the ± 8 per 100,000 declared cases of syphilis: 34.5 per 100,000 male immigrant workers between 1971 and 1974, 72 per 100,000 male detainees during the same period,[78] 65 per 100,000 blood donors between 1975 and 1980.[79]

This is nothing compared to the figures brought to light in systematic surveys of large samples, judged to be representative, of patients of the Sécurité Sociale: although the figures appear modest in absolute terms, rates of 90 per 100,000 in the Centre region[80] and even 1,600 per 100,000 (1.6 per cent) in the Caisse primaire centrals d'Assurance Maladie de la Region parisienne in 1970[81] were obtained. Even if, in the case of Seine, account must be taken of the very high incidence of blood tests in immigrant workers,[82] it is still the case that the rate of latent syphilis in France is between 10 and 100 times greater than that of declared cases of primo-secondary syphilis.[83]

However, the notion of serological syphilis is problematical because it corresponds both to latent syphilis, and thus to an infection which is still evolving, but also, wrongly, to a serological persistance (persistant seroreactors who are no longer infected and are therefore no longer contagious). It follows that the serological index of a population is ultimately a debatable index of morbidity, particularly in the case of immigrants in whom serological persistence is fairly often the result of an infantile treponematosis.

Ping-pong syphilis

There are several reasons why syphilis remains at the unacceptable level which these serological examinations reveal, by far the most important being what the Americans have aptly called ping-pong syphilis: one partner is treated, the other not. In fact, although the ideal would be to systematically treat all the recent partners of a patient found to have syphilis (the notion of 'epidemiological treatment'), things go quite differently in reality; the partner who is diagnosed as syphilitic is not only averse to 'denouncing' his or her partners to the health authority, but ashamed to warn them him or herself. The chain of contaminations therefore remains unbroken, and, in fact, the one who is treated without playing the game of epidemiological treatment not only allows the disease to be passed on from one partner to another but runs the risk of being reinfected himself following receipt of a negative blood test (hence the term ping-pong).

This phenomenon may proceed equally well from an ignorance of the disease, insufficient self-medication or a diagnostic error; each of these possibilities is made more likely by the present atypical and discreet form of the primary chancres and the secondary lesions, particularly when antibiotic treatment for some other disease at an untimely moment has 'decapitated' the syphilis (this phenomenon being particularly common when gonorrhoea is involved). If we add to this the fact that most doctors nowadays have not seen chancres, roseola or mucous plaques during their medical studies, and have consequently lost the habit of thinking of syphilis, it is not surprising that they produce erroneous diagnoses of an allergic reaction, mycosis, acne, ulcers, herpes, eczema etc. This emphasizes the need for serological monitoring – examinations which are neither onerous nor difficult to perform.

As to the armoury of weapons for the repression of syphilis, it is not only limited, particularly in France, but also unused. We have seen how private doctors baulk at the simple (anonymous) declaration. There was no question of making a nominal declaration of refractory patients and, as a possible consequence, requiring that they be hospitalized. Another weapon, and a considerable one at that, involves invoking the crime of contamination, as provided for in the Code de la santé publique (art. L.285), which states that every contaminator who is aware that he has a venereal disease but cannot prove that he is being treated regularly, can be punished with a fine or between two months and a year in prison (other penalties are laid down for those responsible for the contamination of a suckling or a wet-nurse). But this type of judicial action is almost never brought to bear either in France or elsewhere. There is a similar lack of enthusiasm for an alternative which numerous venereologists have called for, namely increasing systematic serological monitoring of high-risk groups: homosexuals and prostitutes.

Such severity on the part of the authorities, such vigilance on the part of doctors and such conscientiousness on the part of patients presupposes that the fear of syphilis persists, if not at the obsessive and disproportionate level of the pre-war period, then at least at a reasonable level. But, things have gone from one extreme to another and now no-one is afraid of syphilis. There are many who think that it has disappeared, and some female school leavers think that the pill is both a contraceptive and an anti-venereal agent! This highlights a lack of information which is astonishing in our day and age, but which says a good deal about the shame which, whatever one might say, attaches to syphilis.

Above all, let's not talk about it

As anxious about this general complacency as about the upsurge in syphilis and venereal diseases in general from the sixties onwards, the Member States of the Council of Europe adopted in 1974 a common policy aimed at setting international standards for anti-venereal prophylaxis.[84] All the participants stressed the magnitude of the problem and expressed concern about the shortcomings of declarations of cases and the epidemiological enquiries. But although all economic, social, legislative and psychological factors were examined in depth, the measures which were recommended contained nothing more than the usual pious wishes: international support for research into the perfection of vaccines and more manageable tests, the harmonization of laws and regulations at an international level, better interdisciplinary cooperation between venereologists, epidemiologists, gynaecologists and general practitioners (now called 'omnipractitioners') – all these categories being required to cooperate with teachers, social workers, etc.

On the other hand, two of the things which were particularly called for seemed *a contrario* rather disturbing. One was a better training for the medical and paramedical professions (hadn't they been trained properly before?), and the other was better health education for the public. It was estimated that 50 per cent of those questioned in France, the United Kingdom, and even Sweden, knew nothing, or next to nothing, about venereal diseases. It was also noted that throughout the world 'despite the current emphasis on sex, the level of knowledge of venereal diseases amongst the young is remarkably low.'[85]

Today, alas, it certainly seems as if we have made no progress, as Dr Siboulet, Director of the Centre DMS–MST of the Alfred Fournier Institute, confirms: 'Public ignorance at all levels of society remains astonishing.'[86] Yes, admittedly, but who is there to inform the public? A poster issued by the Ligue National Française Contre le Péril Vénérien (which still exists) is entitled: 'Sexually transmissible diseases. Let's talk about them.' The trouble is precisely that we don't talk about them! Nothing at school, nothing on TV, nothing from the family doctor, and, of course, nothing from the family, all of which demonstrates that syphilis (and venereal diseases in general) remains – despite liberalization or, if you like, a slackening of moral standards – a culturally conditioned disease, in other words shameful and taboo.

Is this to say that there is nowadays no prophylactic information on syphilis of the sort that was so common between the wars? Of course not, for the Ligue Nationale Française Contre les Maladies Vénériennes and the Société de Prophylaxie Sanitaire et Morale tirelessly pursue a campaign which has been in progress for over half a century.[87] But the least one each say is that the anti-syphilis propaganda of the late twentieth century (like that of the anti-alcohol organizations) is neither clearly illustrated nor outstandingly original. Some leaflets are too simple for the general practitioners at whom they are aimed (an astonishing choice of target, since one would hope that most doctors would have at least some knowledge of the subject) and too complicated for the general public. Others, it must be said, are disturbingly naive, and border on the unwitting farce, *mezza voce*, found in pre-war publications. Even worse are the few ageing films in which we see nothing but the patients' backs,[88] and the series of stills in a format which is impossible to use, perhaps in this case because the images are so realistic![89]

Those leaflets which are a little better done[90] are in any case only distributed through confidential outlets such as the dispensaries,[91] far from the major media like the press, the radio and the television. When will we have a twenty-four hour telephone

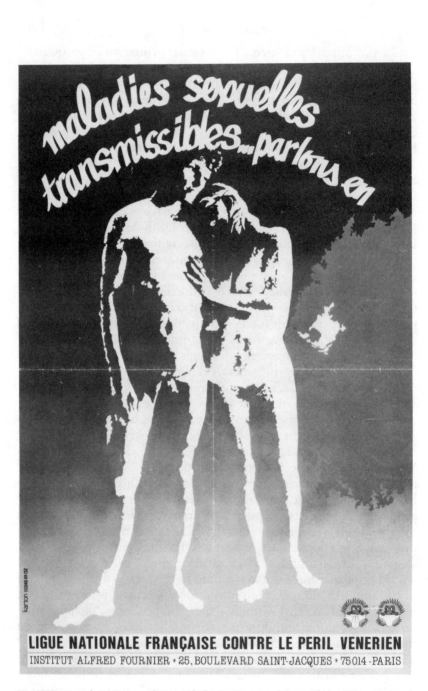

PLATES 21 and 22 Present-day prophylactic poster and logo of the Ligue Nationale Française Contre le Péril Vénérien. Very nice, very clean, but it doesn't sell'.

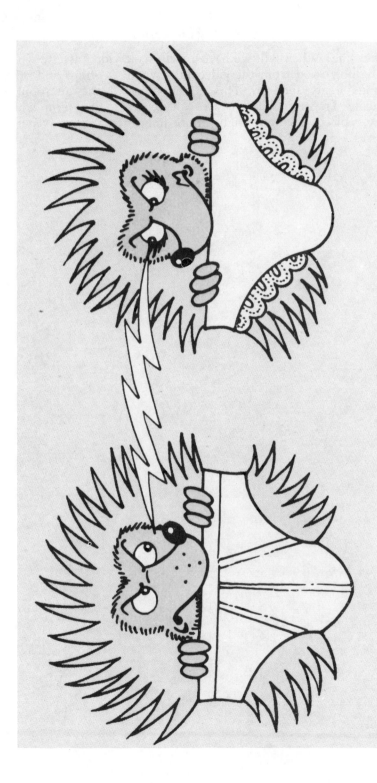

answer line? When will we have a well-made videocassette which can be borrowed from the videoclubs where 'X'-films and other dubious items abound? This is the heart of the question of 'Sexually Transmissible Diseases' in general – the term which today replaces the supposedly more judgemental term 'venereal diseases'.

Conclusion: From Syphilis to AIDS

The world-wide resurgence of syphilis (70 million cases declared – and, of course this is just the tip of the iceberg)[1] is not an isolated phenomenon, but part of a general upsurge of STDs. Thus those two old travelling companions of syphilis, soft chancre and gonorrhoea, (diseases which had often been confused with syphilis), are making a forceful comeback. The former, which had been forgotten, is prevalent amongst prostitutes and immigrant workers; the second is universal, and occurs particularly in summer, as a result of casual encounters. As regards the latter, moreover, a growing number of strains of gonococcus resistant to antibiotics have been appearing. But we have also had to reckon with newcomers, first and foremost urethro-genital infections with *Chlamydia trachomatis*,[2] which have become the commonest of the STDs (especially in women) despite the fact that people are often unaware of its development. There is also genital herpes. Although it was described two centuries ago, it has only recently been classified as a STD. In the last twenty years it has assumed epidemic proportions in the United States (one million new cases a year, and 13 per cent of the total number of cases of STDs). Its virus, like the syphilitic spirochaete, can survive for a very long time in a latent form. There is also urethro-genital trichomoniasis, which is still poorly understood, mycoplasmic infections, urethro-genital candidiasis, which is being seen increasingly frequently, hepatitis B, etc. (see table 4).

But despite their upsurge, all these sexually transmissible diseases pale into insignificance beside the newest of the newcomers, AIDS, which has taken over syphilis's role as the terror of the masses. Let us briefly recap on its history, although for such a recent phenomenon the word 'history' is hardly appropriate. In June 1981, five cases of pneumocystis carinii were detected in Los

Angeles thanks to the Atlanta centre of epidemiology. This pneumonia, found in those with depressed immune systems, had in these cases the peculiarity that it struck young men with no medical antecedents, but who were homosexuals.[3] The term AIDS (Acquired Immune Deficiency Syndrome) was coined after the recording of several hundred identical cases, all characterized by infectious diseases resulting from opportunist germs, with or without cutaneous tumours, and Kaposi's sarcoma. The disease spread via epidemic foci. In the United States, the great urban centres of New York, San Francisco and Los Angeles alone accounted for 60 per cent of cases; likewise, the majority of cases in Europe were concentrated in the British, French and West German capitals. In 1982 it was noted in the United States that AIDS was particularly common in people of Haitian origin, whereas almost all cases in Belgium, and 15 per cent of the cases observed in France were discovered in people originating from equatorial Africa. This suggested that the diseases was of central African origin, a conjecture confirmed by investigations carried out in these countries. The groups at risk were identified: people with many sexual partners, haemophiliacs, homosexuals, and heroin addicts. Only the hypothesis of an infectious agent transmitted via sexual intercourse or via blood could account for all of these characteristics. Researchers were thus directed towards the retroviruses,[4] organisms responsible for leukaemias, but also known to provoke immune deficiencies.

At the Pasteur Institute in Paris in January 1983 Professor Montagnier's team isolated a new human retrovirus christened LAV (Lymphadenopathy Associated Virus) from the ganglion of a patient; a year late Professor Gallo of the 'National Cancer Institute' discovered the same retrovirus which he named HTLV III. Despite disagreement between the two teams as to which had discovered the retrovirus first and what it should be called, it was undoubtedly the same pathogenic agent (today called HIV), that of AIDS. From the summer of 1983, serological tests have made it possible to detect AIDS antibodies, but it was not until 1985 that the industrial production of the reagents necessary to the tests allowed systematic identification, starting with blood donors; this resulted in the discovery of thousands of asymptomatic but contagious carriers, thus giving the disease one of its most unusual characteristics.

There were around 38,000 recorded cases throughout the world in December 1986[5] (an overwhelming majority of which were in the United States and Western Europe), but it was estimated that there were a hundred seropositive cases for every one case of

Table 4 Sexually transmitted diseases (STDs)

Pathogenic agent	Name of disease	Clinical manifestations
Bacteria		
Neisseria gonorrhoeae (gonococcus)	Gonococcal gonorrhoea (clap)	Purulent urethritis, cervicitis (leucorrhoea), epididymitis, bartholinitis, inflammation of the rectum, pharyngitis, conjunctivitis, salpingitis (sterility, ectopic pregnancy) periphepatitis, ophthalmia neonatorum, generalized gonococcal infection
Chlamydia trachomatis	Chlamydial urethro-genital infections	Usually subacute urethritis, epididymitis, cervicitis, bartholinitis, inflammation of the rectum, otitis, salpingitis perihepatitis, pneumonia in adults and children, Fiessingen Leroy-Reiter syndrome, generalized forms
	Lymphogranuloma venereum Nicolas Faure's disease	Microchancre, inguinal adenopathy periadenitis complications: esthiomena, genital elephantiasis anorectal syndrome
Mycoplasma H and T Ureaplasma urealyticum	Mycoplasmic urethro-genital infections	Subacute urethritis, cervicitis, salpingitis, sterility
Haemophilus Ducreyi	Soft chancre	Genital ulceration (skin), painful adenopathies, phagedaena
Gardnerella vaginalis (Haemophilis vaginalis) Gram negative bacillus	Feminine genital infections by Gardnerella vaginalis	Leuchorrhoea, painful adenopathie complications: phagedaena
Calymmatobacterium granulomatis	Donovanosis (inguinal granuloma)	Ulceration (cluster of cicatricial spots), tumoural mass, complications: elephantiasis, stenosis, phageadaena
Shigella salmonella	Shigellosis salmonellosis	Especially in male homosexuals, neonatal septicaemia, neonatal meningitis
Streptococcus Gram positive cocci of group B Gram negative bacilli: E. coli, proteus, etc.	Genital infections by pyogenic bacteria	Subacute urethritis, subacute vulvovaginitis
Spirochaetes	Syphilis	Early syphilis: lesions of the skin and mucous membranes Latent syphilis Symptoms of advanced syphilis: gummas, cardio-vascular and nervous complications Congenital syphilis

Table 4 (cont.)

Pathogenic agent	Name of disease	Clinical manifestations
Protozoa		
Trichomonas vaginalis	Genital trichomoniasis	Urethritis, prostatitis, vaginitis
Entamoeba histolytica	Amoebiasis	Particularly in male homosexuals
Giardia lamblia	Lambliasis	Particularly in male homosexuals
Fungi		
Candida albicans	Urethro-genital candidiasis	Vulvo-vaginitis, balanitis, urethritis
Viruses		
Herpes types 1 and 2	Primary and recurrent genital herpes	Skin vesicles, painful genital ulcerations, clear-liquid meningitis, encephalitis of the newborn
Hepatitis B virus, Hepatitis A virus, and non-A, non-B	Acute or chronic hepatitis	Particularly in male homosexuals
Cytomegalovirus	Genital infections with cytomegalovirus	Serious and fatal infantile malformations, infectious mononucleosis, neonatal retardation, deafness
Papilloma virus	Candyloma acuminatum (venereal vegetations)	Genital vegetations, laryngeal papillomae in breastfeeding babies. Factor in dysplasia
Pox virus	Molluscum contagiosum	Small genital papules
Retrovirus	AIDS	Diverse infectious manifestation pulmonary, intestinal, meningeal, cerebral, etc. Adenopathies, cutaneo-mucous lesions, etc. Kaposi's sarcoma
Ectoparasites		
Phthirus pubis	Phthiriasis	Pubic irritation
Sarcoptes scabiei	Scabies	Pruritis

AIDS. This large group is continuing to grow (even though many predictions are excessive) and, it should be repeated, every one of these cases is contagious. Moreover, given that it is impossible to know which of this number will develop AIDS (or when), that the disease can take between six months and five years to develop (unlike syphilis which takes between fifteen days and three weeks), that it has no particular symptoms, and above all that five years after the disease has been identified only 15 per cent of patients will survive in the absence of specific treatment and a vaccine, it is understandable that attention should be focused on AIDS as has been demonstrated by the international congress on STDs which was held in Paris in June 1986 (following the Puerto-Rican Congress of 1981).

It is impossible to give a detailed description of a disease which, as everyone knows, results from HIV parasitizing the T4 lymphocytes, producing various forms of infection of which the most serious by far is AIDS, the collapse of the immune system leading to a succession of opportunist diseases. Our only concern here is to compare the epidemiology and prophylaxis of this terrible disease with those of other STDs, syphilis in particular. The first question is whether AIDS is an STD. The answer is yes if we consider that HIV is transmitted mainly through sperm, but it is also transmitted through the blood and thus contaminates haemophiliacs, recipients of blood transfusions, and heroin addicts. However, given that contamination of haemophiliacs and recipients of blood transfusions has virtually ceased since the introduction of strict controls in 1985, and also that the proportion of heroin addicts is small (around 15 per cent), it is clear that most cases of AIDS are caused by sexual contamination, particularly in the case of homosexuals, who are undeniably the group most at risk (65–75 per cent); contaminations due to heterosexual relations remains small (5–10 per cent), although they are increasing (likewise that of women, and consequently breastfeeding babies). It is also interesting to note that syphilis is often associated with AIDS in people in high-risk groups such as homosexuals and heroin addicts; the treponema sets in or is reactivated in people who, like AIDS victims, are immunodeficient.

From these few data the cultural aspect of the disease becomes patently obvious as soon as we broach the questions of epidemiology, detection and prophylaxis. In these respects AIDS, like syphilis, is a true 'venereal' disease, in other words it is shameful – although in the case of AIDS the word takes on a particularly strong resonance because of the seriousness of the disease. And here AIDS raises a serious dilemma: on the one hand, the authorities repeat that we must inform, monitor and prevent. But what actually happens? Publicity campaigns dare to do no more than recommend that good old protective of which Ricord said, as regards syphilis, that it was a suit of armour against pleasure, but no more effective than a spider's web against danger. The height of audacity in an age of pornographic films was, in France at any rate, to show on TV a folded protective which might easily have been taken for chewing gum. The message delivered, far from being informative, was confined to the proud battle cry inherited from the 'poilus' of the First World War ('Ils ne passeront pas', it was said at the time, referring to the Germans: 'AIDS will never get past me' a girl says idiotically, offering the famous folded protective to her companion. We find here the same paucity of information that we have already noted as regards syphilis. The measures recommended are limited, given the present state of therapeutic research, to the improved monitoring of the diseases. However, there is no question of monitoring everybody systematically for fear of unleashing a panic which is already smouldering. Nor is there any question of monitoring the high-risk groups for fear of being accused of persecuting sexual minorities, and homosexuals in particular. On this subject we have witnessed many strange scenes, like that of the Strasbourg prostitute literally attacking transvestites suspected of having AIDS. Isa, the Swede, (such was her 'nom de guerre') even telephoned the Ministry of Health to express her indignation. Thus in one of those paradoxes so beloved by history, prostitutes, that age-old high-risk group which has constantly defied all sanitary supervision by the authorities, are ready today to demand it for another high-risk group, namely homosexuals.

This digression has shown that we are not far from the question of syphilis, though we should keep a sense of proportion about the relative seriousness of each disease. The epidemiology of STDs and prophylaxis against them are linked, and their upsurge, like that of the newcomer AIDS poses a general problem which it is not clear that our health systems are adapted to resolve. What good now are our ageing anti-venereal dispensaries which virtually no one visits any more?[6] Increasing numbers of doctors are calling for the campaign against STDs to be taken on by the teaching hospitals, which are more efficient at every level: doctors who are better qualified and who work full time, better equipment, better team work between dermatologists, gynaecologists, biologists, epidemiologists, etc. (not forgetting general practitioners) and, moreover, closer links with teaching and research.[7] Moreover, it would be absurd to overlook the fact that, with this type of disease more than with any other, patients prefer the discreet atmosphere of the private consulting room, whether it be that of the GP or that of the dermatologist. But the doctor is no different, culturally speaking, from the rest of society. What should he do and what can he do when faced with someone who is suffering from gonorrhoea, syphilis or AIDS and refuses to inform or name his partners? Admittedly, it must be emphasized, these cases are not comparable in point of seriousness, but the necessary and sufficient conditions for establishing a chain of contamination are the same. But who today would venture to establish a chain of contamination?

But where is syphilis in all this? Is it ultimately a disease destined, if not to disappear, then at least to become a museum piece? Or will it, on the contrary, hide behind AIDS and begin a new career, as the recent increase in cases of congenital syphilis seems to indicate? From its first appearance in Europe and throughout its history of comebacks, syphilis has demonstrated its capacity to adapt itself to circumstances, deserving more than any other the epithets which our forefathers generously conferred on it; proteiform, insidious, deceitful, underhand and capable of lying dormant for years, ready to strike suddenly when it is no longer expected. Syphilis has long fed on an hysterical panic which has ill-served the cause of prophylaxis. People are so busy crying wolf that they fail to spot the wolf when it is really there. Nowadays, by contrast, syphilis feeds on the carefree disdain of the general public. Can penicillin vanquish it? Of course, but one still has to know that one is contaminated. The treponema is a tiny fragile thing, a vulgar protozoon, not even a virus. But this fragility which has so far made it impossible to make an *in-vitro* culture of it, and thereby gain a sufficient understanding of its modes of operation, assures its survival.

To these physiopathological considerations we may add that syphilis nowadays remains the most socioculturally conditioned of diseases, despite a greater permissiveness which ultimately defines its limits. AIDS strikes too hard and evokes too much fear, at least for the moment, for things to stay as they are. Whatever we may say, syphilis remains a shameful disease which is not spoken of or, what is even worse, is scoffed at. This is perhaps the last and greatest *tour de force* of this disease, since it had found the means of perpetuating itself. As I observed at the beginning of this work, syphilis endures; once it made a great stir, but now it is more discreet, sparing us in order to spare itself. As Thomas Mann writes, 'the spirilla (have been) domesticated for a long time now . . . . In the old countries, where they have been established for centuries, they no longer indulge in the crude pranks of yesteryear – gaping chancres, pestilence, rotting noses.'[8] Let us hope that we don't have to wait another five centuries to say the same thing about the AIDS virus.

Notes

Chapter 1 A Terrifying Affliction (1495–1519)

1 Observations of Marcellus Cumanus reported by C.-G. Gruner, *Aphrodisiacus, sive de lue venerea* . . ., Jena, 1789. (Gruner's compilation completes that of the same title by Aloysius Luisinus (2 vols, 1728).

2 Alexandri Benedicti, *Veronensis physici historiae corporis humani* . . . (1497).

3 'A cultural category which brings to mind a deadly threat ready to swoop down on a nation to weaken or, more often, destroy it', Florence Dupont, 'Pestes d'hier, Pestes d'aujourd'hui' in the special issue of *RHES*, 1984.

4 Veronensis Natalis Montesauri, *De dispositionibus quas vulgares Mal Franzoso appelant, tractatus*, 1498.

5 Nicolo Leoniceno, *De morbo gallico* (Venice, 1497 and Milan, 1497).

6 Collection des Chroniques nationales françaises, vol. XLVII: *Chroniques de Jean Molinet*, by J.-A. Buchon, vol. V (Paris, 1828).

7 '*Universitatis Manuascae Commentarii* . . .', cited in Gruner, *Aphrodisiacus*.

8 A. Péricaud, 'Notice sur André d'Espinay, cardinal, archevêque de Lyon et de Bordeaux', *Rev. du Lyonnais*, VIII, 1854.

9 Archives municipales de Besançon, cc55, fol. 69.

10 *Registers of the Council of Geneva*, Soc. d'hist. et d'archéol. de Genève, V, 1914. See also Wickersheimer, *La syphilis à Genève, à la fin du XVᵉ siècle*, 5th International Congress of the History of Medicine (1925) (Geneva, 1926).

11 Anton Philipp Segesser, *Die Eidgenössichen Abschiede aus dem Zeitraume von 1478 bis 1499* Zurich, 1858.

12 Brièle, *Collection de documents pour servir à l'histoire des hôpitaux de Paris*, vol. III, 'Collection des comptes de l'Hôtel Dieu ' (ledger for 1 October 1495 to 30 September 1496) (Paris, 1883).

13 'Délibérations du chapitre de Notre-Dame de Paris relatives à l'Hôtel-Dieu de Paris (1326–1539)', in E. Coyecque, *L'Hôtel-Dieu de Paris au Moyen-Age – Histoire et documents*, vol. II.

14 Von H. Michelant, *Gedenkbuch des Metzer Bürgers Philippe Von Vigneulles aus den Jahren 1471 bis 1522* (Stuttgart, 1852).

15 A considerable number of incunabula are devoted to the outbreak of the *morbus gallicus* in Europe. See *The Earliest Printed Literature on Syphilis, Being Ten Tractates from the Years 1495–1498*, Karl Sudhoff (Florence, 1925).

16 J. Rohrbach's chronicle of 1496, cited by W. Sticker, 'Zur Geschichte der Syphilis in Deutschland', *Virchows Archiv*, vol. XXXI, 1864.

17 Bibliothèque Nationale, department of engravings and photographs.

18 Bartholomaüs Steber, *A Malafranzos morbo Gallorum, praeservatio ac cura . . .*, Vienna, 1498.

19 Proclamation of King James IV, in the registers of the Edinburgh City Council, 22 September 1497, in Gruner, *Aphrodisiacus*.

20 Parvi Rosaefontani, *Chronicon Johannis Regis Daniae*, 1560.

21 *Tractatus de pestilentiali Scorra Sive Mala de Franzos. Originem, Remediaque ejusdem continens, côpilatus a vene rabili viro Magistro Joseph Grunpeck de Burckausen sub carmina quedam Sebastiani Brant utriusque juris professoris*, 1496.

22 *Libellus Josephi Grunpeckii de mentalagra, alias morbo gallico*, 1503.

23 The term is too modern. (It means to make the symptoms of syphilis, particularly the cutaneous ones, disappear without in any way curing the disease.) The terms 'primary, secondary and tertiary' are also too modern in this context.

24 Amongst the works which have highlighted the importance of Spanish contributions to the study of syphilis following its appearance in Europe, particular mention should be made of Marcel Morel's medical thesis: *Essai critique sur la syphilis en Espagne au temps de la Renaissance*, Faculty of Medicine and Pharmacology of Lyons, 1936. In a work of modest dimensions it is obviously impossible to cite, in the present chapter or in those which follow, all the authors who have written about syphilis, or even to give a biography of those who are mentioned. One attempt to do so, though it is incomplete, is '*Notable Contributors to the Knowledge of Syphilis*', Herman Goodman (New York, 1943).

25 Gasparis Torellae, *Tractus cum consiliis [contra] Pudendagram, seu morbum Gallicum* (Rome, 1497).

26 Gasparis, Torellae, *Dialogus de dolore, cum tractatu de ulceribus in pudendagra evenire solitis* (Rome, 1500).

27 Petrus Pintor, *Agregator sententiarum doctorum omnium de preservatione et curatione pestilentiae*, Rome, 1499, and *De morbo foedo et occulto (morbo gallico) . . .* (Rome, 1500).

28 Juan Almenar, *Libellus ad evitandum et expellendum morbum gallicum, ut nunquam revertatur . . .* (Venice, 1502). There were numerous editions of this work in the first half of the sixteenth century.

29 *Sumario de la Medicina en romance trovado con un tratado sobre las pestiferas Bubas por el lecenciado Francisco Lopez de Villalobos . . .* (Salamanca, 1498). The 'treatise on the *bubas*' follows the *Sumario de la Medicina*, according to Avicenna's 'canons'. People were unaware of the existence of Villalobos' treatise for a long time. Dr F. Lanquetin recognized its worth and translated it into French in 1890. It was edited by Masson.

30 Quoted in Morel, *Essai critique sur la syphilis en Espagne . . .*

31 Coradinus Gilinus, *De morbo quem gallicum nuncupant* (Ferrara, 1497).

32 *Tractatus clarissimi medicinarum doctoris Johannis Widman dicti Meichinger, de pustulis et morbo, qui vulgato nomine mal de franzos appellatur* (Strasbourg, 1497 and Rome, 1497).

33　Antonio Scanaroli, *Disputatio de morbo gallico* (Bologna, 1498).

34　Torella, *op. cit.*

35　Villalobos, *Sumario de la Medicina.*

36　Torella, *Tractus cum consiliis.* This demanding remedy was reproduced, with variations, from the sixteenth century to the eighteenth: 'Take a chicken or pigeon and immediately cut it down the middle, push the ulcerated penis into the warm flesh and keep it there for as long as the flesh exercises its calorific action' Gruner, *Aphrodisiacus sive de lue venerea*, quoted from the 1728 edition. Thus it was thought that the bloody flesh of the animal which had been sacrificed would, by its vital warmth, help to disperse, and even consume, the poison which had entered the male member.

37　This date is problematic. Jeanselme, (*Traité de la syphilis*, chap. VIII) following Anstruc, tried to demonstrate that because at that time the year began at Easter we should take the date to be 1497, not 1496. However, the decree refers to 'the great pox' as a disease 'which for two years and more has been rampant in this kingdom'. This would seem to suggest that the disease began before the return of Charles VIII. Quibbles of this sort have fuelled the controversy over the origin of syphilis (see chapter 2).

38　Archives Nationale XIA (Parlement, Conseil XL, fol. 74ff).

39　On the corner of what are now the Rue de Sèvres and the Rue du Dragon.

40　18 May 1498, Coyecque, 'Délibérations du chapitre de Notre-Dame'.

41　Bibliothèque Nationale, département des manuscrits, FF 21629.

42　Jacobi Catanei de Lacumarino, *De Morbo Gallico Tractatus* (1504).

43　Johannis Benedicti, *De morbo gallico libellus . . .* (1508).

44　Petri Mainardi, *De morbo gallico tractatus duo . . .* (Verona, 1506).

45　Antonii Benivenii, *Forentini Medici et Philosophi, de Morbo Gallico tractatus, ex libro ejus ed abditis morborum causis exceptus.*

46　Juan De Vigo, *Practica copiosa in arte chirurgica . . .* (Rome, 1514).

47　Vulgar Latin uses *variola*, but also *vayrola*, for smallpox. But initially the new disease was called 'the great pox' ('*la grosse vérole*') rather than 'pox', and variola was called 'small pox' ['*la petite vérole*'] to distinguish it from syphilis.

48　Ulrich von Hutten, *De guaiaci medicina et morbo gallico* (Mainz, 1519). The work was translated into German the same year (*Von der wunderlichen Arzenei des Harzes, Guaiacum genannt, und wie man die Franzosen heilen soll*, (Strasbourg, 1519), and into French in the following year (*L'expérience de approbation de Ulrich de Hutten touchant la médecine du bois dit guaiacum pour circonvenir . . . la maladie de Naples* (Paris, c.1520).

49　Ibid.

50　The gaiac is a dicotyledonous plant with evergreen leaves which grows in the Antilles and in Central America. Its resinous wood is one of the hardest in the world. Used in cabinetmaking (and notably for making pharmacists' pestles), gaiac shavings intended for dispensaries were for a long time prepared in prisons because of the difficulty of the work.

51　Grunpeck, *Tractatus de pestilentiali . . .*

52　7 January 1497, Coyecque, 'Délibérations du chapitre de Notre-Dame . . .'.

53　Pintor, *Agregator sententiacum doctorum . . .*

54　Almenar, *Libellus ad evitandum et expellandum . . .*

55　De Vigo, *Practica copiosia in arte chirurgica.*

56 In an ointment. 'Take equal parts of both arsenics, of flowers of sulphur, black hellebore, pine resin and garlic ash; mix with myrrh, incense, aloe, nickel, dull mercury, *axungia*, citron juice and lemon juice; add oil and apply to the scabs', Villalobos, *Sumario de la Medicina*, strophe LXII.

57 Gilinus, *De morbo* . . .

Chapter 2 A Much-disputed Origin

1 Ambroise Paré, *Oeuvres*, 'Le seizième livre traitant de la grosse vérole' (1575).

2 Gonzalo Fernandez de Oviedo y Valdes, *Oviedo de la natural hystoria de las Indias*, (Toledo, 1526).

3 Gonzalo Fernandez de Oviedo y Valdes, *La historia general de las Indias* . . . (Seville, 1535 and Valladolid, 1557).

4 Fernandez, *Oviedo de la natural hystoria* . . .

5 Rodrigo Diaz de Isla, *Tractado cõtra el mal serpentino: que vulgarmente en España el llamado bubas g̃ fue ordenado en el ospital de todos los santos d'Lisbona* . . . (Seville, 1539).

6 Bartolomé de las Casas, *Historia general de las Indias* . . . (first edn, Madrid, 1876).

7 Bartolomé de las Casas was in his twenties at the time; his own father, Antonio, had been with Christopher Columbus on his second voyage.

8 Gabriello Falloppio, *Gabrielis Falloppii . . . de morbo gallico liber absolutissimus* . . . (1564).

9 For example: *Natalis Monthesauro Veronensis de Dispositionibus quas vulgares Mal Franzoso appelant*, (c.1496–1497).

10 For example: *Disputatio de morbo gallico* . . ., Antonio Scanaroli (1498).

11 Gui Patin's letters (letter 687, dated 18 September 1665, addressed to Falconet), 1846 edition, vol. III.

12 Jean Astruc, *De morbis venereis libri sex* (Paris, 1736; 2nd edn, 1740; 3rd edn, in French, 1755; 4th edn rev. and ext., 4 vols, 1777).

13 Montesquieu, *L'esprit des lois* (1748; 1958 edition, Classiques Budé).

14 Voltaire, *L'homme aux quarante écus* (1768).

15 Antonio Nunes Ribeiro Sanchez, *Dissertation sur l'origine de la maladie vénérienne, pour prouver que le mal n'est pas venu d'Amérique, mais qu'il a commencé en Europe, par une épidémie* (Paris, 1752; German edn, Bremen, 1775).

16 Charles Musitano, *Traité de la maladie vénérienne* . . . (1711).

17 Philippe-Gabriel Hensler, *Geschichte der Lutseuche, die zu Ende des fünfzehnten Jahrhunderts in Europa ausbrach* (Altona, 1783).

18 M. N. Devergie, *Clinique de la maladie syphylitique* . . . (Paris, 1826).

19 See, for example: Julius Rosenbaum, *Geschichte der Lutseuche, Erster Theil, Die Lutseuche in Alherthume* . . ., (Halle, 1839; French translation: *Histoire de la syphilis dans l'Antiquité*, Brussels, 1847). Also: Dr F. Buret, *Le 'Gros Mal' du Moyen Age et la syphilis actuelle* (Paris, 1894). *NB* Unfortunately, these works are of little value.

20 Iwan Bloch, *Der Ursprung der Syphilis* . . . (Jena, vol. 1: 1901, vol. 2: 1911).

21 Karl Sudhoff, *Graphische und typographische Erslinge der Syphilis-literatur*

aus den Jahren 1495 und 1496, zusammengetragen und ins Licht gestellt . . . (1912). By the same author: *Aus der Frühgeschichte der Syphilis; Handschriften und Inkunablestudien, epidemiologische Untersuchungen und Kritische Gänge, mit 16 Tafeln* . . ., 12th International Congress of Medicine, London, 1913. Etc.

22 Wickersheimer, *La syphilis à Genève.*

23 Cited in Mirko D. Grmek, *Les maladies à l'aube de la civilisation occidentale – Recherches sur la réalité pathologique dans le monde grec préhistorique, archaïlique et classique* (Paris, Payot, 1983).

24 Lorenz Michaëlis, *Vergleichende mikroscopische Untersuchungen an rezenten historischen und fossilen menschlichen Knochen, Zugleich ein Beitrag zur Geschichte der Syphilis* . . . (Jena, 1930).

25 See, for example: George Grant MacCurdy, 'Human skeletal remains from the highland of Peru', *Amer. J. Phys. Anthrop.,* July-Sept. 1923.

26 See Grmek, *Les maladies à l'aube* . . ., who cites various fairly recent American works such as: N. G. Gejvall and F. Henschen, 'Anatomical evidence of pre-Columbian syphilis in the West Indian Islands', *J. Occup. Ther.,* 25, (1971); M. Y. Elnajjar, 'Human treponematosis and tuberculosis: evidence from the New World', *Amer. J. Phys. Anthrop.,* 51 (1979); D. Brothwell, and R. Burleigh, 'Radiocarbon dating and the history of treponematoses in man', *J. Archaeol. Sci.,* 2 (1975).

27 See F. Guerra, 'The dispute over syphilis: Europe versus America' in *Clio Medica* no. 13 (1978), cited by Grmek, ibid., F. Guerra, however, is opposed to the 'americanist' theory – which just goes to show that even today the latter is not unanimously accepted.

28 G. Del Guerra and Pier Luigi Mondani, 'I primi documenti quattrocenteschi sulla sifilide', *Scientia Veterum,* Pisa, 1970.

29 Bartolomeo Senarega, 'B. Senaregae de rebus Gennensibus commentaria ab unus 1488 usque ad annum 1514 . . .', in Lodovico A. Muratori *Rerum italicarum scriptores* . . . (vol. 24, 1723).

30 *Journal de Jehan Aubrion, bourgeois de Metz, avec sa continuation par Pierre Aubrion (1465–1512), publié en entier pour la première fois par Lorédan Larchey* (Metz, 1857).

31 All the details of Columbus' voyages are drawn from Jacques Heers' excellent biography, *Christophe Colombe* (Hachette, 1981).

32 David de Planis-Campy, *La vérole reconnue, combattue et abattue sans suer et sans tenir chambre, avec tous ses accidents, Le tout selon l'ancienne et moderne médecine* . . . (Paris, 1623).

33 Oscar Panizza, *Das liebes Konzil,* Zurich, 1895; translated into French under the title: *Le concile d'amour,* ed. Pauvert, collection Libertés, 1964; the extracts which follow are from this edition).

34 Published as an appendix to the Pauvert edition, see n. 33.

Chapter 3 The Great Pox (Sixteenth Century)

1 Paré *Oeuvres*, ch. 2.
2 Jean De Bordigné, *Histoire agrégative des Annales et Chroniques d'Anjou* (1529).
3 Francesco Guicciardini, *Histoire d'Italie, de l'année 1492 à l'année 1532* (Paris, 1836).
4 Alain Briot, 'La Syphilis au Japon à l'époque d'Edo' (Paper given at the Fourth Congress of Japanese Studies in Europe, October 1985). On the question of syphilis in the Far East see also Keizo Dohi's essential text *Beiträge zur Geschichte der Syphilis, insbesondere ueber ihren Ursprung und ihre Pathologie in Ostasien* (Tokyo, 1923). The Japanese edition is dated 1921.
5 Briot *La Syphilis au Japon.*
6 *Des, Erasmi Roterodami, Lingua sive, de linguae usu, atque abusu, Liber unus* . . . (1520; prefatory letter).
7 Girolamo, Fracastor, *Hieronymi Fracastorii Syphilis sive morbus gallicus* (Verona, 1530).
8 French translation in 1753 under the title *Syphilis ou le mal vénérien. Poème Latin de Jérome Fracastor.* But it was Auguste Marseille Barthélemy who in 1840 produced the most elegant translation, after having himself composed in the same mode a remarkable poem in two cantos entitled *Syphilis* (see ch. 5). Here is an extract of his translation of Fracastor's poem:

> *Chose étrange! ce mal, introduit dans le corps,*
> *Parfois avec lenteur se trahit au-dehors,*
> *Et souvent, sans qu'il donne un signe manifeste,*
> *La lune, quatre fois, forme son plein céleste:*
> *Il se cache, il hésite, il couve sourdement,*
> *Et semble en notre sein prendre son aliment.*
> *Cependant le malade, en proie à ses atteintes,*
> *Sous un poids inconnu sent ses forces éteintes:*
> *Une torpeur de plomb s'appesantit sur lui,*
> *Aux travaux journaliers il vaque avec ennui:*
> *Les symptômes fâcheux ne tardent pas d'éclore:*
> *L'oeil perd de son éclat, le front se décolore,*
> *La hideuse carie, étendant ses progrès,*
> *Porte sa lime sourde aux organes secrets,*
> *Ronge les lieux voisins et s'étend jusqu'aux aines,*
> *Le mal n'est plus douteux, ses marques sont certaines.*

9 Girolamo Fracastori, *Hieronymi Fracastorii . . . Liber I de sympathia et antipathia rerum, de contagione et contagiosis morbis* . . . (1550).
10 Jacques de Béthencourt, *Nova penitentialis Quadragesima, nec non purgatorium in morbum Gallicum, sive Venereum* . . . (Paris, 1527). There is a French translation and commentary by A. Fournier entitled *Nouveau carême de pénitence et purgatoire d'expiation à l'usage des malades affectés du mal français ou mal vénérien* . . . (Paris, 1871).
11 Thierry de Héry, *La méthode curatoire de la maladie vénérienne, vulgairement appelée grosse vairolle, et de la diversité de ses symptômes* . . . (Paris, 1552; there was a new edition in 1634).

12 Guillaume Rondelet, *Traité de la vérole* (Bordeaux, 1576).

13 Antonii Musae Brassavoli, *Ferrarensis, de morbo gallico* . . . (1551).

14 Niccolo Massa, *Niccolai Massae . . . Liber de morbo gallico* . . . (1532).

15 Jean Fernel, *Joannis Fernelii . . . de Abditis rerum causis* . . . (Paris, 1548). By the same author: *Joannis Fernelii . . . Febrium ac luis venereae curatio methodica* . . . (1580). A French translation by Michel Le Long entitled *Traité de Maître Jean Fernel, jadis conseiller et premier médecin du Roy, de la parfaite cure de la maladie vénérienne.*

16 Vidius (Vidus, the elder), *Vidi vidii . . . De curatione generatim* . . . (1587).

17 Falloppio, *Gabrielis Falloppii*, ch. 2.

18 Niccolo Massa, *Nicolai Massae, Epistolarum medicinalium* . . ., vol. 1, letter 30 (Venice, 1558).

19 Paré *Oeuvres*, ch. 2.

20 Briot, *La Syphilis au Japon.*

21 Ibid.

22 Massa, *Liber de morbo gallico* . . .

23 Falloppio, *Gabriellis Falloppii*, ch. 2.

24 Briot, *La Syphilis au Japon.*

25 Béthencourt, *Nova penitentialis Quadragesima* . . .

26 Fracastori, *Hieronymi Fracastorii.*

27 Rabelais, *Gargantua* and *Pantagruel*; the 1542 edition is the definitive one.

28 Botal, *Lues venereae curandi ratio* (Paris, 1563).

29 Petrus Andreas Matthiolus, *De morbo gallico liber unus* (Venice, 1535).

30 Diaz de Isla, *Tractado côtra el mal serpentino*, ch. II.

31 'Libro de las cuatro enfermedades cortesanas que son: catarro, gota artetica sciatica, mal de piedra y rinones e hijada, y mal de buas. Dirigido al muy illustre Sr. Dn. Juan de Zurriga' (Toledo, 1544), in C.-G. Gruner, *Aphrodisiacus.*

32 Niccolo Campana, *Lamento di Strascino, sopra il male incognito* . . . (Venice, 1521).

33 Briot, *La Syphilis au Japon.*

34 Procès-verbaux, 23 Feb. 1507, destroyed in the town hall fire of 1871, but mentioned by Husson in *Inventaire des archives hospitalières* . . .

35 For example, we can read in the registers of the Hôtel-Dieu accounts for 1509: 'A poor woman sick with the so-called Naples sickness, and to get her to go home six sous . . . to another ill of the said sickness who wished to stay, two sous given by force to go away.'

36 From the time that the two buildings belonging to the abbey of Saint-Germain were put in operation, women began to be set apart in a house in the Saint-Honoré district. The question was then raised of putting the victims of venereal disease in the house of the Croix de la Reine in the Saint-Denis district, but this establishment, formerly reserved for pilgrims returning from Palestine, had been progressively transformed into a theatre where, initially, the mysteries of the Holy Places were performed. The 'Confrères de la Passion' resisted, and the people of the district with them. Similarly, a former leper colony which, for the purpose, became Saint-Eustache hospital, was unable to keep the pox-victims intended for it because the ill-will of the churchwardens was so great. Another establishment in a little 'hospital' of the Saint-Nicolas parish failed in its turn, and the buildings soon fell into ruin.

37 Arch. Nat., XIA, 1528 fol. 583 (Parlement, Conseil).
38 B. N., ms FF 18606, appendix I bis ('Abrégé du nombre des pauvres qui dépendent du Grand Bureau').
39 E. Wickersheimer, 'Les débuts, à Strasbourg, de l'hospitalisation des syphilitiques', extract from *Le Scalpel*, 5 March 1960.
40 Torella, *Tractus cum consiliis*.
41 Rondelet, *Traité de la vérole*.
42 Erasmus, *seu conjugium impar* (1524; translated into French as *L'union mal assortie*).
43 According to tradition, this tyrant of Agrigentum, famous for his cruelty, had his enemies roasted alive in an iron bull.
44 *Le triumphe de haulte et puissante Dame Verolle, Royne du Puy d'Amours . . .* (Lyons, 1539), anonymous.
45 In the *Dialogue entre le mercure et le gaiac* by J. De Béthencourt, *Nova penitentialis Quadragesima*, mercury can say to its rival, not without vanity: 'Today I keep company with kings, princes, generals, prelates, bishops, and all the important figures of this world.'
46 Drouyn (Jean), *La ballade de la grosse vérolle* (Lyons, 1512).
47 *Les trois comptes, intitulez, de Cupido et d'Atropos, dont le premier fut inventé par Seraphin, poète italien, le second et le tiers, de l'invention de Maistre Jean Le Maire* (1525).
48 'La Patenostre des vérollez', in *Recueil de poésies françaises des XVᵉ and XVIᵉ siècles . . .*, selected and annotated by A. de Montaiglon, vol. 1, Paris, 1855).
49 Ibid., vol. 3.
50 On this whole question I follow Yvonne David-Peyre's noteworthy thesis *La peste et le mal vénérien dans la littérature ibérique du XVIᵉ et du XVIIᵉ siècle*, Fac. des lettres et sciences humaines de Poitiers, 1967.
51 Gaspar Lucas Hidalgo, cited by David-Peyre.
52 The author, Francisco Delicado, had himself contracted the pox, cited by David-Peyre.
53 *El Criticon*, cited by David-Peyre.
54 *Paradoxa en loa de las bubas*, cited by David-Peyre.
55 See ch. 7: 'Madmen and hérédos'.
56 Cited by David-Peyre.

Chapter 4 From Pestilence to Disease

1 Planis Campy, *La vérole reconnue*.
2 Ibid.
3 'Harangue faicte au charlatan de la place Dauphine . . . avec une salade . . . pour la guérison de sa maladie napolitaine' from *Pièces tabariniques . . .* (Paris, undated, beginning of the seventeenth century). A very rare pamphlet (Bibl. Mun. de Rouen, Fonds Leber).
4 Marie de Maupeou, Fouquet, Mme François), *Recueil des remèdes faciles et domestiques . . . recueillis par les ordres charitables d'une illustre et pieuse dame . . .* (1678, with the author's name omitted). (There were numerous editions in the reigns of Louis XIV and Louis XV).

5 Jean-Baptiste Lalli, *La Francéide ou le Mal français, poème burlesque* (translated into French from the Italian, original edition, 1629).

6 Traité de la maladie vénérienne . . . par le Sieur de la Martinière, médecin chimique et opérateur du Roy et de plusieurs princes (Paris, 1664).

7 B. N., Département des estampes et de la photographie.

8 Pierre Chaunu, *La civilisation de l'Europe classique* (Paris, 1966).

9 G. R. Le Fébure de Saint-Ildephont, *Le médecin de soi-même ou méthode simple et aisée pour guérir les maladies vénériennes avec la recette d'un chocolat aphrodisiaque aussi utile qu'agréable par M. Lefebvre de Saint Il . . .* (1775).

10 See P. Morel and C. Quétel, *Les médecines de la folie* (coll. Pluriel, 1985), p. 44ff: 'Non à la masturbation'.

11 Caen medical thesis (1772) by Joanne-Francisco-Renato de Parfourru: *An in aestimandâ mercurialum anti-venerae vi, ratio ipsorum solubilitatis habenda* ('Must we take account of the solubility of mercurial compounds in order to evaluate their antivenereal powers?').

12 Astruc, *De morbis venereis*. (The quotation is taken from the preface to the 4th edn (1777), which appeared under the title *Traité des maladies vénériennes*.)

13 See, for example, Everard Maynwaringe, '*The history and mystery of the venereal lues, concisely abstracted and modelled (occasionally) from serious strict perpensions, and critical collations of divers repugning sentiments and contrary assertions of eminent physicians, English, French, German, Dutch, Spanish and Italian dissenting writers, convincing by argument and proof the traditional notions touching this grand evil, and common reputed practice grounded thereon, as erroneous and unsound*' (London, 1673).

14 François Ranchin, 'Traité de l'origine, nature, causes, signes, curation et préservation de la vérolle' from *Opuscules ou traités divers et curieux en médecine* (Lyons, 1640).

15 Briot, *La Syphilis au Japon*.

16 Gervais, Uçay, *Nouveau traité de la maladie vénérienne* (1699).

17 In 1606, in Nicot's *Trésor de la langue française*, and likewise in Furetière's *Dictionnaire universel*.

18 *Dictionnaire universel de médecine . . . James*, vol. IV, translated by Diderot, Eidous and Toussaint (Paris, 1747).

19 Preface to the 1728 edition of C.-G. Gruner, *Aphrodisiacus*. (This preface appeared separately in London in the same year, and was then translated into French by de La Mettrie in 1735, and into German in 1783.)

20 Nicolas Andry, *De la génération des vers dans le corps de l'homme* (Paris, 1700).

21 Antonie Deidier, *Dissertation médicinale sur les maladies vénériennes* (1735, 6th edn.; 1st edn in Latin in 1713).

22 Pierre Desault, *Dissertation sur les maladies vénériennes . . .* (Bordeaux, 1733).

23 Astruc, *De morbis venereis*. (All references are to the 1777 edition).

24 Paul-Joseph Barthez, *Nouveaux éléments de la science de l'Homme* (Montpellier, 1778).

25 John Hunter, *A treatise on the venereal disease* (London, 1787).

26 This theory is mentioned in the *Encyclopédie méthodique* (surgery, vol. II, 1792), but only as a point of interest, for 'the truth is that no-one knows, and

perhaps no-one will ever know, the ultimate nature of the pox virus.'

27 Joseph Lieutaud, *Synopsis universae praxeos medicae* (1765).

28 The *Encyclopédie méthodique*, touches on the question as follows: 'The virus, once received, does not always produce its effects immediately at the place at which it has been admitted; it is sometimes four to five days, and at other times eight, before the part in question shows evidence of its action . . . . But also, in some cases, it has an unusually prompt effect.

29 Antonio Nunes Ribeiro Sanchez, *Observations sur les maladies vénériennes . . .* (Paris, 1785).

30 One of the first medical works to use the word syphilis in its title is an English work: D. Turner, *Syphilis. A practical dissertation on the venereal disease . . .* London, 1727, (3rd edn).

31 For example: Jacques Gautier D'Agoty, *Exposition anatomique des maux vénériens sur les parties de l'homme et de la femme, et les remèdes les plus usités* (Paris, 1773).

32 There were 1,912 exactly, according to Ch. Girtanner, *Abhandlung ueber die Venerische Krankheiten* (1793, 2nd edn).

33 *Dictionnaire universel de médecine.*

34 F. Balfour, *Dissert. de Gonorrhoea virulenta* (Edinburgh, 1767).

35 Benjamin Bell, *A Treatise on Gonorrhea and Lues venerea*, 2nd edn, 2 vols, Edinburgh, 1797.

36 F. X. Swediaur, *Practical observations on venereal complaints . . .* (1784; French edition in 1785, and many subsequent editions in English, French and German in the following three decades).

37 D. R. De Horne, *Exposition raisonnée des différentes méthodes d'administrer le mercure dans les maladies vénériennes, précédé de l'examen des préservatifs* (Paris, 1775).

38 De Horne, *Observations faites et publiées par ordre du Gouvernement sur les différentes méthodes d'administrer le mercure dans les maladies vénériennes* (Paris, 1779).

39 1 *gros* = 72 grains (1 grain = 0.053 g.).

40 Planis-Campy, *La vérole reconnue* (arsenic is recommended in the *Antidotaire* appended to the work).

41 Torella, *Tractus cum consiliis*, first chapter.

42 Bibliothèque Nationale, Réserve des Imprimés (Prospectus), Te. XVIII, 665.

43 L. S. Mercier, *Tableau de Paris* (new edn, corrected and extended, 12 vols, 1782 to 1788).

44 Le Fébure de Saint-Ildephont, *Le Médecin de soi-même.*

45 For example, 'Letter from M. Thomas to M. de Lonche, surgeon of Meulan': 'Monsieur Gabon and I beg you to tell us if you know M. Keyser, who boasts of having an infallible secret cure for the venereal sickness and who has performed over one thousand amazing cures in his birthplace, Gisors. He would have us believe that he is equal to none, and yet he often fails to satisfy those who entrust themselves to him. We have heard a good deal about him, and we would like to know whether his supposed miracles at Gisors have as little foundation in fact as those he claims to perform here' (see n. 46 for reference).

46 'Lettre de M. Keyser à M . . ., docteur en médecine, servant de réponse à un faux article inséré dans le journal économique' (Paris, 1757).

47 Laffecteur, *Rapport sur l'analyse du rob anti-syphilitic du Sieur Laffecteur* (Paris, 1779).

48 Andrieu, *Agenda antisyphilitique* . . . (Paris, 1786).

49 Fabre, *Traité des maladies vénériennes* (Paris, 1782, 4th edn).

50 British Museum, Prints Department.

51 Saint-Simon, *Mémoires* (La Pléiade edn, vol. 1, XLIV).

52 'Sometimes the chancres are so malignant and corrosive that they produce an aqueous humour on the surrounding skin, which shines like crystal, hence the name cristalline' (Ranchin, 'Traité de l'origine . . .'). Boerhaave saw the cristalline as a more benign form of the venereal disease, and his description is somewhat reminiscent of genital herpes: 'The spot which is infected first is always characterized by a reddish blotch, rather like a flea-bite, a measle, or nascent smallpox. The patient feels a slight itch there, a hot sensation which is uncomfortable rather than painful. The surface of the skin rises over this spot and forms a small blister which can be completely cured be evacuating the limpid humour which fills it . . . . These small blisters, called cristallines by common surgeons, can easily be gotten rid of by the simplest of remedies.'

53 Uçay, *Nouveau traité*.

54 Voltaire, *Candide ou l'optimisme* (1759).

55 Voltaire, *L'homme aux quarante écus*.

56 Translated from the French, Casanova, *Histoire de ma vie* (Brockhaus unabridged edn, Plon, 1960).

57 James Boswell, '*Boswell's London Journal, 1762–1763*', F. A. Pottle, *The Yale Editions of the Private Papers of James Boswell* (1952).

58 James Boswell, '*Boswell in search of a Wife 1766–1769*', ed. F. Brady and F. A. Pottle (1957).

59 See the recent edition in vol. 3 of *L'enfer de la Bibliothèque Nationale* (anonymous works of the eighteenth century, vol. I; Fayard, 1985).

60 Taken from *Les petits bougres au manège ou Réponse de M*** en l'an second du rêve de la liberté*, B. N., Imp. Réserve (enfer).

61 *Aventures galantes de Rosalie, fille de joie* . . . (London, 1796).

62 Hunter, *A treatise on the venereal disease*.

63 It is more likely to have been named from the Latin *condere* (to protect, hide) than after the hypothetical doctor Condom, though this last explanation had many supporters.

64 Turner, *Syphilis*.

65 This precursor of the IUD seems to have been mentioned for the first time in seventeenth-century Italy.

66 *La cacomonade, ou Histoire politique et philosophique du mal de Naples, traduit de l'allemand de Dr Pangloss* (attributed to Linguet; Cologne (Paris), 1756). Condemned in 1825 as offending moral standards.

67 Restif de La Bretonne, *La pornographe, ou idées d'un honnête homme sur un projet de règlement pour les prostituées, propre à prévenir les Malheurs qu'occasione le Publicisme des Femmes* . . . London (The Hague), 1769. (There were many editions in the years which followed. There is a recent edition in vol. 2 of *L'enfer de la Bibliothèque Nationale*.

68 'Poverty-stricken mendicants afflicted with leprosy, or with a contagious disease, or with venereal disease will not be received by the above-named General Hospital and those Houses which constitute it.' (Regulation following the edict of 1656 creating the general hospital of Paris, art. VI.)

69 'The Hôtel-Dieu of Paris receives, feeds and tends all poor sufferers, wherever they come from and whatever ailment they may have, even plague victims, though not if they have the pox, because of the abuses and problems which could result . . . . As for those pox-victims who have caught the sickness in question by ill-fortune and through no fault of their own, as, for example, a good woman given it by her bawdy husband, or a husband by his unchaste wife, or a suckling child by its wet-nurse, or a wet-nurse by a child, the aforementioned Commissioners of the Poor will have them tended and cured by barbers at public expense, and give them help from a certain fund provided by the Hôtel-Dieu, following the decrees of the Court.' (R. P. F. Jacques Du Breul, *Le Théâtre des Antiquitez de Paris*, 1639).

70 (Mirabeau), *Observations d'un voyageur anglais sur la maison de force appelée Bicêtre* . . . (1788).

71 See, for example, *Médecine militaire ou Traité des maladies tant internes qu'externes auxquels les militaires sont sujets, dans leurs différentes positions de paix ou de guerre, par ordre du Gouvernement* (vol. V, Sec. IV: 'Préservatifs contre le mal vénérien', anon. (Paris, 1778).

72 In 1789, 32 out of 226 beds were for sufferers of venereal disease (seven beds for French Guards, seven for Swiss Guards and eighteen 'reserved for individuals who have contracted the shameful disease'). From Tenon, *Mémoire sur les hôpitaux de Paris*, printed by the King's order (1788).

73 Hardy (*Mes loisirs*), B. N. ms FF 6062, cited by Erica-Marie Benabou in 'La maladie antisociale: le danger vénérien à Paris au XVIII^c siècle' (*Mélanges Goubert*, Privat, 1984).

74 An idea advanced by J.-L. Flandrin in *Familles – parenté, maison, sexualité dans l'ancienne société* (Hachette, 1978).

75 *L'antisyphilitique ou la santé publique* . . . (1772).

76 Turmeau de la Morandière, *Représentations à M. le lieutenant de Police sur les courtisanes à la mode et les demoiselles de bon ton* Paris 1760; cited by E. M. Benabou, 'La maladie antisociale'.

77 Joseph Raulin, *Conservation des enfants, ou les moyens de les fortifier, de les préserver et guérir des maladies depuis l'instant de leur existence jusqu'a l'âge de puberté* (1768).

78 Particularly F. Doublet, *Symptômes et traitement de la maladie vénérienne dans les enfants nouveau-nés* (Paris, 1781).

79 See *Instruction sommaire sur le traitement des maladies vénériennes dans les compagnes, lue dans la séance tenue au Louvre par la Société royale de médecine le 12 septembre 1786, rédigée et publiée par ordre du Gouvernement*, 1787. Note, in particular, the following observation: 'The venereal disease, formerly unknown in the provinces, has recently become fairly common in some areas, because workers whom need has driven to the capital during the summer return home infected with the diseases to which they have exposed themselves . . . and soon an entire canton can find itself infected with an unknown or unrecognized virus which wreaks havoc, degrades the species,

and by imperceptible degrees destroys the future races on which the hopes of agriculture and the forces of the State are founded.'

80 See *Mémoire sur la nécessité d'interdire l'allaitement naturel pour les enfants trouvés et notamment les enfants attaqués du mal vénérien* (extract from the registers of the Société royale d'agriculture, 4 March 1790, Archives Nationales F16.936). Lawsuits initiated by wet-nurses against mothers who had placed their children with them were not uncommon. The following is an example: 'Mlle Adélaïde who formerly danced at the Opéra and who lives with M. de Montbarey, is being sued by her child's nurse, who says that the child has given her the pox and who demands compensation. Adélaïde has been condemned to the Châtelet in respect of 6,000 livres. She is appealing to the Parlement' (B. N., ms FF 11357).

Chapter 5 The Nineteenth-century Impasse

1 J.-S. Mittié, *A l'Assemblée Nationale, Sur le traitement de la syphilis* . . . (1789).

2 Ibid.

3 *Procès-verbaux et rapports du Comité de Mendicité de la Constituante, 1790–1791*, published and annotated by C. Bloch and A. Tuetey (Paris, 1911).

4 On the question of the history of French medicine in the nineteenth century, and especially as regards its foundations, see the excellent *La médecine entre les pouvoirs et les savoirs* by Jacques Léonard Aubier, (1981).

5 *Traité de la maladie vénérienne chez les enfants nouveau-nés, les femmes enceintes et les nourrices (. . .) par M. Bertin* . . . (Paris, 1810).

6 *Dictionnaire des sciences médicales* (60 vols), ed. Panckoucke (Paris, 1821), article on 'Syphilis' by Cullerier and Bard.

7 *Dictionnaire de médecine et de chirurgie pratiques* (21 vols), (1836) article on 'Syphilis' by Cullerier and Ratier.

8 A.-J.-L. Jourdan, *Traité complet des maladies vénériennes* . . . (Paris, 1826).

9 J.-F. Hernandez, *Essai analytique sur la non-identité des virus gonorrhoïque et syphilitique* (Toulon, 1812).

10 Philippe Ricord, *Traité pratique des maladies vénériennes, ou Recherches critiques et expérimentales sur l'inoculation appliquée à l'étude de ces maladies* . . . (Paris, 1838).

'Clinical observation has led me to the following classification of the symptoms of syphilis: (1) The primary manifestation, the chancre, is due to the direct action of the virus, which it reproduces . . . (2) The symptoms which are consecutive, or which follow very soon afterwards, or as a mere extension of the first localized manifestation, such as further chancres . . . (3) Secondary manifestations or manifestations of a general infection . . . . These phenomena can undoubtedly be inherited by children from their mothers . . . without them having any of the primary manifestations . . . . (4) Tertiary manifestations, which occur at various stages, but usually a long time after the primary manifestations have disappeared; most subjects only develop these manifestations when the secondary manifestations have taken place, whether they have disappeared or still persist . . ., manifestations which no longer spread the infection. To this category of tertiary manifestations belong the nodes, the deep tubercules, the tubercules of the cellular tissue, the periostoses, the exostoses, the caries, the necroses, and the syphilitic tubercules of the brain.'

11 Philippe Ricord, *Lettres sur la syphilis, adressées à M. le Rédacteur en chef de l'Union medicale par Ph. Ricord* (Paris, 1851), letter 12.

12 Devergie (the elder) *Première lettre sur la syphilis, ou examen critique des doctrines de M. Ricord* (Paris, 1840).

13 William Wallace, 'Clinical lectures and remarks delivered on diseases of the skin, venereal diseases and surgical cases. Lectures XXII and XXIII, on Syphilis', *The Lancet*, 8 and 22 July 1837.

14 J. Rollet, 'Étude clinique sur le chancre produit par la contagion de la syphilis secondaire, et spécialement sur le chancre du mamelon et de la bouche', *Arch. gén. de méd.*, February, March and April 1859.

15 On this subject see Pierre Darmon's definitive work *La langue traque de la variole* (Perrin, 1985).

16 'De la syphilisation ou vaccination syphilitique', by Dr Auzias-Turenne. Taken from *Arch. gén. de méd.*, June 1851, and subsequent issues.

17 Dr Auzias-Turenne's papers are at the Bibliothèque de l'Arsenal, 25 boxes, mss 6715 to 6739.

18 *Correspondance syphilographique par le Dr Auzias-Turenne* (Paris, 1860), letter 3: to M. Miranda, student of medicine.

19 *Rapport à M. le Préfet de Police sur la question de savoir si M. le docteur Auzias-Turenne peut être autorisé à appliquer ou à experimenter la syphilisation à l'infermerie de la prison Saint-Lazare* (Paris, 1853).

20 *Procès-verbaux et rapports du Comité de Mendicité . . . .*

21 J. Capuron, *Aphrodisiographie, ou tableau de la maladie vénérienne . . .* (Paris, 1807).

22 P. Baumès, *Aperçu médical des hôpitaux de Londres où sont traitées les maladies vénériennes et les maladies de la peau* (Paris, 1835).

23 Briot, *La Syphilis au Japon*.

24 F. Swediaur, *Traité complet . . . des mal. vénér.*, pluviose an IX 4th edn (1801), vol. II, ch. XIII, *De la nouvelle maladie syphilitique qui a paru depuis peu au Canada*.

25 For information on extra-venereal epdemics of syphilis see Lancereaux, 'Traité historique et pratique de la syphilis' (Paris, 1873).

26 See, for example, H. M. J. Desruelles, *Traité pratique des maladies vénériennes . . .* (Paris, 1836).

27 See, for example, G. Hume Weatherhead, '*The history of the early and present state of the venereal disease examined: wherein is shown that mercury never was necessary for its cure, as well as the injurious consequences that result from its employment . . .*'.

28 In *Gazette des médecins practiciens*, no. 26, 1839 (Hôtel-Dieu, service de M. Chomel).

29 Briot, *La Syphilis au Japon*.

30 Brera in Italy, Wallace in Dublin ('Treatment of the Venereal Disease by the Hydriodate of Potash, or Iodine of Potassium's, *The Lancet*, 1835–6), and Ricord (who combined it with mercury) in France.

31 Achille Hoffmann, *La syphilis débarrassée de ses dangers par la médecine homoeopathique, ou conseils aux jeunes gens victimes des erreurs de la médecine ordinaire* (Paris, 1848).

32 H. Crosilhes, *Traité complet des maladies vénériennes* (Paris, 1849).

33 *Dictionnaire encyclopédique des sciences médicales*, ed. A. Dechambre ('Syphilis', vol. XIV, 2 vols.), (Paris, 1884).

34 By Dr J.-P. des Vaux (1862). The foreword begins as follows: 'I address this book to young people. Those who, lured by its title, might open it in search of obscene pictures or smutty anecdotes can close it again without reading it; it is not for them that it was written. My aim has been to forwarn those who are embarking upon life against the imminent perils to which they may be exposed by a moment of pleasure shamefully sought in an illicit companionship to which one blushes to admit, and to give useful advice to those who have unfortunately allowed themselves to be led astray.'

35 By Dr A. Lebel (1855).

36 Dr M. Levy, *Hygiène publique et privée*, 2nd edn (Paris, 1850).

37 J.-B. Venot, *Aperçu de statistique médicale et administrative sur l'hospice des vénériens de Bordeaux* (Paris and Bordeaux, 1837).

38 A. J. B. Parent-Duchâtelet, *De la prosititution dans la ville de Paris considérée sous le rapport de l'hygiène publique, de la morale et de l'administration* (2 vols., Paris, 1836).

39 G. Ferrus, *Des Aliénés* (Paris, 1834).

40 Ibid.

41 P. Yvaren, *Des metamorphoses de la syphilis* (Paris, 1854).

42 Théophile Gautier, *Deuvres érotiques, poésies libertines, lettres à la présidente* (Arcanes, Paris, 1953).

43 It would be a pity not to give another example of the verve, so notable in this instance, of the author of *Le Capitaine Fracasse* and *Emaux et camées*, so rightly acclaimed for their polish and erudition: '(In Florence) There were two flower-girls, very bold, very provocative, and always ready to take a turn on their backs; but the first took a knock once during which she caught the pox. According to some she still has it; according to others she has been cured, but it has made her more difficult to mount than a flayed mule. The second is in love with a robber, which makes her impregnably virtuous. As for the honest women, it is difficult to serve them because they have always got some man or other on the job. The husband, the lover and the servant follow each other with scarcely a pause; you have to wait your chance, and stand by at the cunt's edge, tool in hand, ready to plunge it in the moment it is unoccupied, which it rarely is.'

44 Patrick Wald-Lasowski, *Syphilis – essai sur la littérature française du XIXe siècle* (Gallimard, coll. Les essais, 1982).

45 See Marc Fumaroli's outstanding treatment of this question in the Gallimard edition, collection Folio, 1977.

46 See for example: Moïse Le Yaouanc, *Nosographie de l'humanité balzacienne*, doctoral thesis in literature, Paris, 1959.

47 Is it because Zola, whose method of working is well-known, did not have a syphilologist amongst his medical advisers? (See Y. Malinas, 'Zola et les hérédités imaginaires', *Expansion scientifique française*, 1985.)

48 Jean-Louis Douchin, *La vie érotique de Flaubert* (Carrère-J.-J. Pauvert, 1984).
49 Ibid.
50 Frank Harris, *Ma vie et mes amours*, transl. into French from the English (Gallimard, 1960).
51 This astonishing episode is related in the Goncourts' diary (Sunday 1 February 1891); one of the brothers (Jules) himself contracted syphilis.
52 Sale catalogue of autographs from the Hôtel Drouot (20 November 1984), letter no. 219. (This letter went for the trifling sum of 90,000 F.)

Chapter 6 The Great Turning Point (around 1900)

1 *Dictionnaire encyclopédique des sciences médicales*, edited by Dechambre, 1884.
2 'It is the bubo, then, which very often testifies to the chancre when the latter no longer exists. And, in fact, the chancre often disappears rapidly, especially in women, sometimes leaving no trace. The bubo, by contrast, is very much more persistent. It always survives the chancre. It is there, therefore, when the chancre is no longer, like a posthumous witness to the chancre, testifying both to its previous existence and to its location, like a witness who makes a deposition in the following terms: "Not only have I had a chancre, but this chancre was sited here, within the area covered by my lymphatic network".' (*Traité de la syphilis*, see n. 4.)
3 Fournier classifies the syphilides according to whether they are early (according to Dechambre's dictionary, 'early syphilides open the drama to which the syphilitic chancre is the prologue'), intermediate or late:
I. *Early* syphilides, at the very beginning, or in the early stages of the secondary period; roseola, urticaria, papulous or papulo-squamous with little papules, acneiform syphilides of the scalp.
II. *Late* syphilides, which never, or almost never, appear until a very late stage of the second period, or even later: pustulo-crustaceous syphilide, severe Ecthyma, Rupia.
III. *Intermediate* syphilides, appearing neither as early as the first nor as late as the second: rings of roseola, papulo-squamous syphilide with large papules, palmar and plantar Psoriasis, papulo-crustaceous syphilide, impetiginiform syphilide, acneiform syphilide, Impetigo, superficial Ecthyma, pigmentary syphilide.
4 A publication was dedicated to each of these questions. The works of Alfred Fournier are collected in his *Traité de la syphilis*, 2 vols, compiled in 1899 and 1901 by his son, Edmond Fournier.
5 A. Fournier, *Leçons sur la syphilis tertiare . . .*, (Paris, 1875) and *De l'ataxie locomotrice d'origine syphilitique. Leçons recueillies par F. Dreyfous* (Paris, 1876).
6 A. Fournier, *Traitement de la syphilis* (Paris, 1909).
7 In *Prophylaxie de la syphilis* (1903), Fournier sets out the numerous conditions necessary for the smooth functioning of a community clinic.
8 The two terms were coined in 1842.
9 On this subject, read *L'Hôpital Saint-Louis*, by N. Sant-Fare-Garnot in the Hôpitaux de France collection – Histoire et architecture, éditions de l'Arbre à images (1986).

10 This museum, for the exclusive use of the medical profession, still exists today. With some 2,000 waxworks it is the biggest and most remarkable collection of specimens of skin disease. Chancres and syphilides occupy only one of the ten rows of glass cases which belong to the museum, now required to move into another section of the Hôpital Saint-Louis (with all the dangers which the handling of such fragile waxworks entails).

The museum was created in 1865 when Dr Devergie, before leaving the hospital where he had been head of department for twenty-five years, made a present of a series of watercolours of the various dermatoses to the administration of the Assistance Publique. His successor, Dr Lailler, had added several casts before discovering the rare talent, Baretta, a moulder who until then had manufactured plaster fruits. From 1867 to 1894 Baretta executed 1,800 technically brilliant dermatological studies, to which were added the collections of several doctors, notably, as far as syphilis is concerned, Dr Fournier's collection. Together they formed the only collection of its kind in the world, set out from 1882 to 1885 in a museum built specially for the occasion in the precincts of the Hôpital Saint-Louis. As a testimony to its success, a dermatological and syphilological atlas entitled *Le musée de l'hôpital Saint-Louis* was published at the end of the nineteenth century.

11 A. Fournier, 'Document statistique sur les sources de la syphilis chez la femme – syphilis des femmes mariées – syphilis imméritées', *Bulletin de l'Académie de médecine*, session of 25 October 1887.

12 Edmond Fournier, 'A quel âge se prend la syphilis?', *La presse médicale*, April 1900.

13 L. Queyrat and M. Pinard, 'Résultats de l'inoculation des produits syphilitiques primaires aux sujets atteints d'accidents tertiares', *Bull. de la Soc. de dermat. et de syph.*, 1906. M. Pinard, *L'immunité dans la syphilis. Superinfection and réinfection*, thesis, Paris, 1910.

14 Metchnikoff and Roux, 'Études expérimentales sur la syphilis' (five papers which appeared in the *Annales de l'Institut Pasteur*, 1903, 1904 and 1905). NB After the monkey, which was too costly, and almost always destined for tuberculosis research, rabbits were used from 1906 onwards.

15 Metchnikoff, 'La syphilis expérimentale', *Académie de médecine*, 8 and 15 May 1906. 'Sur la prophylaxie de la syphilis', *Annales de l'Institut Pasteur*, 1905, 1906.

16 Maisonneuve, *Expérimentation sur la prophylaxie de la syphilis*, medical thesis, Paris, 1906.

17 The use of bismuth in the treatment of syphilis had already been anticipated, in 1889, by Balzer, who quickly abandoned it after observing signs of poisoning in dogs injected with salts of bismuth.

18 Sonnet signed R. C. (hospital extern, 1910), appearing in *Anthologie hospitalière et latinesque*, vol. II (Paris, 1913).

19 A. Corbin, 'Le péril vénérien au début du siècle: prophylaxie sanitaire et prophylaxie morale', *Recherches*, 29 Dec. 1977 (devoted to 'L'haleine des faubourgs').

20 Cited by Corbin, ibid.

21 *Bulletin de la Société de prophylaxie sanitaire et morale*, 1903.

22 Draft published in 1902 at the instigation of the Société de prophylaxie

sanitaire et morale. NB The difference in age in the two titles was the result of investigations which concluded that women had their first sexual encounters at an earlier age than men.

23 Émile Pierret, *Le péril de la race – avarie-alcoolism-tuberculose* (Paris, 1907).

24 Cited in Corbin, *Le péril vénérien*.

25 It appeared between two equally evocative titles: *Les accouplements* (1887) and *Les baisers morts* (1893).

26 Michel Corday, *Vénus* (republished under the title: *Vénus, ou les deux risques*).

27 In another novel, *Les demi-fous*, which appeared in 1905, and whose foreword is dedicated to Professor Lacassagne, Michel Corday sets out his notion of the 'physiological novel', a rich and inexhaustible form which consists in mixing art and science, and which will, in the long term, allow us to 'cultivate and improve the human race in the way we have been cultivating and improving vegetable and animal species for centuries'.

28 The author even denies himself the easy option of presenting his message in the classic form of a testament addressed to the young son, telling the reader that the sacrifice has not been in vain. Here, the message is only a draft. 'My son, my dear son, This is for you when you are grown up. Remember. Don't think that love is so pleasant, nor so easy, nor so important in life . . .'. But 'the note stopped at that point, unfinished. What good could it do?'. It is on this darkly pessimistic note that the novel ends – leaving one wondering just what message the author intended to address in his 'physiological novels' in which he claims to 'restore to the physical body the prime importance which it has in our lives'.

29 Syphilomania: 'A mania for receiving anti-venereal treatment exhibited by certain individuals because they believe themselves to be still infected with the syphilis of which they have already been cured' (*Dictionnaire de médecine . . .*, ed. P. A. Nysten, 4th edn (1824; 1st edn 1806).

30 Excerpt from *La vie médicale* (March 1901): 'Kieman, of Chicago (*New York Med. Journ.*) showed that syphilophobia is one of the most depressive of afflictions, particularly when it occurs in neurasthenic subjects; it is accompanied by melancholia, loss of appetite and even a strong tendency towards suicide.'

31 See 'Des méfaits de la syphilophobie, par le Dr Janselme', *La médecine moderne*, 1895.

32 Corbin, *Le péril vénérien*.

33 Prince A. Morrow, 'Publicity as a factor in venereal prophylaxis', *JAMA*, 47 (10 October), cited in Allen M. Brandt, *'No Magic Bullet:* A social history of venereal disease in the United States since 1880 (Oxford University Press, 1985).

34 Brandt, No Magic Bullet.

35 This fine phrase slightly predates the period with which we are presently concerned, for it dates from 1865: *De la santé des gens mariés ou physiologie de la génération de l'homme et hygiène philosophique du marriage*, by Dr Louis Seraine.

36 P. Diday, *Le péril vénérien dans les familles* (Paris, 1881).

37 This phrase is used in a pamphlet by Dr Gaultier-Boissière, *Pour préserver des maladies vénériennes* (Bibliothèque Larousse, around 1910). We may read

there that 'every factory girl, peasant and maid must be told that if she abandons herself to the seducer then not only does she run the risk of having to bring up the child which might result from her transgression, but also that of catching a disease whose consequences can make her suffer for the rest of her life.' (Here too it is noticeable that the daughters of the bourgeoisie are, by implication, exempt.)

38 Alfred Fournier, *Syphilis et marriage*, 2nd edn (Paris, 1890).

39 Edmond Langlebert, *La syphilis dans ses rapports avec le marriage* (Paris, 1873).

40 Raymond Villey, *Histoire du secret médical*, Seghers, coll. Médecine et Histoire (Paris, 1986).

41 See Dr G. Thibierge, *Syphilis et déontologie* (Paris, 1903).

42 Diday, *Le péril vénérien*.

43 In the following case, doesn't Dr Diday well and truly flout medical confidentiality, in spirit if not in letter, even though he believes that he has circumvented it? The parents of a future bridegroom come to see him to question him as to whether their son has syphilis, as they suspect. The doctor does not remember, or does not choose to remember, the name they tell him, but he allows that the mother, if she is unable to bring the person in question himself, should bring a prescription ('the easiest thing in the world for her; the ABC of maternal espionage'). 'Once in possession of the document,' continues Dr Diday, 'I can tell her: "This prescription or prescriptions mean such-and-such a disease, with such-and-such a degree of seriousness, requiring such-and-such abstentions or precautions." And I have given her the information which my conscience told me it was my duty to give, without betraying a professional secret . . . all I did was to make an impersonal judgement, without knowing to whom it applied.'

44 Eugène Brieux (1858–1932) is the author of many plays with social problems as a theme (for example, in 1900, *La robe rouge*, on the magistrature, and, early in 1901, *Les remplaçantes*, which condemned breastfeeding by wet-nurses). He was a favourite of the Théâtre Antoine, and was elected to the Académie Française in 1909 (when he died, his place was given to François Mauriac).

45 Michel Corday, author of *Vénus ou les deux risques*, also supports *Les Avariés*, hailing the theatre as 'a centre of resonance infinitely more powerful than the book'.

46 See *L'illustration* of 16 Nov. 1901: 'M. Brieux has resolved to read his play himself to guests chosen from amongst those whom Paris numbers as serious and distinguished men. Paris has proved him right by listening to him with a sustained interest and applauding the boldness and generosity of the author's ideas.'

47 Six editions in the first year! And a bookshop success which was only halted by the Second World War. (In the *Théâtre complet d'Eugène Brieux* (9 vols published by Stock), *Les Avariés* was curiously placed with two other plays, *Les hannetons* and *La petite amie* – a lot to get one's teeth into.)

48 See *La chronique médicale* (1914). (From the time of the ban in France Brieux had already noted the good reception which the army had given his play.)

49 Cited in Corbin, *Le péril vénérien*.

50 Cited in Brandt, *No Magic Bullet*.

Chapter 7 Madmen and Hérédos

1 J. Haslam, *Observations on Madness and Melancholy: including practical remarks on those diseases* . . . (London, 1809). Cited by Jacques Postel in *La syphilis et ses répercussions en pathologie mentale* (II: 'Histoire et actualité de la paralysie générale'), enquête A.T.P. Santé, CNRS, March 1982.

2 A. L. J. Bayle, *Nouvelle doctrine des maladies mentales* (Paris, 1825). By the same author: *Traité des maladies du cerveau et de ses membranes* (Paris, 1826).

3 L. F. Calmeil, *De la paralysie considerée chez les aliénés* (Paris, 1826).

4 J. B. M. Parchappe, *Des altérations de l'encéphale dans l'aliénation mentale. Recherches sur l'encéphale* . . . (Paris, 1838). Cited in Postel, *La syphilis et ses répercussions*.

5 'Rapport général à M. le Ministre de l'Intérieur sur le service des aliénés en 1874, par les Inspecteurs généraux du Service, MM. les Doctors Constans, Lunier et Dumesnil', Paris, Imprimerie nationale, 1878.

6 Mme Dominique Giraud, in a study of Charenton, makes the interesting observation that even in the capital of organicism the registers of the insane continued to include psycho-social diagnoses (family and professional troubles, etc.).

7 *Dictionnaire encyclopédique des sciences médicales.*

8 At this time, 45–60-year-olds were the age group most affected; they were predominantly widowers and bachelors.

9 Gireaudeau de Saint-Gervais, for example, in a mediocre and pretentious work (*Traité des maladies vénériennes* . . ., numerous editions from 1838 onwards) writes, in a chapter entitled 'Consecutive venereal diseases seated in the nervous system', that 'the sudden suppression of a primitive venereal disease may be followed by a metastasis towards the brain, and give rise to all the nervous ailments which can develop from the irritation of this organ'. (Gireaudeau de Saint-Gervais was one of the late epigones of Broussais.)

10 Notably in 1859 by Hildebrandt, who had detected syphilitic antecedents in almost all general paralyses.

11 Notably Lasèque (*Sur la paralysie générale* (1884): 'There is therefore no syphilitic general paralysis; there can be, and there are, general pseudo-paralyses which overlay it; but in no case has general paralysis been observed.'

12 A. Fournier, *Syphilis du cerveau* (Paris, 1879).

13 Fournier describes six forms of cerebral syphilis, which is 'of an essentially protean nature': cephalic, congestive, convulsive or epileptic, aphasic, mental, paralytic. In the mental form there is excitement or depression. The depressive variety consists of intellectual asthenia or an incoherent hebetude. The variety in which there is excitation is syphilitic madness.

14 Primarily with tabes and general paralysis.

15 *Des rapports de la syphilis et de la paralysie générale, par le professeur Joffroy* (Paris, 1905).

16 In the years which followed, by way of counter-proof, general paralytics who had reached the final stage of the disease were infected with material scraped from very virulent syphilitic lesions – the absence of result proving that they

were syphilitics of long standing (see, for example, E. Jeanselme *Traité de la syphilis* (2 vols, 1931).

17 Cited by Dr Jean Lacassagne in *Guy de Maupassant et son mal* (1951).

18 *Ma vie et mes amours.*

19 Charles Mauriac, *Nouvelles leçons sur les maladies vénériennes. Syphilis tertiare* (Paris, 1889).

20 'Today, 23 February, he still believes that his life is threatened, but that God knows very well that he is immortal . . . He will kill God by giving him the black pox . . . (12 March): One must never pass water in the evening, for urine makes one sleep: these are precious stones which must not be put in the pot. That feeds the body, I tell you! . . . I have a terrible silver in my belly . . . Russia hears me . . . England hears me . . . China hears me . . .' (Georges Normandy, *La fin de Maupassant* (Paris, 1927).)

21 *Souvenirs sur Maupassant* (Rome, 1905).

22 See the last section of chapter 4: 'Saving the race'.

23 Complementing it, Profeta's law (1865) states that a syphilitic mother cannot contaminate a healthy child.

24 Adam Dewre of Christiania opposed it in several papers between 1868 and 1876 (concluding in particular that the sperm of a syphilitic has absolutely no influence on the mother, either directly or indirectly). At the same period, Edmond Langlebert *La syphilis dans ses rapports . . .* declared that he had never encountered a case of hereditary syphilis which was not attributable to the mother.

25 On this question, see Nicole Valleur's comprehensive study ('Le mythe de l'hérédo-syphilis') in Postel, *La syphilis et ses répercussions.*

26 Pr Roux, *La syphilis – ce que doit savoir tout syphilitique – Peut-il devenir vieux? Peut-il créer une famille saine? A quelles conditions?* (Paris, 1918).

27 'Rapport fait au conseil de salubrité de la ville de Marseille, sur l'État et les besoins du service, au dispensaire des filles publiques de cette ville, au nom d'une commission, par M. Pelacy, rapporteur', *Annales d'hygiène publique* (Paris, 1841, XV).

28 A. Fournier, *Syphilis héréditaire tardive* (Paris, 1886).

29 Cited by Nicole Valleur, in Postel, *La syphilis et ses répercussions.*

30 S. Freud, *Cinq psychoanalyses* (French translation 1970, PUF, 4th edn). (Cited by Nicole Valleur, in Postel, above.)

31 S. Freud, *Trois essais sur la théorie de la sexualité* (French translation 1962, Gallimard). (Cited by Nicole Valleur, in Postel, above).

32 Cited by Nicole Valleur, in Postel, above.

33 *Traité des dégénérescences* (1857). *Traité des maladies mentales* (1860).

34 E. Fournier, *Recherche et diagnostic de l'hérédo-syphilis tardive* (Paris, 1907): *Syphilis héréditaire de l'enfance* (Paris, 1921).

35 M. Comby, *Ligue nationale contre le péril vénérien: Conférence de la syphilis héréditaire* (Paris, 1925). Cited by Nicole Valleur, in Postel, above.

36 Roux, *La syphilis . . .*

37 'Remarques sur la syphilis scolaire' by Dr F. Gidon of Caen, *Annales des Laboratoires Clin.*, no. 4, 1926.

38 Alain Corbin, 'L'hérédo-syphilis ou l'impossible rédemption. Contribution à

l'histoire de l'hérédité morbide', in *Romantisme, revue du XIXe siècle*, no. 31 ('Sangs' 1981).

39 Which furnishes, for example, the theme of the golden spot in *Nana*.

40 Jean Moyë, *La vie d'un hérédo* (Paris, Denoël, 1939).

41 Louise Hervieu, *Le crime* (Paris, Denoël, 1937).

42 *Observations sur les maladies vénériennes*.

43 Léon Daudet, *Devant la douleur* (1915 edn).

44 Maurice Phusis, *La grande infection héréditaire (l'hérédo-syphilis)* (coll. Phos-Bibliothèque scientifique de Perfectionnement humain, undated *c*.1920).

45 R. Bellière, *Paralysie générale et génie*, medical thesis, Paris, 1932.

46 J. Audrain, *La syphilis obscure* (Paris, 1911).

47 Daudet, *Devant la douleur*.

48 Marc La Marche, . . . *En vrac* (Paris, 1929).

49 It is true, on the other hand, that the general paralysis of a great military leader did nothing to help sort out France's affairs in 1940.

50 Judith Thurman, *Karen Blixen* (Seghers, 1986).

Chapter 8 Syphilis Everywhere (Between the Wars)

1 For example, Dr L. M. Pautrier, professor in the treatment of cutaneous and syphilitic diseases at the Faculty of Medicine in Strasbourg after the Great War.

2 Phusis, *La grande infection héréditaire*.

3 Dr L. M. Pautrier, *Collec. d'études économiques, médicales et sociales*, no. 12: 'La lutte contre les deux grandes fléaux sociaux: la tuberculose et la syphilis' (1923).

4 Ibid.

5 Whereas in all other countries the number of recorded cases of syphilis increased during the twenties, Belgium continued to show a regular fall thanks to a vigorous health policy: an increase in the number of small dispensaries (there were 400 in Belgian territory) and intensive propaganda (1,500,000 pamphlets and tracts, 50,000 posters etc. in just a few years). On Belgian anti-syphilitic prophylaxis after the First World War see 'La lutte contre la syphilis' by W. Schraenen, General Secretary of the League Against the Venereal Peril. (From *L'Avenir social*, June 1928, Brussels.)

6 Louis Spillman was born in Nancy in 1875. The son of a doctor, he too became a doctor of medicine in 1900, and in 1929 was given the chair in the treatment of syphilitic and cutaneous diseases. Amongst his numerous works on the subject is *Guérir est bien, prévenir est mieux*, a veritable manifesto of anti-syphilitic prophylaxis published in collaboration with J. Parisot in 1925. He set up the first syphilitic dispensaries in his city, attended all the congresses, and soon became Dean of the Faculty of Medicine at Nancy.

7 A. Fournier, *Prophylaxie de la syphilis* (Paris, 1903).

8 Cavaillon, 'L'état actuel de la lutte contre les maladies vénériennes', *Annales des maladies vénériennes*, Dec. 1926.

9 It has been used freely here, particularly because of its wealth of bibliographical

information and the relative accuracy of its quotations, including those relating to the first centuries following the appearance of syphilis in Europe. The work in question is *Traité de la syphilis*, published under the supervision of Ed. Jeanselme, ed. G. Doin (7 vols, Paris, 1931), approx. 8,000 pp.

10 Professor Jeanselme, 'Le dispensaire antivénérien de la clinique de l'hôpital Saint-Lous', *La presse médicale*, no. 32, 20 April 1935.

11 262 cases of primary syphilis, 165 of secondary syphilis, and 28 of tertiary (but also 1,436 assorted dermatoses).

12 The first in France seems to have been the one set up in the Baudelocque clinic in 1919.

13 See, for example, Dr J. Hericourt, *Les maladies des sociétés (tuberculose, syphilis, alcoolisme et stérilité)* (Paris, 1918).

14 L. Spillman, *L'évolution de la lutte contre la syphilis – Un bilan de 25 ans: Nancy, 1907–1932* (Paris, 1933).

15 Dr Léon Legendre (Éditions médicales Maloine, Paris, 1928).

16 Dr Maurice Bernay, *La syphilis et ses conséquences* (Paris, undated).

17 A prophylactic tract to be distributed in dispensaries drafted by the French Society for Sanitary and Moral Prophylaxis and published in the journal *La prophylaxie antivénérienne* in 1933 gives the usual advice on prevention and hygiene (with, in passing, the following argument: 'However, it is not only prostitutes who are infectious; beware of any woman who invites you to become intimate with her; if she does so it is very probable that she has already done it with others, and that she might therefore have become infected in that way.) Curiously enough, this tract was only intended for men who asked for it in dispensaries – which seems somewhat over-scrupulous in view of the intense propaganda effort elsewhere.

18 This poster is featured on the cover of Pierre Guillaume's excellent study of the history of tuberculosis, *Du désespoir au salut: les tuberculeux aux XIXe and XXe siècles* (Aubier – collection historique, 1986).

19 Spillmann, *L'évolution de la lutte contre la syphilis*.

20 In 1932, for example, a poster entitled 'Against the Venereal Peril' placarded on the walls of the town of Saint-Ouen invited needy people to attend the town's prophylactic dispensary without being required to give their names and addresses. On it we read that 'syphilis, like tuberculosis and cancer, is not a shameful disease.'

21 In the monthly journal *Le prophylaxie antivénérienne* (official organ of the French Society for Sanitary and Moral Prophylaxis and the French National League Against the Venereal Peril), 1932.

22 A novel in three volumes by Maurice Landay, *La blessure, L'autre avarié, L'Avarie, tueuse de femmes*.

23 Loïc Le Gouriadec, *Le mortel baiser*, a drama in four acts (dedicated to E. Brieux), played for the first time on 5 April 1920 at the French National Theatre, Montreal.

24 Aline, the nurse, explains her action to the doctor, who is horrified by the scandal, thus: 'She was so white! so white! . . . I, who knew, how could I let her go thus to her monstrous wedding? I wouldn't have been a woman!'

25 *La prophylaxie antivénérienne*, 1932.

26 The author, Albert Nast, was a doctor. The play had been written in 1919, but it was not published until it was performed in 1926 (republished in 1929).

27 RAYMOND (*exaltant*): Ah!, Danièle! (*He moves nearer to her, Danièle's posture betrays a growing emotion. Raymond takes her hands and covers them in kisses; then he leans towards her.*)

    DANIÈLE: *close to fainting, gently pushing him away*): No, Raymond! Your misfortune is too recent; you need to recuperate.

    RAYMOND: How beautiful you are! (*He leans towards her once more.*)

    DANIÈLE: No, not yet, not yet!

    RAYMOND (*mystical*): Why refuse me the kiss of the Ideal which would refresh my soul and help me to live again! Why?

    DANIÈLE (*in a feeble voice*): A day will come . . . A day will come, perhaps, when you will understand me!

28 'Keeping fit to fight' (Washington, 1918, lecture to troops), cited in Brandt, *No Magic Bullet*.

29 In Brandt, ibid.

30 André Gide, *Si le grain ne meurt* (Paris, 1926).

31 Julien Green, *Jeunesse* (Paris, Plon, 1974).

32 Letter of October 1933 to Jean Schlumberger, cited in the latter's edition of the complete works of Roger Martin du Gard, vol. VII, p. 178.

33 *Correspondence between A. Gide and R. Martin du Gard* 2 vols, (Gallimard, 1968), letter of 30 August 1942, vol. 2, p. 263.

34 J. Green, *Jeunesse*.

35 H. Roger, J. Alliez and J. Cain, *Syphilis et troubles mentaux – a propos d'une expérience de trente années à la clinique des maladies nerveuses*, inaugural sessions (13 and 15 October 1950) of the Marseilles branch of the French Society of Dermatology and Syphilology.

36 Dr Ch Fiessinger, *Souvenirs d'un médecin de campagne* (Paris, 1933).

37 There are many cases in which someone in whom syphilis is diagnosed by a venereologist refuses even to notify his GP.

38 See, for example, Dr V. Scheikevitch, *Suis-je syphilitique?* (Paris, 1928).

39 Its author was Dr H. Bourges.

40 Dr Louis Bory, *Essai sur les douleurs morales de la syphilis . . .* (Paris, 1918).

41 Ibid.

42 Ibid.

43 L. Bizard, J. Bralez, *Existe-t-il des signes de certitude de la guérison de la syphilis?* (1923).

44 Dr H. Mathias, *Autour du drame vénérien* (Paris, 1930).

45 The principle of syphilitic reinfection – admitted at this period, though it had been fiercely denied by Ricord – obviated the need to describe as 'quaternary' a roseola manifested by a former syphilitic.

46 From an article by Henri Bouquet in *Le monde médical*, 1 August 1927.

47 *Annales d'hygiène publique et de médecine légale*, 1882.

48 Dr Louis Queyrat, 'Le délit pénal de contamination', in *La prophylaxie antivénérienne*, January 1933.

49 Especially the Billon novarsphenamines from the Specia laboratories.

50 Weissenbach and Basch, *Les traitements de la syphilis* (Paris, 1934). See also A. Sezary, *Le traitement de la syphilis* (Paris, 1930).

51 J. Crozet, *Guide intime pour la cure des maladies spéciales* (Paris, 1917).

52 Dr Arthur Vernes, *La syphilis est un facteur incalculable d'incapacité et de sous-production qui peut être supprimé* (Paris, 1928). Jacques Bernstein, *Contrôle par la syphilimétrie de l'efficacité des différents médicaments au cours du traitement de la syphilis*, medical thesis, Paris, 1933. Dr Arthur Vernes, *Mesure et médecine* (Paris, 1943).

53 The theory which made syphilis responsible for numerous cancers was widely held in the thirties. See Jeanselme, *Traité de la syphilis*, and also, though it is somewhat more far-fetched, Vernes, *La syphilis est un facteur incalculable* . . .: 'For syphilis, on account of its hereditary consequences alone, is a very ugly phenomenon; whether or not it is associated with alcoholism and tuberculosis it causes the multiplication of human defects and the most unfortunate moral and physical predispositions, and it even plays such an important role in the production of cancer that those who specialize in this other scourge recently went so far as to say that there is no cancer without syphilis. Syphilologists, for their part, have long been of the opinion that to be handsome, upright and long-lived, and to bring descendants of the same calibre into the world, is clear proof that hereditary syphilis has not been transmitted.' There were some, however, who denied all links between syphilis and cancer. One such was Dr William Bainbridge, who in 1914 ('The problem of cancer') informs us in passing that cancer, like syphilis, was at that time regarded as a shameful disease by some families, especially amongst poor people in the United States.

54 E. Jeanselme, *La syphilis, son aspect pathologique et social* (Paris, undated (1925)).

55 Dr A. Vernes, *SOS pour la défense de la race* (Paris, 1936). Vernes cites the *Journal officiel*, annexe no. 809, p. 1156, Rapport de la Commission des Finances, Chambre des Députés.

56 Dr Marcel Leger, *Les méfaits de la syphilis dans les colonies françaises*, *Revue d'hygiène*, 1926.

57 There was a reduction in the number of cases in Switzerland, Austria, Spain (see, Marcel Petit, *Contribution à l'étude comparée de la syphilis en France et à l'étranger*, medical thesis, Paris, 1926) and, in particular, in Belgium; here, thanks to the sterling efforts which had been made, official statistics showed a 90 per cent reduction in syphilis, and the Belgians even set as their target nothing short of the complete eradication of syphilis. (See Pr. A. Bayet, *La lutte contre la syphilis en Belgique* . . . Ligue nationale belge contre le péril vénérien, 1929.)

58 Source: Dr Cavaillon, head of the Central Service for Prophylaxis of Venereal Diseases of the Ministry of Health, secretary-general of the International Union against the Venereal Peril.

59 Robert Szigeti, *Essai de statistiques sur la date de début clinique et la fréquence des syphilis nerveuses*, medical thesis, Paris, 1932.

60 Hemiplegia, meningitis, optical neuritis, facial paralyses etc. must also be taken into account.

61 The anti-venereal departments which increased in number from 1,349 in 1929 to 1,580 in 1930, broke down as follows: 580 anti-syphilitic departments *per se*, 80 rural departments, 168 departments in prisons, 604 departments for the

detection and treatment of hereditary syphilis, 85 anti-gonorrhoeal departments, and 63 analytical laboratories.

62 William Allen Pusey, *The History and Epidemiology of Syphilis* (Springfield and Baltimore, 1933).

63 Ibid.

64 Vernes, *Mesure et médecine*.

65 See the extracts from her novel, *Le crime*, in the previous chapter.

66 Dr J. Payenneville, *Le péril vénérien*, vol. 58 of the collection *Que sais-je?* (PUF, 1942). (It has, as an epigraph, Charles Maurras' aphorism: 'Savoir pour prévoir afin de pourvoir'.)

67 For example, the Rue d'Assas dispensary recorded an increase from 5–10 recent contaminations per 100 new patients in 1939, 1940 and the first part of 1941 to 10–15 and above in the second part of 1941 and in 1942 (Vernes, *La syphilis*).

68 Modifying article 63 of the civil code.

69 Law published in the *Journal officiel* of 3 March 1943.

70 The Vichy government completed these provisions with a certain number of prescriptions, including one which, by the order of 25 February 1943, introduced consultant venereologists into every health region.

71 *Paris-Soir*, 6 December 1937 (interview with Pr Pautrier).

72 *Du délit impuni* (Paris, 1870).

73 'Rapport adressé á M. le préfet de Police au nom de la sous-commission sur la réglementation de la prostitution à Paris', from *Journal de médecine de Paris*, 8 June 1887.

74 Queyrat, 'Le délit pénal de contamination'.

75 Quoted in *La prophylaxie antivénérienne* (1932): 'Article 155 of the Soviet code – Knowing contamination of another person with a serious venereal disease is punishable by the deprivation of freedom for a maximum period of three years.'

76 Queyrat, 'Le délit pénal de contamination'.

Chapter 9 The Pox and the Prostitute

1 There were numerous calls for 'houses of prostitution' to be suppressed, but in the name of morality rather than to protect people against venereal diseases.

2 Quoted by Alain Corbin in his seminal work on this subject, *Les filles de noce – misère sexuelle et prostitution (XIXᵉ siècle)* (Aubier-Montaigne, 1978).

3 In Paris from 1812 to 1830 the total number of registered prostitutes increased from 1,293 to 3,000 (and 'house' prostitutes alone increased from 700 to around 1,000), whereas the number of regulated brothels remained constant at around 200. All of these figures declined sharply at the beginning of the 1820s, reflecting the influence of those in power: at the end of the empire and the beginning of the Restoration the authorities had encouraged the proliferation of regulated brothels to counteract the proliferation of clandestine ones. But in 1820 the 'ultras' returned to power and a large

number of prospering brothels had to close (those which were too close to churches, for example) and the number of registered prostitutes decreased. However, the consequent increase in the number of unregulated prostitutes led to a return to the previous policy.

4 Cullerier, *Dictionnaire des sciences médicales* . . . (1821), article entitled 'Syphilis'.

5 Paris, 1836, chap. V (new editions in 1837 and 1857). Parent-Duchatelet was a doctor, a member of the Academy of Medicine and also of the City of Paris Council of Health. In the expanded edition of 1857 he appealed to two collaborators: one was chairman of the Health Office and secretary of the Council of Health, the other was a secretary of the Prefecture of Police.

6 Ibid., vol. I, ch. XVI: 'Des soins sanitaries donnés aux prostituées de Paris'.

7 An idea put forward by Corbin, 'Le péril vénérien'.

8 Ibid.

9 'Debauchery is a delirious fever of the senses; it leads to prostitution (or to premature death) without being as demeaning or as incurable as this latter' (A. Béraud, *Les filles publiques de Paris et la police qui les régit* (Paris, 1839), cited by A. Corbin, 'Le péril vénérien').

10 See, for example, Giraudeau de Saint-Gervais, *Traité des maladies vénériennes* . . . (Paris, 1838 and numerous subsequent editions).

11 'Congrès scientifique de France, 14ᵉ session (Marseille, septembre 1846), Mémoire en réponse à la 9ᵉ question de la section 3 (sciences médicales) du programme, ainsi conçue: Comment s'opposer aux ravages de la syphilis? Les mesures d'hygiène publique auxquelles on soumet les prostituées sont-elles suffisantes? Dans la négative, en indiquer de plus efficaces', by Dr J. Venot, Bordeaux, 1846.

12 Many proposals went further, demanding, for example, that prostitutes should be issued with a booklet containing advice and health regulations, or that keepers of official brothels should receive a rudimentary medical training which would allow them to examine prostitutes and clients and thus take responsibility for the health of their charges (see, for example, Lagneau the younger, 'Mémoire sur les mesures hygiéniques propres à prévenir la propagation des maladies vénériennes' in *Annales d'hygiène publique et de médecine légale*, 1856.

13 In Brest, weekly medical examinations were instigated in 1830.

14 Cited by Corbin, 'Le péril vénérien'.

15 Ricord, *Traité pratique* . . .

16 This division was caused by a dispute between the hospital doctors as to the best method of treatment. The supporters of the sublimate held sway at the Hôpital des Vénériens, and those of mercurial frictions at Saint-Louis.

17 336 beds, with 415 single men.

18 In the 12th arrondissement (276 beds).

19 The annual 'turnover' was around 1,200.

20 Dr A. Potton, *De la prostitution et de la syphilis dans les grandes villes, dans la ville de Lyon en particulier* . . . (Paris and Lyons, 1842).

21 Ibid.

22 Venot, *Aperçu de statistique médicale*.

23 Dr E. Strohl, *Coup d'oeil sur la prostitution publique à Strasbourg* (1856).

24 Cited by Corbin, 'Le péril vénérien'.

25 Bourneville, 'Quelques notes sur l'hospitalisation des vénériens en province' in *Le progrès médical* (1877), cited by A. Corbin.

26 Michael Ryan, *Prostitution in London, with a comparative view of that of Paris and New York, as illustrative of the capitals and large towns of all countries; and proving moral depravation to be most fertile source of crime and of personal and social misery: with an account of the nature and treatment of the various diseases caused by the abusus of the reproductive function* (London, 1839).

27 There is a large bibliography on the contaminating role of prostitutes – see William Acton, '*Prostitution, the greatest of our social evils, as it now exists in London, Liverpool, Manchester, Glasgow, Edinburgh and Dublin; an enquiry into the cause and means of reformation based on statistical documents; by a physician*' (London, 1857). Also, G. Dolmage, 'Remarks on prostitution, with a view to the adoption of measures for the checking of venereal diseases', in *Med. Circular*, London, 1864. As regards the United States, see W. Boeck, 'Prostitution in relation to national health', *Amer. J. of Syph. and Dermat.*, New York, 1870, also Edmund Andrews, *Prostitution and its sanitary management* (Chicago, 1871), and 'The supervision of prostitutes and the control of venereal diseases', *Med. News*, New York, 1897. As regards Canada, see C. A. Wood, 'The question of prostitution and its relation to the public health', *Canada Med. Record*, Montreal, 1880–1, and other articles from 1885–6.

28 Charles-Louis Philippe (1874–1909) published *Bubu de Montparnasse* in 1901.

29 Letter to a friend dated 26 October 1898 (published in the Garnier-Flammarion edition of 1978).

30 See the remarkable account of the personality and works of Jean Lorrain (1855–1906) by Hubert Juin in the 10–18 edition of *Monsieur de Phocas*.

31 The first edition appeared in 1943, and the novel enjoyed a great success. Its hero, Michel Doutreval, has an edifying medical career, giving up a promising hospital career to devote himself to being a GP in a small industrial town (and to the love of Evelyne, a working-class prostitute with – as one might have expected – tuberculosis).

32 This evocation soon turns into a meditation on the dangers of sex, in an outrageous piece of purple prose: 'Even Chavasse, who was not in the habit of exaggerating, told me, one morning, how upset he had been by these sights. We had just witnessed the taking of a sample of pus from the neck of a womb. "These things were awful to see," he said to me, "it makes me ill to cold-bloodedly watch a woman, her legs spread and her speculum in place like a round eye which stares at you with a drop of pus in its depths . . . . It hurts me just to think of that messy thing, pickled with the treponema or with gonorrhoea. The saddest thing is that when they have their legs in the air they all look the same, you can't tell them apart. And the more you see in the speculum the more you realize that it is stopping up holes like these which makes you so excited! Why one rather than another? Why not the hole in the stove? I have tried to think about this matter, but it made me ill, it was too much for me and I had to stop." '

33 Neisser, *Dans quel sens peut-on réformer la réglementation de la prostitution?*, report presented to the German Society for Prophylaxis, 1904.

34 See, for example, Dr Chery, *Syphilis maladies vénériennes et prostitution* (undated, *c.*1910).

35 8,940 to be precise (including 71 deaths), making a total of 361,629 days of hospitalization (41 days per patient, on average). From *Situation administrative et financière des hôpitaux et hospices de l'Empire* (Imprimerie impériale, vol. I, 1869).

36 Survey by Dr Jullien (cited by Corbin, 'Le péril vénérien').

37 In 1939 the Nice Centre for Prophylaxis recorded what is effectively an identical percentage of cases of syphilis in prostitutes (46%). The figures also bring out the extreme rarity of neurosyphilis (1% had GPI, and there were no cases of tabes), whereas 22% of the other syphilitics who attended the dispensary had nervous symptoms (there were twice as many men as women).

38 Lacassagne and Lebeuf, 'Considérations sur la métallo-prévention chez les prostituées', *Bulletin de la société française de dermatologie et syphiligraphie*, June 1936.

39 Jean Lacassagne, *A Lyons avec les filles*, albums du crocodile publiés sous le patronage de l'association générale de l'internat des hospices civils de Lyon (Lyons, 1937).

40 Jean Lorrain, *La maison Philibert* (Paris, 1932).

41 Unfortunately, Nana dies of smallpox rather than pox. Constrained, as ever, by the documentary evidence, Zola must have had in mind the smallpox epidemic which claimed numerous victims in Paris in the spring and early summer of 1870. However, the description of the pustules that disfigure and rot away Nana's face is virtually identical to the description given at the time of certain syphilides which ate away the face. But smallpox killed more swiftly and more surely than syphilis, thus giving the novel, says Flaubert admiringly, an epic conclusion.

42 *L'agonie* (aquatint), Bibliothèque Nationale, prints department.

43 In London, for example, prostitutes long refused to allow medical inspectors to use the speculum.

44 An American, Abraham Flexner, in a work (1913) translated into French as *La prostitution en Europe* (Payot, 1919), gives figures which speak volumes as to the chimerical nature of medical supervision of prostitutes. Out of 845 prostitutes known to be syphilitic in Stockholm between 1885 and 1906, 77.6% disappeared after initial treatment. In Berlin between 1888 and 1901 more than 50% missed their appointments, etc.

45 Léo Taxil, *La prostitution contemporaine* (Paris, undated, *c.*1900).

46 Dr Patoir, 'La prostitution à Lille', in *L'écho médical du Nord*, 7 September 1902.

47 This was the name given to the inmates of the brothels, which were known as 'maisons à numéro' or 'à gros numéro' because of the enormous number which signalled to clients the precise nature of the establishment, which was in other respects highly discreet (though it is true that shutters which were closed, even during the day, were another way of attracting attention).

48 Taxil, *La prostitution contemporaine.*

49 *Mémoires de M. Gisquet, ancien préfet de police, écrits par lui-même*, vol. IV (Paris, 1840).

50 Potton, *De la prostitution.*

51 Venot, *Aperçu de statistique médicale.*

52 Dr Barthélemy 'Exposé des mesures en vigueur en France, et d'un projet de réorganisation de la surveillance de la prostitution' in *Communications relatives à la prophylaxie de la syphilis et à la surveillance de la prostitution* (proceedings of the Congress, published by H. Feulard, Paris, 1890).

53 Dr Butte, 'De la prophylaxie de la syphilis par la surveillance médicale des prostituées. Action du dispensaire de salubrité de la ville de Paris pendant les trente dernières années', in *Communications . . .* (ibid.). In another article the same author, who was a doctor at the health clinic, observes that in the years of the Great Exhibitions (1855, 1867, 1889 and 1900) the incidence of syphilis soared amongst all prostitutes, registered or otherwise (See *Annales de thérapeutique dermatologique et syphiligraphique*, 20 January 1901).

54 Touraine and Chon, 'Les sources de contamination syphilitique, (statistique personelle d'après deux dispensaires)', in *Bulletin de la Société française de dermatologie et de syphiligraphie*, no. 4, April 1937.

55 Unfortunately the figures for the sources of contamination for women (same dispensaries, same years) make no distinction between prostitutes and 'honest women'. However, they show that 17.7% of contaminations were due to the legitimate husband.

56 Dr Jullien's survey (cited by Corbin, 'Le péril vénérien').

57 Dr E. Maréchal, 'La Syphilis dans les Lupanars . . .' *Révue médicale de Franche-Comté*, Besançon, 1923.

58 See, for example, Dr Bergeret, 'La prostitution et les maladies vénériennes dans les petites localités' (*Annales d'hygiène publique et de médecine légale*, January 1866), which contains, amongst others, the following case history: 'In the summer of 1853 I saw what was obviously an epidemic of buboes. In less than two months more than thirty young people, both from the town and from the rural communities around it, consulted me with cases of inguinal adenitis, all of which had the same characteristics. All of these young people owed their disease to the same source, namely Julie A——. Six of them had caught it on the same evening; Julie A. had been brought in . . . secretly to a private room in the café d'Arbois, and each of these young people had paid her a visit in turn. The prostitute often plied her trade in this café, and the police had never been aware of this.' See also Payenneville, 'Augmentation des cas de syphilis dans la région rouennaise. Ses causes probables. Difficultés d'interpretation des statistiques', *Bulletin de la Société française de dermatologie et de syphiligraphie*, June 1933, which gives the history of a chain of contamination in a large town on the outskirts of Rouen: 'A tavern prostitute appeared in a hotel where a dance party was taking place and contaminated a number of young people, the result being that in this area, which up until this point had been almost free of syphilis, a full-scale epidemic of syphilis broke out, affecting all classes of society; in the space of three months, with the help of my colleagues, whom I had alerted, I brought

to light twenty-five new cases of syphilis. I was able to have the woman in question hospitalized fairly rapidly, but the damage had already been done, and the disease continued to spread.'

59 Dr Lardier, *Les vénériens des champs et la prostitution à la campagne* (Paris, 1882).

60 Flexner, *La prostitution en Europe*.

61 In Rouen, for example, twenty 'women of low repute' were arrested 'in the wake of the regiments' during the second half of 1788 and taken to the beggars' prison 'for military discipline'. The Extraordinary Council of War paid for their board, and even for boxes of Keyser's anti-venereal dragées – obviously in the mind of the authorities all these prostitutes were afflicted with venereal diseases (see Archives départementales de la Seine-Maritime C1019).

62 Archives départmentales des Bouches-du-Rhône.

63 Doctors deplored the use of the crude quack remedies which were widely used by soldiers with venereal disease: 'Soldiers thought they would be less exposed to contagion if they drank eau-de-vie with a little gunpowder in it; I doubt if this drink has ever preserved anyone from venereal infection' (Dr M. L. Tournier), *Manuel de siphilixie ou Notice sur le virus, les préservatifs et les erreurs populaires de la maladie vénérienne* (Paris, 1817).

64 Philippe Avon, *Contribution à l'histoire des maladies vénériennes dans l'armée française – Prophylaxie et traitement*, medical thesis, Lyons, 1968.

65 In France these orders often remained no more than pious wishes, but in Belgium, which passed similar measures the same year, they were applied more severely.

66 Dr J. Rochard, *De la prostitution à Brest* (1856).

67 In Caen, for example, nightly patrols were organized to back up policemen whose mission it was to arrest prostitutes found in the company of military personnel. When these latter refused to cooperate they were threatened with court martial, no less (this formal severity reflects the inefficacy of the measures) (Letter from the commander of the 17th Infantry Brigade of Caen to the Prefect of Calvados, dated 8 July 1875).

68 William Acton, *Prostitution in relation to public health, forming the introductory chapter to the second edition of the treatise on syphilis. Reprinted for private circulation* (London, 1851); and, by the same author, 'Observations on venereal diseases in the United Kingdom from statistical reports in the army, navy and merchant service, with remarks on the mortality from syphilis in the metropolis, compiled from the official returns of the registrar-general', *The Lancet*, 1846, I, p. 703; II, p. 369.

69 George R. Dartnell, 'On the prevalence and severity of syphilis in the British army; and its prevention', *British Medical Journal*, 28 April 1860.

70 Avon, *Contribution à l'histoire* . . .

71 Flexner, *La prostitution en Europe*, cited in Corbin, *Le péril vénérien*.

72 'Men who up until then had been faithful to their wives, finding themselves suddenly separated from their families and knowing themselves to be continually risking their lives, forgot their peacetime prudence. Venereal infection was the result of casual and dubious encounters which these men, in civilian life, would have been careful to avoid.' (paper on venereal diseases

during the war at the Villemin military hospital by Professor Gaucher, *Bulletin Académie de Médecine*, 28 March 1916).

Military statistics give the following figures for primary syphilis per 1,000 men. 1916: 14.16; 1917: 21.19; 1918: 20.29; 1919: 11.51; 1920: 6.43; 1921: 2.68; 1922: 3.02; 1923: 2.38; 1924: 2.49; 1925: 1.84; 1926: 1.95; 1927: 1.98.

73 E. Bénichou, *La lutte contre la syphilis dans l'armée métropolitaine*, medical thesis, Lyons, 1933.

74 Commission on Training Camp Activities, cited in Brandt, *No Magic Bullet.*

75 Brandt, ibid. But, as has already been emphasized, the statistics are inconsistent. So, for example, Pusey in *History and Epidemiology of Syphilis*, which appeared in 1933, hails the success of the anti-venereal prophylaxis in the American army, due to which the incidence of syphilis fell from 2.68 per thousand in 1909 to 1.17 per thousand in 1919.

76 As early as 1913 Flexner wrote 'Certain venereal afflictions have been popularly considered to be a badge of maturity. Dr Magnus Möller talks of a club of army officers which existed in Stockholm between 1890 and 1900 and admitted no-one who could not prove that they had had syphilis.'

77 M. Carle, *Conseils d'un médecin, Comment se défendre des maladies vénériennes* (Lyons, undated, c.1920).

78 A survey of the Val-de-Grâce military hospital dating from the beginning of the thirties gives the following breakdown of the sources of soldiers' infections. Clandestine prostitutes: 47.82%; girlfriends: 32.18;% brothel prostitutes: 17.39%; legitimate wives: 2.29% (Jame, *Archives de Médecine et Pharmacie militaires*, c.1933)).

79 Ministère de la Défense nationale – Direction centrale des services de santé des armées, 4ᵉ Bureau matériel et pharmacie. Object: préservatifs. Letter no. 110 of 12 February 1953 relating to the reprovisioning of the Depôt avancé for sanitary supplies.

80 See, for example, Alfred Hall, *Essay on great Prevalence of Venereal Disease* (Glasgow, 1847), or Horatio Prater, 'Considerations on the action of preventions of venereal diseases considered physically, chemically and morally', *The Lancet*, 17 June 1843.

81 De Meric, '*Rapport succinct sur les visites hebdomadaires faites dans une maison de tolérance de Londres*' (International Medical Congress of Paris, 1867).

82 Acton, *Prostitution in relation to public health*, which in 1857 became *Prostitution considered in its moral, social and sanitary aspects in London and other cities, with proposals for the mitigation and prevention of its attendant evils* (11 edns between 1857 and 1870).

83 J. Jeannel, 'Étude sur la prostitution et sur la prophylaxie des maladies vénériennes en Angleterre', *Annales d'hygiène publique et de médecine légale*, (XLI, 1874).

84 *Some remarks on a recent contribution to the literature of regulated and supervised immorality*, by the Rev. C. S. Collingwood, rector of Sontwick, and formerly fellow of University College, 2nd edn (Durham, 1874).

85 See, for example, Professors James Stuart and J. V. Laborde: 'Les Acts sur les maladies contagieuses en Angleterre et leur influence réelle au point de vue sanitaire', paper to the Académe de médecine, 29 March 1898, in which the

authors claim, with supporting figures, that the repeal of the Acts was accompanied by a decrease, not an increase, in cases of syphilis.

86 Mrs Scheven, in *Der Abolitionnist*, 1 May 1902.

87 The Salvation Army, founded during this period, was one of the most active agents in the abolitionist movement.

88 Louis Fiaux, *Les maisons de tolérance – leur fermeture* (Paris, 1892). The work is dedicated to Professor Fournier, though the latter, laments the author, was an opponent of abolitionism. See, by the same author, *La police des moeurs devant la Commission extra parlementaire du régime des moeurs* (Paris, 1909).

89 Louis Fiaux, *L'armée et la police des moeurs – Biologie sexuelle du soldat – Essai morale et statistique* (Paris, undated, c.1913).

90 *La Fédération et l'hygiène* (Geneva, 1905), report by Mrs E. Pieczynska published to mark the thirtieth anniversary of the International Abolitionist Federation.

91 Ibid.

92 See in particular the battle waged by Yves Guyot in 1876 and 1877 in the columns of the *Droits de l'Homme* (in Corbin, *Les filles de noce*) or the press campaign in *La lanterne, La police des moeurs*, which ran from 14 to 31 October 1878.

93 See on this subject Corbin, *Les filles de noce*.

94 Fiaux, *Les maisons de tolérance*.

95 Flexner, *La prostitution en Europe*.

96 Herbert Spencer, *The Study of Sociology* (1873).

97 Dr A. Guichet, *Les Etats-Unis – notes sur l'organisation scientifique, les facultés de médecine, les hôpitaux, la prostitution, la syphilis, l'hygiène, etc.* (Paris, 1877).

98 Quoted in Brandt, *No Magic Bullet*.

99 Pompe Van Meerdervoort, *Vijf jaren in Japan (1858–1863)* cited in Briot, *La Syphilis au Japon*.

100 Dassy De Lignières, *Prostitution et contagion vénérienne* (Paris, 1900) cited in Corbin, 'Le péril vénérien'.

101 All the information concerning the failure of Sellier's bill is taken from a forthcoming work of Gérard Massés: *1936: La santé à un tournant* (Henri Sellier, Minister of Health, June 1936 to June 1937).

102 Bernay *La Syphilis et ses consequences*.

103 M. L. Bizard, 'Statistique des cas de syphilis observés dans les maisons de tolérance de la région parisienne de 1917 à 1926', *Bulletin de la Société française de dermatologie et de syphiligraphie*, (no. 2, February 1927).

104 Cited by Corbin, 'Le péril vénérien'.

105 Ibid.

106 Dr Grandier-Morel, *Voyages d'étude physiologique chez les prostituées des primcipaux pays du globe* (Paris, undated (1901)).

107 Reported in *Bulletin de la Société française de dermatologie et de syphiligraphie*, June 1937.

108 As early as 1856, Lagneau the younger, in *Mémoire sur les mesures hygiéniques propres à prévenir la propagation des maladies vénériennes*,

proposed to mark the stomach or thighs of quarantined prostitutes with a mark which would remain indelible for a long time.

109 J. Bénech, 'Le dispensaire de salubrité publique de la ville de Nancy', in *Annales des maladies vénériennes*, February 1932.

110 In 1924, a first upsurge of syphilis (290 new cases at the dispensary as opposed to 125 the previous year) had been attributed to the arrival of numerous foreign workers. The epidemic of 1930, to which the authors here are alluding (188 cases as opposed to the 100 of the previous year) was blamed on more or less casual prostitutes.

111 J. Bénech and A. Spillmann, 'L'épidémie de syphilis de Nancy, 1929–1930, valeur de la réglementation', *Annales des maladies vénériennes*, March 1932.

112 Touraine and Fouassier, 'Dix ans d'"abolitionisme" à Strasbourg', in *Bulletin de la Société française de dermatologie et de syphiligraphie*, November 1937.

113 The idea had already been set out by Dr H. Mireur, an assistant to the mayor of Marseilles (*La syphilis et la prostitution dans leurs rapports avec l'hygiène, la morale et la loi*, (Paris, 1887): To bring prostitutes back within common law, argues Mireur, would be the best way to combat clandestine prostitution, which would be more likely to be scotched by the reformatory than by regulation. On the other hand, Mireur was in favour of keeping regulated prostitutes – which paradoxically made him a hyper-regulationist.

114 See ch. 8.

115 At Caen, for example, the Minister of the Interior's model decree was followed by a Prefect's decree of 28 January 1941; in April 1942 the mayor of the city proposed to the Prefect of Calvados to grant the status of soliciting-place to five cafés, and that of place of prostitution to three hotels (see Marie-Claude Guinchard, *Prostitution et maladies vénériennes à Caen et dans le Calvados durant la période 1939–1945*, Caen medical thesis, 1983).

116 Ibid. Guinchard cites this detail and numerates other equally interesting details of the regulation: a prohibition, as was to be expected, on Jews and half-castes, but also the chaperoning of prostitutes leaving the establishment, a ban on abnormal relations and obscene pictures, on prostitutes possessing photographs of German soldiers, etc.

117 See ch. 8.

118 A figure from the Seine health authority cited by J. Bataillard, 'Prostitution et maladies vénériennes', in *Informations sur les maladies vénériennes* (the official organ of the Société française de prophylaxie sanitaire et morale, and of the Ligue nationale française contre la péril vénérien), May–June 1975.

119 *La super-réglementation de la prostitution au service des tenanciers – un arrêté type scandaleux*, undated (1942?) edited by the Ligue française pour le relèvement de la moralité publique.

120 On this subject see Alphonse Boudard's work, *La fermeture*, collection Ce jour-là (R. Laffont, 1986) which is interesting as a testimony to this great moment in the history of prostitution in France.

121 Maxence Van der Meersch, in *Femmes à l'encan*, which appeared in 1945, gives a good insight into the prevailing outlook. To guarantee that brothels met acceptable sanitary standards it would be necessary to preserve the system adopted by the German army during the Occupation: 'An officer at

the foot of the stairs in every brothel . . . . If we adopt this system, the registered brothel would, as far as hygiene goes, deserve the highest praise!' But this was impossible, and it was therefore necessary to put an end to an absurd situation by closing them.

122 *Extrait du décret du 5 novembre 1947 portant application de la loi du 24 avril 1946 tendant à instituer un fichier sanitaire et social de la prostitution: Art. 8.* – Every woman entered on the health and social records of prostitution must submit to a twice-weekly medical examination . . . . The first visit following registration must include the following examinations: (a) clinical; (b) serological; (c) bacteriological (of the genital exudations). If the examination takes place in the dispensary, it will also be followed, wherever possible, by a radioscopic and psychopathological examination. These last examinations will be clinical ones, and will be accompanied by: (1) a weekly bacteriological examination; (2) a monthly serological examination.

123 L. Laporte, 'L'état actuel de la lutte antivénérienne', *Revue du praticien*, 1 November 1953.

124 Bataillard, 'Prostitution et maladies vénériennes'.

Chapter 10 The End of the Terror

1 See for example an article in *Le Monde*, 10 July 1947 which reports a recrudescence of venereal diseases following the closure of regulated brothels, a recrudescence which stimulated a debate in the Conseil général de la Seine.

2 This law was discussed in the National Assembly from 10 May 1948 onwards, the aim being to 'perfect our sanitary weaponry' by improving the organization and functioning of the anti-venereal dispensaries. Alcoholism was also on the agenda.

3 At national level a Commission on prophylaxis distributed grants, coordinated activities and studied the various reform projects, with the help of twenty-seven regional consultants. In every 'département' an anti-venereal organization under the authority of the director of health for the 'département' was directed by a senior doctor assisted by doctors from anti-venereal dispensaries qualified in dermato-venereology and one or more specialist social workers. Every small town possessed a secondary dispensary, a satellite of the main dispensary in the capital of the 'département' or in the most important town. Certain specific dispensaries were also set up in ports and factories, etc. There were approximately 600 of these various centres at the beginning of the fifties, to which must be added the 200 anti-venereal departments which operated in penal establishments.

4 Syphilis, gonococci, soft chancre and Nicolas-Favre disease (see Conclusion).

5 It is INSERM (Institut national de la Santé et de la Recherche médicale – Unité 165) which is responsible for statistics on STDs (Sexually Transmissible Diseases) on behalf of the Ministry of Health.

6 A test involving the immobilization of the treponemas, using the treponemic antigen which is itself pathogenic and living.

7 Archives départementales du Calvados M16202–2.

8 See, for example, Dr Vernes (*Pour que ceux qui n'ont pas compris comprennent*

pourquoi ils n'ont pas compris (1950) who refers to 'arsenoprovocation' in which the treponemas are attacked without being destroyed – the effect of which is to 'dope' the survivors . . . . There were more serious criticisms by numerous practitioners who deplored the toxicity of the arsenicals and, to a lesser extent, bismuth.

9 'Long-term studies of results of penicillin therapy in early syphilis', in *Bulletin de l'OMS*, 10 (1954), no. 4.

10 Certain doctors long continued to pose themselves this question, even though pencillin was used on its own in the treatment of syphilis in France in 1947 (by Dr Marc Bolgart at the Hôpital Saint-Louis, for example). However, as late as 1968, although only in a treatise (*Petite encyclopédie médicale de Hamburger*, Flammarion) we find bismuth, novarsphenamine and even cyanide of mercury being recommended in the treatment of syphilis, even though pencillin was the main prescription.

11 See the *Revue du praticien*, November 1953 (foreword by P. Harvier): 'There are some who remain faithful to penicillin in aqueous solution, but the majority have adopted slow-release penicillin, in particular P.A.M. in a solution of oil. The same treatment can be applied to primary or secondary syphilis, but the techniques recommended are different: some use a daily injection of a million U. of P.A.M., up to a total dose of between 6 and 15 million. Others confine themselves to 3 weekly injections of 3 million U. of P.A.M. There are yet others who reduce the treatment to a single injection of between 2,400,000 and 3 million U. of P.A.M.'.

12 Laporte 'L'état actuel de la lutte.

13 In Calvados, for example, declared cases of primo-secondary syphilis dwindled sharply after the brief flaring up due to the Liberation: 1941: 159; 1945: 271; 1946: 252; 1948: 72; 1950: 37; 1951; 26. (See Dainville de la Tournelle, directeur départemental de la Santé, 'L'état sanitaire du Calvados et les causes de mortalité', *Revue des études normandes*, 2nd quarter, 1953).

14 *La fin de la syphilis nerveuse*, G. Boudin in collaboration with L. Durupt.

15 Charles Clayton Dennie, *A History of Syphilis*, ed. Ch. C. Thomas (Springfield, 1962). The author notes that 'Few books have been written upon the modern treatment of syphilis for the very good reason that penicillin has so simplified the treatment of that disease that large books upon this subject are unnecessary. One of the most complete books in this field is *Syphilis: Its Course and Management* by Evan W. Thomas, and a handbook upon syphilis published by the United States Public Health Service.'

16 This was one of the five dispensaries at the Hôpital Saint-Louis (See 'Étude de 1,929 cas de syphilis primo-secondaires observés à la clinique des maladies cutanées et syphilitiques de la faculté de médecine de Paris', *Bulletin de l'INSERM*, May-June 1968).

17 Avon, *Contribution à l'histoire*.

18 *Bulletin de la Société française de dermatologie et syphiligraphie*, November 1970.

19 *Annales de médecine et de pharmacie de Reims*, February 1970.

20 Dr D. Heyne, *Maladies vénériennes en Belgique, année 1976* (ministère de la Santé publique et de la famille, inspection de l'hygiène).

21 'La syphilis à Genève au cours des deux dernières années . . .' (group

authorship) in *Praxis*, 60 (1971). (After a peak in 1962, a new diminution in cases was followed by a further resurgence in cases from 1968 onwards.)

22 'Maladies vénériennes et tréponématoses: activités internationales (1948–1963)', *Chronique DMS*, 18 (1964).

23 Dennie, *A History of Syphilis*. On this subject the author gives an interesting example of what one might call bourgeois syphilitic contamination, something which is far less easy to discern than that of prostitutes and servicemen: 'A fair sized city with one large high school was a target of interest for the Committee for the Control of Venereal Diseases. A frantic call for aid came from the town's general practitioner. He had examined three high school girls in one week, each of whom was suffering from early syphilis. An investigator was sent posthaste to this community and in three days found the source of the trouble. An unmarried high school teacher was infected with early latent syphilis. There had been forty-one contacts from this source and twenty-one of the contacts had developed syphilis. Certainly not all of the contacts were uncovered. People of that social status would not universally admit to such social errors'. (*Author's note*: Kinsey estimated that 20% of female students had had sexual intercourse in 1953, and 44% in 1967.)

24 The WHO is an institution based in Geneva that was created by the UN in 1946.

25 A. Duval, *Aspects épidémiologiques de la syphilis*, medical thesis, Bordeaux, 1970.

26 See *Santé, Sécurité sociale – statistiques et commentaires*, November–December 1980, 1981, 1982.

27 Since the war this was by far the most common form of tertiary syphilis: there were 444 cases in Lille in twenty years, of which 150 were tabes and 148 GPI. (See C. Huriez, 'Bilan de deux décenniés de lutte contre la syphilis . . .', *Bulletin de l'Académie de Médecine*, 1965, nos 9–10), 115 cases in Strasbourg between 1960 and 1968, 55 of which were tabes and 14 GPI. (See 'Aspects actuals de la morbidité syphilitique en Alsace' (joint authorship), *Journal de Médecine de Strasbourg*, March 1971).

28 *La syphilis et ses répercussions en pathologie mentale*, report presented in March 1982 to the CNRS (ATP Santé) by the Centre d'études psychiatriques historiques critiques (EPHC) (Postel, Quétel).

29 Ph. Lorteau, *Aspects actuels de la paralysie générale*, medical thesis, Caen, 1978.

30 The same attenuation of symptoms has been observed in tabes.

31 See R. R. Willcox and T. Guthe, *Treponema Pallidum – A bibliographical review of the morphology, culture and survival of I. pallidum and associated organisms*, (WHO, Geneva, 1966).

32 The rarity of textbook cases was mentioned in the 1940s in Van der Meersch *Corps et âmes*.

33 The laboratory diagnosis is either bacteriological (direct observation of the treponema in primary and secondary lesions using an ultramicroscope), or serological. Some of the serological tests are tests for antilipidic antibodies, or reagents, using a non-treponemic antigen (the first of these was the Bordet-Wassermann test, which is still being used despite the criticism that positive results are unreliable); others are tests using specific treponemic antigens (the

most widely used is the Nelson and Mayer test perfected in 1949, and the most reliable is the TPHA). On the complex question of these different techniques see, for example, A. Paris-Hamelin, 'Les problèmes particuliers du diagnostic direct et sérologique de la syphilis', *Médecine et maladies infectieuses*, 1980, no. 11 bis.

34 Gjestland, 'The Oslo studies of untreated syphilis', *Acta Derm. Venereol.*, 35 (1955), supplement 34.

35 A. Siboulet, *Maladies sexuellement transmissibles* (Paris, Masson, 1984).

36 The goal of the WHO is to 'bring all peoples to the highest possible state of health'.

37 This distinction has been questioned on the grounds that it is difficult to make a clinical distinction, and impossible to make a serological distinction, between yaws and endemic syphilis.

38 The classic example is that of Bosnia at the beginning of the fifties. Here there raged an endemic syphilis which was contracted during infancy and which was not considered by those infected to be a venereal disease. It was characterized by lesions of the secondary type, usually found in the buccal region, and late lesions of the tertiary type. Due to widespread promiscuity, and in particular to the fact that everyone drank from the same 'ibrik' contagion remained at very high levels, despite campaigns waged by the Yugoslav government from 1948 onwards. The WHO launched a mass campaign there, centred on systematic penicillin therapy as a stop-gap measure until higher standards of living led to better hygiene.

39 Ridet, Idsoe, Guthe, 'Épidémiologie actuelle de la syphilis', *La revue de médicine*, 1 June 1970.

40 A. Fasquelle, *A propos de la syphilis endémique – Notions classiques – Enquête sur l'endémicité tréponémique dans un groupe de population nomade des régions sahéliennes de Haute-Volta*, medical thesis, Paris, 1971.

41 'Nature et ampleur du problème des tréponématoses', *Chronique de l'OMS*, February–March 1954.

42 J. Ruffié and J. C. Sournia, *Les épidémies dans l'histoire de l'homme* (Flammarion, 1984).

43 On this important question, which falls outside the scope of the present work on venereal syphilis, see R. R. Willcox, 'Evolutionary cycle of the treponematosis', *Brit. Journ. Vener. Dis.*, 36 (1960), (on the fundamental notion of the cycle of treponematoses). Also T. Maleville, 'La syphilis et les tréponématoses endémiques', *les Cahiers d'Outre-Mer*. January–March 1976. (A resurrection of the unicist theory, according to which the various treponematoses constitute a universal disease caused by a single pathogenic agent, whose clinical manifestations vary according to local conditions: pinta in Latin America, yaws in the humid tropical regions, endemic syphilis in the dry regions, and venereal syphilis in affluent societies. This geographical spread has considerable implications, for the endemic forms of the treponematoses, whilst consisting of a huge reservoir of pathogenic agent, protect populations against contagion by the venereal form.)

44 Delacrétaz and Nicollier, 'Problèmes actuels posés par le dépistage des sources de contamination vénérienne', *Dermatologica*, 131 (2) (1965).

45 A. Cheseaux-Rihtar, *Épidémiologie de la syphilis primaire et secondaire chez*

les malades hospitalisés dans le service de dermato-vénériologie de Lausanne de 1960 à 1973, medical thesis, Lausanne, 1976.

46 A. Sage, *Considérations épidémiologiques sur la syphilis vues à travers les statistiques du dispensaire de Saint-Quentin de 1930 à 1975 . . .*, doctoral medical thesis, Reims, 1976.

47 B. A. Gerber, *Épidémiologie de la syphilis récente à Strasbourg*, medical thesis, Strasbourg, 1973.

48 Certain conditions for success are rather amusing, as, for example, in a work translated from English (C. B. S. Schofield, *Maladies sexuellement transmissibles* (undated, 1970), which recommends that the patient be questioned by a woman who is 'kindly and representable, but not provocative' (as if it were the moment for provocation!). The same work raises the old question: 'What should be said to the spouse?' The answer: once again, nothing.

49 R. Hy, 'Une enquête épidémiologique particulièrement fructueuse tirée du Rapport du service antivénérien départemental de Maine-et-Loire pour 1971', *La prophylaxie sanitaire et morale*, January–February 1974.

50 M. Vieu, *L'importance de l'enquête épidémiologique dans le dépistage de la syphilis récente contribution à l'étude de la recrudescence de la syphilis dans la région toulousaine au cours des années 1962–1963*, medical thesis, Toulouse, 1964.

51 J. P. Rouge, *Bilan d'activité du dispensaire antivénérien d'Amiens en ce qui concerne la syphilis de 1953 à 1972*, medical thesis, Amiens, 1975.

52 Duval, *Aspects épidémiologique*.

53 Ridet, Idsoe, Guthe, *Épidémiologie actuelle*.

54 Delacrétaz and Nicollier, (*Problèmes actuels*) point out that in a study presented to the 'World forum on syphilis and other treponematoses' held in Washington in December 1962, 25% of sexual contacts mentioned by American syphilitics had taken place outside their town or district of residence.

55 *La syphilis à Genève . . .*

56 Cheseaux-Rihtar, *Épidémiologie de la syphilis*.

57 'Étude de 1,929 cas'.

58 For example, *Le Monde* of 13 April 1965 ('An upsurge of venereal disease in young people has been noted by the WHO') and of 26 January 1968.

59 Ridet, Idsoe, Guthe, *Épidémiologie actuelle*.

60 Sage, *Considérations épidémiologique*.

61 Ph. Cambier, *Épidémiologie de la syphilis au dispensaire de Valenciennes (1965–1981)*, medical thesis, Lille, 1982.

62 For example, Achten, Moriame and Wanet, 'Aspect de l'épidémiologie de la syphilis à Bruxelles', *Archives belges de dermatologie et de syphiligraphie*, 22 (1968).

63 'Continued and indiscriminate sexual vagabondage is something quite different. If it is excessive it can be considered as a psychopathological phenomenon. In men it is usually associated with immaturity or an inability to adapt emotionally . . . . Some take up drinking, then become heavy drinkers (which is probably linked to their impotence), and finally alcoholics. In other cases they take up drugs, if these are easily available. Women also practise chronic sexual vagabondage if they are immature . . . . They tend to be very

emotional, and often lie without reason; they sometimes live in a dream world. In these circumstances it is not surprising that many of them drink heavily or take drugs (or both), or that a large proportion of them are psychotic' (Schofield, *Maladies sexuellement transmissibles.*

64 Vieu, *L'importance de l'enquête épidémiologique.*

65 Garber, *Épidémiologie de la syphilis.*

66 'La syphilis à Genève.'

67 To which we should add 9.3% who declared themselves to be bisexual (Cheseaux-Rihtar, *Épidémiogie de la syphilis*).

68 J. Richard, *Situation épidémiologique des MST dans le Doubs – 1970 à 1980*, medical thesis, Besançon, 1982.

69 62.1% in London, and as much as 73.3% in five West End clinics (*British Journal of venereal diseases*, 49 (1973)).

70 In Strasbourg 24% of women were contaminated by their husbands as opposed to 3% the other way round (Gerber, *Épidémologie de la syphilis.*) In Toulouse (Vieu, *L'importance de l'enquête épidémiologique*) the proportion was 54% (excluding prostitutes) as opposed to 3% vice versa.

71 B. Cantaloube, *Syphilis et prostitution dans la région toulousaine – l'expérience I.*, medical thesis, Toulouse, 1966.

72 Vieu, *L'importance de l'enquête épidémiologique.*

73 Duluc, Labouche, Barreau, 'Le visage clinique actuel de la syphilis récente dans la Marine – IIIᵉ Région', *Revue des Corps de santé des Armées*, February 1964.

74 P. R. Rouilleaut, *La syphilis au dispensaire Brocq de l'hôpital Saint-Louis de 1963 à 1970*, medical thesis, Paris, 1971.

75 'And here the notion of the provincial mentality enters for the first time. Whereas before the closure of regulated brothels patients were relatively open about their relations with prostitutes, they now speak of chance encounters who are, in fact, most often prostitutes in disguise' (Sage, *Considérations épidémiologiques*).

76 56.4% of the 4,517 cases of syphilis monitored in Lille (Huriez 'Bilan de deux décennies'. This record was beaten at the Saint-Denis dispensary on the Island of Réunion with 72.4% of syphilis in blood tests as opposed to 10.7% of primary syphilis and 16.9% of secondary syphilis (See Ph. Dreux), *Évolution de la sérologie chez les malades syphilitiques traités au dispensaire d'hygiène sociale de Saint-Denis de la Réunion*, medical thesis, Tours, 1980).

77 J. D. Fritsch, *La syphilis – Son dépistage à l'hôpital Pasteur de Colmar, Problèmes médico-sociaux*, doctoral thesis in medicine, Strasbourg, 1975.

78 Statistics produced by INSERM.

79 Statistics produced by the Centre national de transfusion sanguine.

80 F. Bardot, *Dépistage systématique de la syphilis – étude d'après 138,250 examens de santé faits à l'IRSA de janvier 1973 à juin 1974*, medical thesis, Tours, 1975.

81 J. P. Bardelli, *Le dépistage de la syphilis aux examens de santé de la Caisse primaire centrale d'Assurance Maladie de la Région parisienne en 1970*, medical thesis, Paris 1971. See also Ph. Franceschini, 'Persistance de la syphilis', *Gazette médicale de France*, 8 December 1972.

82 Rouilleaut, *La syphilis au dispensaire Brocq.*

83 A systematic enquiry is presently being carried out by the research laboratories of the Institut Alfred Fournier.

84 See the issue of *Informations sur les maladies vénériennes* which is devoted to this subject (January–February 1975) and in particular 'Les maladies transmises dans les rapports sexuels – ampleur du problème et mesures de lutte', European Council on Public Health, and also 'Résolution (du Comité des ministres) sur la lutte contre les maladies transmises dans les rapports sexuels'.

85 Ridet, Idsoe, Guthe, *Épidémiologie actuelle*.

86 Editorial ('L'amour, pas la maladie') in the special edition of *Quotidien du médecin*, 18 August 1985, devoted to STDs.

87 These two organizations are based at the Institut Alfred Fournier, 25 bd Saint-Jacques, Paris, as is the Union Internationale Contre les Maladies Vénériennes et les Tréponématoses.

88 For example, *Le risque vénérien en croissance*, produced by the Sécurité Sociale and available from the Institut Fournier.

89 For example, a series of Army stills whose format (18 × 24 mm) means that special apparatus is required to view them!

90 For example, Drs Coulon and Siboulet, *Maux d'amour . . .*, available from the Institut Fournier. This leaflet is fairly comprehensive, despite its appalling illustrations.

91 In the special issue of *Quotidien du médecin* of August 1985, Dr Siboulet mentions 24,700 pamphlets on STDs distributed at the last Paris exhibition. Why at an exhibition and not in schools, universities and businesses?

Conclusion: From Syphilis to AIDS

1 In the United States, for example, the number of new cases of early syphilis is put at 100,000 a year. The residue of untreated cases, however, is estimated to be at least 350,000.

2 On this subject, and in particular on the astonishing history of the long-misunderstood infectious agent, see Dr Jeanine Henry-Suchet, 'Chlamydia féminine', *Temps médical*, November 1981.

3 As early as 1980, an article in the *New England Journal of Medicine* reported the existence of Kaposi's syndrome and opportunist infections in American homosexuals.

4 Retroviruses, which were discovered in 1911 (viral transmission of sarcoma in poultry), have inverted genetic material: in other words, instead of genetic information initially coded in the form of DNA being translated into RNA and then into proteins, retroviruses are initially coded in RNA, which is retrotranslated to DNA, thanks to an enzyme, inverse transcriptase, which was brought to light in 1970. This first human retrovirus, discovered in 1980, has a particular tropism towards T-lymphocytes.

5 Figures given in F. Vachon, 'Epidémiologie compréhensive du SIDA Du mode sporadique et du mode épidémique' *Médecine et maladies infectieuses*, 1987, no. 4.

6 The figures produced by antisyphilitic monitoring in the dispensaries are

increasingly often inferior to those of the hospitals. In Colmar, for example, in the early seventies, twenty cases a year were diagnosed in the dispensary as opposed to forty in the hospital (see Fritsch, *La Syphilis – Son dépistage*). This is particularly true of the newly-arrived STDs, for which most dispensaries are not prepared.

7 See in particular the proposals made by the dermatologist Professor P. Morel and the biologist Professor Y. Perol of the Centre clinique et biologique des MST, Hôpital Saint-Louis, Paris (internal document of the 27 May 1986).

8 Cited by Patrick Wald-Lasowski in '*Syphilis. Essai sur la littérature française au XIXe siècle*' (Gallimard, 1982).

Bibliographical Note

The bibliography for this subject is so vast that, apart from the works and articles given as references in the text, a general bibliography cannot be given. For works prior to 1889, see J. K. Proksch's imposing international bibliography, '*Die Litteratur über die venerischen krankheitein* . . .', Bonn, 1889 (plus a supplement, by the same author, for the years 1889–99).

Chronology

1495 First allusions (following the battle of Fornovo) to the 'French sickness' at the time of Charles VIII's Italian campaign.

1496 (autumn) The first pox-victims flock to the Hôtel-Dieu in Paris.

1497 Torella's treatise on the French sickness.

1498 Villalobos' treatise on the 'bubas'.

1503 Joseph Grunpeck's book.

1514 Juan de Vigo is one of the first to give a complete description of the 'French sickness'.

1519 Ulrich Von Hutten's book.

1526 Fernandez de Oviedo is the first to mention the 'American' origin of the new sickness.

1527 Jacques de Béthencourt's '*Nouveau Carême de pénitence . . .*' comparing the therapeutic properties of mercury and gaiac is published in Latin.

1530 Jérôme Fracastor publishes a poem ('*Syphilis sive morbus gallicus*') which was to give syphilis its name.

1539 '*Le triomphe de haute et puissante dame vérole . . .*'.

1548 Jean Fernel's first writings on the venereal disease.

1557 The construction of the Petites Maisons on the site of the Saint-Germain leper colony, to which victims of venereal disease and the insane were to be sent.

1690 Victims of venereal disease of both sexes are admitted to Bicêtre (general hospital).

1713 Deidier defends the parasitic theory of the pox.

1736 First edition of Jean Astruc's treatise on the venereal disease (first French edition, 1755).

1759 Start of the monopoly for the sale of Keyser's dragées in the French armies.

1767 Balfour of Edinburgh is the first to attack the unicist theory by distinguishing between gonorrhoea and the pox.

1769 '*Le Pornographe, ou idées d'un honnête homme sur un project de règlement pour les prostituées . . .*', by Restif de La Bretonne.

1780 The Vaugirard Hospice is founded 'for new-born children afflicted with the venereal sickness'.

1785 Sanchez produces a theory of 'chronic venereal disease', a precursor of the theory of hereditary syphilis.
A hospital for victims of venereal disease is set up in Paris (it became fully functional in 1792).

1787 *Instruction sommaire sur le traitement des maladies vénériennes dans les campagnes . . . publiée par ordre du Gouvernement.*

1812 Hernandez: *Essai analytique sur la non-identité des virus gonorrhoïque et syphilitique.*

1822 Bayle defends his thesis on chronic arachnitis.

1831 Ricord enters the Hôpital des Vénériens.

1836 Regulationism is sanctioned by the publication of Parent-Duchatelet's *De la prostitution dans la ville de Paris* . . . (and the creation of the Infirmarie Spéciale de Saint-Lazare).
A question is put before the Société des Sciences Médicales de Bruxelles: 'What measures of medical policing are most suitable for halting the spread of venereal disease?'.

1837 William Wallace proves that secondary manifestations are contagious.

1852 Léon Bassereau asserts the separateness of the soft chancre.
The Académie Impériale de Médecine condemns Dr Auzias-Turenne's method of syphilization.

1864 The first of the 'Contagious Diseases Prevention Acts'.

1876 Alfred Fournier asserts the syphilitic origin of tabes.

1877 First International Abolitionist Congress in Geneva (against the regulation of prostitution) 'I have got the pox! at last! the real thing! . . .' (letter by Maupassant dated 2 March).

1879 Alfred Fournier asserts the syphilitic origin of GPI.
Creation of the first chair of dermatology and syphilology at the Hôpital Saint-Louis (incumbant: Alfred Fournier).

1884 '"There is nothing but syphilis", reflected des Esseintes' (Huysmans, *A Rebours*).

1889 First international congress on dermatology and syphilology (in Paris).

1899 First international congress on the prophylaxis of syphilis and venereal diseases (in Brussels).

1901 Foundation (on the initiative of A. Fournier) of the 'Société française de prophylaxie sanitaire et morale'.

1902 Second international congress on the prophylaxis of syphilis and venereal diseases.

1905 (22 February) Premiere, at the Théâtre Antoine in Paris, of *Les Avariés* by Eugène Brieux.
(3 March) Discovery of Treponema Pallidum by Schaudinn and Hoffmann in Berlin.

1906 Perfection of the Bordet–Wassermann serological test.

1909 Ehrlich creates Salvarsan, or '606', thus inaugurating the treatment of syphilis using arsphenamines.

1913 Noguchi and Moore discover the treponema in the cerebral cortex of general paralytics, thus verifying Fournier's theory.

1917 (17 April) The 'Commission on Training Camp Activities' (CTCA) is set up in the United States. Wagner von Jauregg (1857–1940) invents malariatherapy for the treatment of general paralysis.

1919 Inter-Allied congress on social hygiene (Paris).

1920 (December) Pan-American congress on venereal diseases, on the initiative of the Red Cross.

1921 Sazarac and Lavaditi reveal the treponemicidal power of bismuth.

1922 (4 May) Resolution of the Commission de prophylaxie des maladies vénériennes inviting the French Minister of Hygiene to ask the 'Parlement' for the funds required to create anti-syphilitic dispensaries.

1922 (June) First 'Congrès des dermatologistes et syphiligraphes de langue française' at the Hôpital Saint-Louis.

1923 Foundation of the Ligue national française contre le péril vénérien.
Premiere of the play *Le mortel baiser*.

1932 Inauguration of the Institut Fournier in Paris.

1939 Model decree of 29 November introduces stricter prophylactic measures against venereal diseases.

1940 The film *Dr Ehrlich's Magic Bullet* starring Edward G. Robinson, is released in the United States. Order of 24 December from the Minister of the Interior to the Prefects reinforcing the regulation of prostitution.

1942 Law of 31 December 'relating to the prophylaxis of and the struggle against venereal diseases', introducing, amongst other things, the declaration of cases of syphilis to the health authorities by doctors.

1943 Mahoney, Arnold and Harris treat four cases of early syphilis with penicillin and obtain complete success.

1946 Law of 13 April (known as the 'Marthe Richard law') ordering the closure of brothels, and law of 24 April introducing a sanitary and social record system for prostitutes.

1948 Laws of July and August revising the organisation of the anti-venereal struggle.

1949 Nelson and Mayer perfect the treponemic immobilization test.

1960 Order of 25 November suppressing the health record system for prostitutes in France (victory for the abolitionists).

1964–1965 Beginning of the world recrudescence of syphilis, putting paid to hopes of eradicating the disease raised by the success of penicillin.

Index

Note: references in *italics* are to illustrations.

204–5; post-war period 248-72; propaganda 7, 145–9, 180–92; prophylaxis 135–6, 141, 143–9, 159, 177–80, 204, 205–10, 268–72, 325; recrudescence (1960s) 251–5, 256, 257; treatment 138, 142–3, 153, 195–9, 249–51; turning point in early 131–59; Vichy régime 205–10; *see also* dispensaries typarsamide 198

Uçay, Gervais 77–8, 94
Ulsen, Theodoricus 34
unicist theory 5, 38, 82–3, 96, 97, 109, 113; destroyed 5, 111, 324
Union of Soviet Socialist Republics 210
United States of America: AIDS 274; antibiotics 249, 251; army 188–9, 192, 231–2, 325; between wars 203–4; blood tests 207–8; compulsory treatment 240; epidemiology 262; genital herpes 273; homosexuality 265; morality 192; Pan-American conference (1920) 178, 325; prophylaxis 141, 149, 157–8, 188–9, 192; prostitution 231–2, 239–40; Public Health Service 250, 251, 252, 253; return of disease (1950s–60s) 252, 262, 263
urban nature of modern syphilis 262
urethro-genital infections 273–4
uvula, destruction of 26

vaccination 112, 131; attempts to develop syphilis vaccine 7, 140; *see also* syphilization
Vade-mecum des jeunes gens (Lebel) 119
Vagensburg, Count of 96
Val-de-Grâce 311
Val d'Oise 254
Valencia 66
Valenciennes 263, 265
Valentius, Nicolas 20
Valleur, Nicole 168
vamianine 198
Van Swieten, Gerard 85, 103–4, 116, 166
Vannes 229
Vaudemont, M. de (courtier) 94
Vaugirard hospice 103, 104, 106, 107, 324
vegetations, venereal 276

Velasquez, Diego Rodriguez de Silva 173
Vendôme, Louis Joseph, duc de 93–4
venereal disease, concept of 3, 54, 272
venereology 218
Venot, J.-B. 120 n. 37, 255 n. 51
Vergery de Velnos (charlatan) 90
Vernes, Arthur 198
Vérola, Paul 145–6
'vérolle, la grosse' 78
Verona 10–11
Vesalius, Andreas 53
Vichy régime 205–10, 244, 325
Vidius, Vidus 56
Vienna 14–15, 32, 227
Vigneulles, Phillipe de 12
Vigo, Juan de 26, 31, 34, 323
Villalobos, Francisco Lopez de 21–2, 23, 31, 34, 86, 323
Villey, Raymond 151
vinegar, washing in 58–9
virulence of disease, initial: Canada 108, 116; Europe 28, 50, 55–6, 63
visceral symptoms 57, 256
Voltaire, François Marie Arouet de 39, 95

Wagner von Jauregg, Julius 198, 325
Wald-Lasowski, Patrick 124
Wallace, William 112, 324
War, First World 141, 158, 231
War, Second World 189, 192, 207, 248; *see also* Vichy régime
wars of Revolution and Empire 123, 229
Wassermann, August Paul von 141
waxworks, dermatological 137
wet-nurses 55, 104–5, 107–8, 131, 155
Widman, Johann 23
wigs 57
Wilson, Thomas Woodrow (US President) 158
wine, washing in white 23, 58–9
women: nineteenth century associations 240; as contaminators 23, 28; incidence of syphilis 109, 262, 263; as victims of ignorance 196
Woodward, George Moutard 93
workhouses, religious 102
World Health Organization 252–3, 254, 258, 317

Xenophon 38

yaws 258, 259
Yin and Yang 117